Ethics in Psychiatric Research

A Resource Manual for Human Subjects Protection

Ethics in
Psychiatric Research

*A Resource Manual for
Human Subjects Protection*

Edited by

HAROLD ALAN PINCUS, M.D.
JEFFREY A. LIEBERMAN, M.D.
SANDY FERRIS

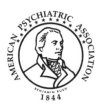

Published by the
American Psychiatric Association
WASHINGTON, DC

Copyright © 1999 American Psychiatric Association
ALL RIGHTS RESERVED
Manufactured in the United States of America on acid-free paper
First Edition
02 01 00 99   4 3 2 1
American Psychiatric Association
1400 K Street, N.W., Washington, DC   20005
www.appi.org

Library of Congress Cataloging-in-Publication Data
Ethics in psychiatric research : a resource manual for human
   subjects protection / edited by Harold Alan Pincus, Jeffrey Lieberman,
   and Sandy Ferris. —1st ed.
        p.   cm.
   Includes bibliographical references and index.
   ISBN 0-89042-281-8
   1. Psychiatry—Research—Moral and ethical aspects—Handbooks,
manuals, etc.   2. Human experimentation in medicine—Moral and
ethical aspects—Handbooks, manuals, etc.   I. Pincus, Harold Alan,
1951–   . II. Lieberman, Jeffrey A., 1948–   .   III. Ferris, Sandy.
   [DNLM: 1. Research—standards.   2. Psychiatry—standards.
3. Ethics, Medical.   4. Human Experimentation.   WM 20 E835 1998]
RC337.E84   1998
174'.28—dc21
DNLM/DLC
for Library of Congress   98-17948
                                                              CIP

British Library Cataloguing in Publication Data
A CIP record is available from the British Library.

Editorial Advisory Board

Contents

Contributors

Paul S. Appelbaum, M.D.
A. F. Zeleznik Professor and
    Chairman, Department of
    Psychiatry, University of
    Massachusetts Medical School,
    Worcester, Massachusetts

Robert W. Baker, M.D.
Associate Professor of Psychiatry,
    University of Mississippi Medical
    Center, Jackson, Mississippi

Jessica Wilen Berg, J.D.
Director, Academic Affairs,
    American Medical Association
    Institute for Ethics, Chicago,
    Illinois

Frederick O. Bonkovsky, Ph.D.
Institut fuer Medizin, University of
    Vienna, Vienna, Austria

Arthur L. Caplan, Ph.D.
Director, Center for Bioethics,
    University of Pennsylvania,
    Philadelphia, Pennsylvania

William Carpenter, M.D.
Professor of Psychiatry and
    Pharmacology, University of
    Maryland School of Medicine,
    Maryland Psychiatric Research
    Center, Baltimore, Maryland

Ruth Dukoff, M.D.
Senior Staff Fellow, Geriatric
    Branch, National Institute of
    Mental Health, National Institutes
    of Health, Rockville, Maryland

Sandy Ferris
Assistant Director, Office of
    Research, American Psychiatric
    Association, Washington, D.C.

Celia B. Fisher, Ph.D.
Professor and Director, Doctoral
    Specialization in Applied
    Developmental Psychology,
    Fordham University, Bronx, New
    York

Laurie Flynn
Executive Director, National Alliance
    for the Mentally Ill, Arlington,
    Virginia

Alan Gelenberg, M.D.
Professor and Head, Department of
    Psychiatry, University of Arizona
    Health Sciences Center, Tucson,
    Arizona

David A. Gorelick, M.D., Ph.D.
Chief, Pharmacotherapy Section,
    Intramural Research Program,
    National Institute on Drug Abuse,
    National Institutes of Health,
    Baltimore, Maryland

Laura Lee Hall, Ph.D.
Director of Research, National
   Alliance for the Mentally Ill,
   Arlington, Virginia

Kimberly Hoagwood, Ph.D.
Associate Director for Child and
   Adolescent Translational Research
   Services, Research and Clinical
   Epidemiology Branch, Division of
   Services and Intervention
   Research, National Institute of
   Mental Health, National Institutes
   of Health, Rockville, Maryland

Peter S. Jensen, M.D.
Associate Director, Child and
   Adolescent Research, National
   Institute of Mental Health,
   National Institutes of Health,
   Rockville, Maryland

Richard S. E. Keefe, Ph.D.
Associate Professor of Psychiatry,
   Duke University Medical Center,
   Durham, North Carolina

Eugene Laska, Ph.D.
Chair, Statistical Sciences and
   Epidemiology Division, Nathan
   Kline Institute for Psychiatric
   Research, Orangeburg, New York

Jeffrey A. Lieberman, M.D.
Professor of Psychiatry,
   Pharmacology, and Radiology,
   Vice Chair Research, and Director
   of Mental Health Clinical
   Research Center, Department of
   Psychiatry, University of North
   Carolina Medical School, Chapel
   Hill, North Carolina

Joseph P. McEvoy, M.D.
Deputy Clinical Director, John
   Umstead Hospital, Butner,
   North Carolina

Jonathan Moreno, Ph.D.
Kornfeld Professor of Biomedical
   Ethics and Director of the Center
   for Biomedical Ethics, University
   of Virginia, Charlottesville,
   Virginia

Roy W. Pickens, Ph.D.
Chief, Clinical Neurogenetics
   Section, Intramural Research
   Program, National Institute on
   Drug Abuse, National Institutes
   of Health, Baltimore, Maryland

Harold Alan Pincus, M.D.
Deputy Medical Director and
   Director, Office of Research,
   American Psychiatric Association,
   Washington, D.C.

A. John Rush, M.D.
Professor of Psychiatry, Betty Jo Hay
   Distinguished Chair in Mental
   Health, Department of Psychiatry,
   University of Texas Southwestern
   Medical Center, Dallas, Texas

Nina R. Schooler, Ph.D.
Professor of Psychiatry and
   Psychology, University of
   Pittsburgh Medical School,
   Pittsburgh, Pennsylvania

Katherine Shear, M.D.
Professor of Psychiatry, Western
   Psychiatric Institute and Clinic,
   Pittsburgh, Pennsylvania

David Shore, M.D.
Acting Deputy Director, Division of
    Clinical Treatment Research,
    National Institute of Mental
    Health, National Institutes of
    Health, Rockville, Maryland

Jane A. Steinberg, Ph.D.
Associate Director for Special
    Projects, National Institute of
    Mental Health, National Institutes
    of Health, Rockville, Maryland

Scott Stroup, M.D.
Assistant Professor of Psychiatry,
    Department of Psychiatry,
    University of North Carolina
    Medical School, Chapel Hill,
    North Carolina

Trey Sunderland, M.D.
Chief, Geriatric Psychiatry Branch,
    National Institute of Mental
    Health, National Institutes of
    Health, Bethesda, Maryland

Jan Volavka, M.D., Ph.D.
Chairman, Clinical Research
    Division, Nathan Kline Institute
    for Psychiatric Research,
    Orangeburg, New York

Paul Root Wolpe, Ph.D.
Faculty Associate Center for
    Bioethics, Assistant Professor of
    Sociology in Psychiatry,
    Department of Psychiatry and
    Department of Sociology,
    University of Pennsylvania,
    Philadelphia, Pennsylvania

Introduction

BACKGROUND AND PURPOSE

The past decades have witnessed unprecedented advances in health care and in the science of medicine. This astonishing progress is due in part to the advent of scientific methods, the advances in technology, and the increasing specification of biomedical research disciplines. As we approach the twenty-first century, the biomedical research community finds itself poised before a watershed of opportunity.

At the same time, the phenomenal growth of scientific discovery confronts medical scientists in general and clinical investigators in particular with vexing ethical dilemmas. These dilemmas extend from placebo-controlled trials to issues of genetic cloning and gene therapy. Recently, both the public and the medical community have begun focusing on these ethical issues in biomedical research because of abuses that have come to light. The broad awareness of human experimentation by Nazi physicians, the Tuskegee Syphilis Study, and radiation research by the U.S. Department of Energy conducted on human subjects during the cold war has raised the level of scrutiny of medical research with human subjects. Over the years the federal government and the medical community have taken a variety of steps to address ethical concerns, through the Nuremberg Code, the Declaration of Helsinki, the Belmont Report, and the current federal regulations (Department of Health and Human Services 1991, 45 *Code of Federal Regulations [CFR]* 46) contained in *Protecting Human Research Subjects: The Institutional Review Board Guidebook*. However, these steps have not been sufficient to wholly ensure the protection of human subjects in medical research. Conducting research on human subjects clearly demands more than just fulfilling the requirements of 45 *CFR* 46. Moreover, new scientific discoveries continually pose new questions and potential ethical problems in medical research. A recent example relating to the ethical implications of clinical trials in HIV patients illustrates this phenomenon (Cohen 1997a, 1997b). Given the newly demonstrated efficacy of combined drug therapies, how should future clinical trials be designed? If new drugs that are not superior in efficacy to combined treatment are tested monotherapeutically, could they cause the development of treatment-resistant strains that might pose a risk, not just to patients participating in the trial but to society at large?

Not surprisingly, the increased complexity of ethical issues in medical research and the growing concern about these ethical dimensions have engendered numerous activities and articles in the biomedical research community, governmental agencies (e.g., National Institutes of Health [NIH], U.S. Food and Drug Administration [FDA]) and the lay public, culminating in President Clinton's appointment of a National Bioethics Advisory Commission.

The American Psychiatric Association's Committee on Research on Psychiatric Treatments (CRPT) is charged with assessing and responding to broad scientific issues of psychiatric treatment. In recent years the CRPT has focused increasingly on ethical issues in psychiatric research. After consultation with the National Institute of Mental Health (NIMH), members of the scientific community, and lay advocacy organizations (National Alliance for the Mentally Ill [NAMI], National Depressive and Manic Depressive Association [NDMDA], Anxiety Disorders Association of America), the committee concluded that understanding and agreement were lacking on many of the critical questions and issues in clinical research, including informed consent, subject competence, institutional review, placebo-controlled trials, and subject risks and benefits. A resource manual containing the relevant information on these issues for clinical investigators was clearly needed. Therefore, the committee established an editorial board with broad expertise to oversee the compilation of a document that would provide useful information to established investigators and could also be used as a training tool for young investigators.

Although efforts from the American Psychiatric Association may have prompted the initiation of this manual, concerns about the issues are shared by many. The federal government requires that applicants for Public Health Service Research Grants, Research Career Awards, and Institutional National Research Service Awards (training grants) safeguard the rights and welfare of individuals who participate as subjects in research activities. NIMH has played a major role in developing the manual; its collaborative efforts have included both financial support and a critical review of all chapters. Patient and family groups such as NAMI, which support the biomedical research enterprise, have provided the important perspective of patients and their families on these issues.

Although regulations and safeguards focus on protecting research volunteers with severe mental disorders, we should not forget that these individuals are really the ultimate beneficiaries of the research. Clinical investigators conduct research because they are concerned about mental disorders and the many individuals affected who do not respond well to currently available treatments. Although it might be simpler or more convenient to study only mildly affected individuals (for whom issues of competency and substituted judgment are the least troublesome), such an approach would be a disservice to severely ill patients.

Indeed, there have been important and dramatic recent advances in available treatments. We must remember that such improvements in treatment (and therefore clinical outcome) have resulted directly from clinical research. Without it, far more individuals would remain institutionalized, impaired, or unable to work or interact with others. Nonetheless, the current arsenal of treatments is imperfect, and our understanding of the causes and mechanisms of mental disorders is limited. Only when we better understand the etiologies of these disorders will we be able to rationally design better treatments and predict who will respond to a given intervention. Therefore, the most ethical approach is to ensure the proper functioning of safeguards to prevent abuse of vulnerable individuals yet encourage continuation of research to shed light on conditions making such individuals potentially vulnerable. If we fail to pursue the causes of and develop treatments for the most severe disorders, we will be failing the next generation of patients.

About This Manual

When working with human subjects, investigators must realize that every situation is unique. However, certain fundamental principles can be generalized to all of medicine. Our intention here is to provide a sensible document for all investigators while highlighting the special issues researchers must consider when working with individuals who may be cognitively impaired.

Early in its discussions, the editorial board agreed to develop a practical manual for investigators that was neither an esoteric discussion of broad ethical principles nor a description of specific regulatory guidelines. Instead, our strategy is open-ended, and the manual reviews the pros and cons of different approaches when considering informed consent and other ethical issues. Rather than specifically direct the investigator to a prescribed course of action, we focus on issues in the conduct of research and informed consent and include examples from not only the field of psychiatry but also other areas of medicine.

Although this volume is intended to be comprehensive, some issues and perspectives have not been specifically addressed. For example, some special issues relate to individuals with HIV. (Some of these issues are addressed by Igor Grant in Appendix G.) The volume is not intended as a how-to manual that lays out specific rules and paths that must be followed by every investigator; rather, it is intended to provide broad guidance, an elaboration of basic principles, and access to other resources in the published literature and through federal and other information sources.

This manual is not a policy document of the American Psychiatric Association. The opinions and conclusions do not necessarily represent the views of the officers, trustees, or all members of the American Psychiatric Association. It does, however, represent the thoughtful judgment and findings of the authors of the individual chapters that constitute the manual.

Summary of Chapters

Each chapter is divided into subsections that address specific issues of relevance and provide concrete recommendations for investigators. A summary of the chapter appears at the end, followed by a list of references and other resource documents for background reading. The appendixes provide additional background and reference material.

Chapter 1, "Ethical Principles and History," by Paul Root Wolpe, Jonathan Moreno, and Arthur L. Caplan, reviews the history of human subjects research and provides the framework for today's federal regulations governing these issues.

Chapter 2, "Issues in Clinical Research Design: Principles, Practices, and Controversies," by Jeffrey A. Lieberman, Scott Stroup, Eugene Laska, Jan Volavka, Alan Gelenberg, A. John Rush, Katherine Shear, and William Carpenter, focuses on experimental designs that involve considerable potential risks to subjects, including medication-free research and research requiring invasive procedures. The authors review ethical principles relevant for research design, statistical design issues, specific issues related to major mental disorders, and ethical implications in the design of nontherapeutic research protocols.

Chapter 3, "Providing Quality Care in the Context of Clinical Research," by Nina R. Schooler and Robert W. Baker, looks at approaches to assessing and monitoring the provision of clinical care both during the conduct of a protocol and after a subject's participation has ended.

Chapter 4, "Subjects' Capacity to Consent to Neurobiological Research," by Jessica Wilen Berg and Paul S. Appelbaum, looks at the complexities related to the capacity to consent and provides practical guidance to policy makers and researchers.

Chapter 5, "Surrogate Decision Making and Advance Directives With Cognitively Impaired Research Subjects," by Trey Sunderland and Ruth Dukoff, reviews the two major mechanisms for addressing informed consent with cognitively impaired research subjects—surrogate decision making and advance directives. The authors show how combining surrogate decision making with a durable power of attorney, a model currently utilized at the NIH Clinical Center, can be applied to other research facilities.

Chapter 6, "Informing Subjects of Risks and Benefits," by Joseph P. McEvoy and Richard S. E. Keefe, comprehensively reviews the issues and information to be covered in an informed consent discussion and summarizes factors that may influence a patient's reception of the information. The authors also provide methods for helping patients understand the information being conveyed.

Chapter 7, "Special Issues in Mental Health/Illness Research With Children and Adolescents," by Peter S. Jensen, Celia B. Fisher, and Kimberly Hoagwood, reviews special regulatory protections that apply to mental health research in children and adolescents, identifies ethical challenges in the conduct of this research, and proposes a reconceptualization of the relationship between investigators and families to address these challenges.

Chapter 8, "Clinical Research in Substance Abuse: Human Subjects Issues," by David A. Gorelick, Roy W. Pickens, and Frederick O. Bonkovsky, reviews research involving subjects who use (or have used) psychoactive substances and research investigating the actions of substances with abuse liability in human subjects.

Chapter 9, "Consumer and Family Concerns About Research Involving Human Subjects," by Laura Lee Hall and Laurie Flynn, presents the patient and family perspective on research involving human subjects and looks at NAMI's role in this area.

Chapter 10, "Administrative Issues and Informed Consent," by David Shore and Jane A. Steinberg, offers the researcher guidance in negotiating the administrative hurdles in the research enterprise, including obstacles in the researcher's home institution, the funding agency, the research team, and the community of potential research subjects and family members.

The APA Council on Research and Office of Research

The Council on Research is the body within the American Psychiatric Association that seeks to ensure continued expansion of the science base and the application of research findings. The council oversees a variety of committees and task forces whose work provides the basis for many of the association's activities related to scientific affairs including the CRPT, whose efforts led to this document.

Through the efforts of the Council on Research, in 1985 the American Psychiatric Association established the Office of Research to provide leadership to the psychiatric research community, strengthen the research infrastructure, and improve the care of patients by encouraging the development of new knowledge and translating that knowledge into practical applications for clinicians (e.g., through the development of evidenced-based practice guidelines, the use of the *Diagnostic and Statistical Manual of Mental Disorders,* and the inception of the Practice Research Network). One important function of the office is to serve as a locus of information that affects the conduct of research in psychiatry, including not only human subjects research but also areas such as animal research, scientific misconduct, and other ethical issues. Many of these issues are covered in *Psychiatric Research Report (PRR)*, a quarterly newsletter published by the office. To receive *PRR*, write to the American Psychiatric Association Office of Research, 1400 K Street, N.W., Washington DC 20005; fax (202) 789–1874; e-mail sferris@psych.org.

One focus of the office has been to ensure the future intellectual development of psychiatry by recruiting talented young people into psychiatric research careers through the Program for Minority Research Training in Psychiatry, the mentoring network, publication of the *Directory of Research Fellowship Opportunities in Psychiatry*, operation and maintenance of the Psychiatric Research Training Clearinghouse, publication of the *Research Funding and Resource Manual: Mental Health and Addictive Disorders*, and activities held at American Psychiatric Association annual meetings for young investigators (e.g., the Research Colloquium for Young Investigators, the Breakfast for Young Investigators, and the New Research Young Investigators' Poster Session). These programs have helped to strengthen the research infrastructure and develop a cadre of researchers who are cognizant of social and ethical issues. For more information, contact Harold Alan Pincus, M.D., American Psychiatric Association Office of Research, 1400 K Street, N.W., Washington DC 20005; fax (202) 789–1874; e-mail hpincus@psych.org.

REFERENCES

Cohen J: AIDS trials ethics questioned. Science 276:520–523, 1997a

Cohen J: Ethics of AZT studies in poorer countries attacked. Science 276:1022, 1997b

Department of Health and Human Services: Rules and Regulations for the Protection of Human Research Subjects, 45 Code of Federal Regulations, part 46 (1991)

Penslar RL: Protecting Human Research Subjects: The Institutional Review Board Guidebook, 2nd Edition. Bethesda, MD, National Institutes of Health, 1993

Acknowledgments

This manual is the result of the combined efforts of many. In particular, we applaud the primary authors and other contributors who donated their time and energy to develop the content of this manual. Special recognition should also go to members of the editorial board who reviewed the numerous drafts of this document.

We want to express our deepest gratitude to the National Institute of Mental Health for providing both financial support and their crucial review of chapters. We are particularly indebted to Steven Hyman, M.D., Andrea Baruchin, Ph.D., David Shore, M.D., Richard Nakamura, Ph.D., and the other NIMH reviewers for their efforts. We would also like to thank the leaders of the National Alliance for the Mentally Ill for their participation. Our thanks to members of the American Psychiatric Association Committee on Research on Psychiatric Treatments who helped to formulate the initial planning for this effort: Alan Gelenberg, John Gunderson, Henrietta Leonard, Jeffrey Lieberman, Henry Nasrallah, Paul Summergrad, Ellen Frank, and Elizabeth Weller.

A very special thanks goes to Jennifer Carpenter, who spent many hours correcting drafts, checking on details, and providing her invaluable administrative support. Elizabeth Tornquist did a wonderful job copyediting the final drafts. Finally, a number of Office of Research staff deserve special note, including Julie Kuzneski, Sarajane Foster, and particularly Emily Anderson for their unfailing assistance and support.

CHAPTER 1

Ethical Principles and History

PAUL ROOT WOLPE, PH.D., JONATHAN MORENO, PH.D., AND
ARTHUR L. CAPLAN, PH.D.

M odern clinical medicine depends on research to elucidate the nature of the disease process, to explore the social and psychological underpinnings of illness, and to develop technological and pharmaceutical responses to illness. Only through pharmaceutical research can we discover and test new psychotropics, only through neuroscientific studies can we understand the physiological dynamics of mental illness, and only through psychosocial studies can we comprehend the lived experience of mental illness. Recent advances in mental illness treatment illustrate the tremendous potential for medical progress using the tools of modern research. Yet by its very nature, clinical research is ethically complex, and the potential vulnerabilities of the psychiatric patient pose a particular challenge for the investigator. It is therefore important for psychiatric clinical researchers to fully understand the regulatory, legal, ethical, and procedural standards that have been developed to ensure that human subjects are protected from undue harm.

Whereas clinical care is intended for the direct benefit of the patient, research has the broader goal of generalized knowledge and requires special attention to possible harm to subjects in pursuit of that goal. In the past few years concern has arisen about the ethics of experimentation with subject populations who may not be able to make informed, voluntary choices about participation in research, either because they have impairments in cognition and reasoning ability or because they live in circumstances or settings that restrict their opportunities for voluntary choice (Levine 1986). Pregnant women, prisoners, members of the armed forces, students, and the institutionalized elderly are all groups whose involvement in research raises difficult issues. In the 1980s the federal government mandated special protections for a number of "vulnerable" populations and imposed extra requirements on those conducting research on children and fetuses, pregnant women, and prisoners. However, for a variety of reasons, discussed later in this chapter, the mentally ill—though cited as a vulnerable population by a number of advisory committees, professional organizations, and articles in the psychiatric literature—were not accorded any formal regulatory protections beyond those existing for any subject recruited to participate in clinical research (Grodin and Glantz 1994; Levine 1986).

In recent years researchers, regulatory agencies, and private companies engaged in human research have proposed increased ethical standards for conducting studies involving the mentally ill and other groups who, while vulnerable, lack special formal regulatory protection. On the other hand, ethical debate about the involvement of persons unexpectedly incapacitated by the sudden onset of disease or trauma led to the promulgation of new rules on the part of the U.S. Food and Drug Administration (FDA) in the fall of 1996 that weakened protections for this vulnerable population (Department of Health and Human Services 1996; Wolpe and Merz 1997).

A number of recent high-profile cases have revived debate about the status of psychiatric patients as a vulnerable population. Some patient advocacy groups and clinicians have voiced concern that too much nontherapeutic research is being conducted on the mentally ill, and subjects with severe chronic mental illness are not adequately protected in studies that use inactive placebos or require washout periods. They suggest that in an increasingly competitive and privately funded research climate, the mentally ill require greater protection.

Other groups, including both patient advocates and researchers, note that significant protections, such as standardized informed consent procedures, the use of surrogates, and local peer review by institutional review boards (IRBs), already exist. These groups argue that the creation of special regulations may inhibit research that could lead to long-sought advances in prevention, diagnosis, and therapy. They also note that treating the mentally ill as a vulnerable population in need of special protection may further stigmatize or disempower a group that is already often denied rights and status in society.

Many also disagree about the kinds of research that ought to be done. Patients who are involuntarily institutionalized, or who are undergoing court-ordered treatment for substance abuse or in response to criminal behavior, live in an atmosphere that by its very nature is coerced, which makes problematic the idea of "freely" consenting to research participation. The vulnerability produced by limits in competence, societal stigma, and potential pressures of psychiatric treatment may also render problematic any research that does not directly benefit the patient. On the other hand, some argue that taking this view would virtually close down psychiatric research—ultimately harming the very patients being protected—and that risk can be minimized through adequate subject or surrogate informed consent, thorough peer review, and adequate supervision of the research process.

The history of abuses in medical research in general, and in research on the mentally ill in particular, is a major factor in the attitudes that many patients and families bring to psychiatric research. Tragic abuses of human subjects, often under government auspices, have led to suspicion on the part of communities who have been subjected to unethical research. Recent historical studies by national advisory panels and national scientific organizations have revealed heretofore unknown instances in the 1950s and 1960s in which mentally ill, mentally retarded, or mentally incapacitated people were used in clinical research without adequate informed consent by either the subjects or their surrogates (Advisory Committee 1995). The mentally ill were a convenient subject pool for a host of nonpsychiatric experiments in European and American medical research, such as the World War II influenza studies that used mentally ill subjects and the 1953 secret United States Army studies of mescaline overdoses at the New York Psychiatric Institute. Recent cases involving subjects with schizophrenia and other disabling diseases in which informed consent procedures were not adequate have triggered a great deal of controversy in Congress, the media, and scientific circles about the conduct of research involving those with mental illness.

Coming to some agreement about the standards for clinical research, as well as providing assurances of adherence to existing standards, would help diffuse some of the controversy. The vast majority of modern researchers choose their careers with the intent to ease suffering, care about the protection of their subjects, and comply with institutional regulations regarding informed consent procedures and IRB review. Yet in modern, high-pressured academic, pharmaceutical, and other research environments, it is important to remember that human subjects research is a privilege, and that through the generosity of subjects researchers' careers and incomes are enhanced. Because regulatory codes place the responsibility for the ethical conduct of research squarely on the shoulders of the researchers, researchers owe a duty to their subjects and themselves to meet the highest standards of integrity and accountability.

One way in which researchers can show their concern for human subjects protection is to familiarize themselves with the basic principles of research ethics that have been articulated by physicians, bioethicists, legislatures, and the courts over the last 40 years. Respect for the self-determination and dignity of all subjects in research, the need for free and informed consent, the importance of protecting subject confidentiality, equity in the selection of subjects and in the distribution of any risks associated with research, and the rights of subjects to withdraw from participation at any time without penalty are the foundations of contemporary research ethics.

Such values and principles have special implications for psychiatric populations, and we explore them in depth in this chapter. Let us begin, however, with a brief history of the development of modern research ethics. Ethical codes and regulations tend to be developed in reaction to scandals and improprieties, and so histories of research ethics often paint a fairly bleak picture of the treatment of subjects at the hands of researchers. It is important to remember that although the scandalous cases make the news, alongside them are the stories of the countless researchers who conducted their experiments with integrity and care for their subjects and through whose work the empirical basis for modern medical practice has been established.

REGULATING HUMAN SUBJECTS RESEARCH

The Nuremberg Code and the Declaration of Helsinki

It is debatable whether the exploitation of human beings in the concentration camps during the Nazi regime should be dignified by calling it medical research. Nonetheless, a defining moment in the history of the ethics of human experimentation in medicine came as a result of the post–World War II trial of 20 physicians and 3 Third Reich administrative officials who had collaborated in the unspeakable victimization of concentration camp inmates in the name of medical research. They picked their victims because they were Jews, homosexuals, twins, and, in some cases, mentally ill. Debates about the nature of medical research and its guiding principles that arose at the ensuing trial inspired the judges to draft the Nuremberg Code (Appendix E), the seminal document in the history of standards for the use of human subjects in research.

The first principle of the Nuremberg Code is that the voluntary consent of the subject is "absolutely essential." (It is both interesting and ironic that the German Interior Ministry had itself drafted model regulations in 1931 that established strict controls over human experimentation, including consent requirements, but these principles were disregarded in Nazi medical research on disfavored minorities.) A medical adviser to the Nuremberg judges, Leo Alexander, drafted language for the code that permitted use of the mentally ill in research "on the treatment of nervous and mental illness" under certain conditions, including permission of the next of kin or legal guardian and, when possible, of the patient him- or herself. The recommendation was dropped by the judges, presumably because they did not intend to deal with research on patients but only on prisoners.

The code lists 10 basic principles, including mandates that subjects be competent; that experiments be performed first on animals and reflect a knowledge of the natural history of the disease under study; that experiments result in a good for society not attainable by other means; and that experiments avoid unnecessary physical and mental suffering and injury, balance the degree of risk with the humanitarian importance of the project, and be conducted with proper safeguards and adequate facilities. The code places the responsibility for the ethical design and competent application of the experimental protocol directly with the researcher (Shamoo and Irving 1993).

Almost as soon as the Nuremberg Code was promulgated, authorities in the world of medical research recognized its shortcomings as a practical guide. Henry Beecher, a prominent professor of anesthesiology at Harvard and a pioneer in research ethics, commented that the code's requirement for subject consent "would effectively cripple if not eliminate most research in the field of mental disease" (Beecher 1959, p. 50). Indeed, any subject population incapable of giving voluntary consent, including young children and the mentally ill, would have been excluded from study.

To address this and other shortcomings of the Nuremberg Code, the World Medical Association formally adopted its own code, the Declaration of Helsinki, in 1964. The declaration distinguished between therapeutic research, which offers some potential for diagnostic or therapeutic benefit to the subject, and nontherapeutic research, which is purely investigational. In nontherapeutic research, the declaration holds, consent can never be waived. However, for incompetent patients for whom participation in therapeutic research is an option, "consent should be procured from the legal guardian" (Katz 1972, p. 312). Allowing surrogate consent for some forms of research ensures that the mentally ill can benefit from clinical research into their condition. The declaration has been revised four times over the years since it was first adopted, and the American Medical Association, the American Society for Clinical Investigation, the American Federation for Clinical Research, the Department of Defense, and the FDA are among the organizations that have either adopted the declaration outright or used it as the basis for their own statements. The declaration helped standardize ethical procedures in research on human subjects and thus made it easier for researchers to conform to ethical guidelines. Yet a number of factors, such as the increasing focus on individual rights that characterized the 1960s, critical articles by scholars, occasional scandals, and the establishment of patients' rights groups, continued to provoke scrutiny of research on those incapacitated by mental illness.

Scandal and Reform in the 1960s

In 1964 issues of informed consent were still inchoate enough that an article in the *Journal of Psychiatric Research* could argue against telling psychiatric subjects about placebo-controlled trials, because such information "would engender suspicion and perhaps hostility in subjects, making them undesirable, if not unwilling, candidates for placebo research" (Liberman 1964, p. 233). In the general climate of distrust of established institutions that characterized the 1960s, however, this attitude changed.

A seminal publication was undoubtedly Henry Beecher's 1966 article in the *New England Journal of Medicine* in which he identified 22 instances of published research that involved patently unethical practices in the use of human subjects. These studies included the injection of live cancer cells into patients with dementia at the Brooklyn Jewish Chronic Disease Hospital without their knowledge or consent and the deliberate exposure of severely mentally disabled children and adolescents to hepatitis virus at the Willowbrook State School in Staten Island, New York. The researchers in these cases were not studying mental illness. Mentally ill populations were being used for studies of other disorders because they were an institutionalized population who could be accessed, in many cases, simply through the permission of the institution's director. The reaction to Beecher's exposé was strong and widespread, and the resulting discussions were instrumental in further reforming the ethics of medical research, including psychiatric research.

Beecher's proposed solution to research ethics violations was more and better voluntary peer oversight among physicians. Yet it was those very physicians, often well respected and working under federal grants and presumed governmental oversight, who had conducted most of the research Beecher cited. Others, therefore, were less sanguine about the medical profession's ability to monitor and reform itself and began to press for legislation.

James Shannon, director of the National Institutes of Health (NIH) from 1955 to 1968, drafted new standards for the Public Health Service, which Surgeon General William Stewart signed in 1966. The new policy required prior committee review for all human subjects research, focusing on subjects' rights and welfare, the methods used to obtain informed consent, and the risk-benefit balance. The policy did not officially come into effect until 1974 (PL 93-348), by which time the new regulations included a somewhat more stringent informed consent requirement, eliminated most exceptions to documenting consent, and required that all research undergo prior review, regardless of the level of subject risk. That same year, the Department of Health, Education, and Welfare (DHEW; now the Department of Health and Human Services [DHHS]) published regulations for the protection of human subjects in the *Federal Register* (under Title 45, *Code of Federal Regulations [CFR]*, part 46), which codified the rules and procedures by which IRBs must operate at any institution receiving federal funding.

Tuskegee and the National Commission

Perhaps no incident during this period aroused more public concern about the ethics of human research than the 1972 revelation of the so-called Tuskegee Syphilis Study. For 40 years researchers had been following the disease progression of 400 African American males living in rural Alabama who were known to have syphilis. The subjects in the study, which was sponsored by the U.S. Public Health Service, were not told of their disease and were offered no treatment except for annual physicals to collect biological information on the progression of the disease. The study directors informed local doctors not to treat the subjects, intervened whenever subjects tried to obtain outside treatment, and even blocked the subjects' conscription into the army during World War II for fear their disease would be treated. Treatment was withheld even after penicillin became widely used to treat syphilis in the late 1940s.

Public and professional outrage at the study led to the establishment of a special advisory panel by the DHEW in 1973. The Tuskegee panel recommended that the Tuskegee study be terminated immediately and found that governmental policies for reviewing scientific procedures and consent processes in federally funded research were inadequate.

From 1974 to 1978 a federal advisory body titled the National Commission for the Protection of Human Subjects of Biomedical and Behavioral Research was chartered to complete the Tuskegee panel's unfinished inquiry into what was wrong with existing protections for human beings involved in research. Congress charged the commission to investigate the use of vulnerable groups as research subjects, including the "mentally handicapped," and to determine the effectiveness of the emerging IRB system. In the commission's famous Belmont Report (National Commission 1978), three ethical principles were held to be central to the research enterprise: 1) the principle of respect for persons (autonomy), which is reflected by obtaining informed consent; 2) the principle of beneficence, which requires that a risk-benefit assessment be made of every research protocol; and 3) the principle of justice, which requires fairness in the selection of subjects. The commission explicitly stated that each class of incompetent patients, including the mentally ill, must be considered on its own terms; that third parties, whose primary goal is to protect the subject from harm, should be used; and that these third parties must be allowed to observe the actual research to determine whether it is in the subject's best interest.

Of special importance for research involving those with diminished capacity was the commission's introduction of the idea of *assent* to refer to the agreement of a person who has impaired capacity but is generally functional. Impaired subjects have the right to assent or not to assent, but only with the subjects' assent can their legal representatives give official consent to research on the subjects' behalf.

The Common Rule and the Federal Regulatory Framework

The commission was followed by other panels, most notably the President's Commission for the Study of Ethical Problems in Medicine and Biomedical and Behavioral Research (1980–1983), and by other DHHS regulations. Yet in the mid-1980s there was still no standard government policy that coordinated the diverse regulations of federal agencies. The situation was finally remedied by the "Common Rule," which was first proposed in 1986 but not codified until 1991. The Common Rule was identical to the basic 1981 DHHS policy (45 *CFR* 46, subpart A) but by executive order extended that basic structure to the regulations of 15 federal agencies and the Central Intelligence Agency. By the early 1990s, then, after more than 25 years in the making, a comprehensive regulatory framework was finally in place that formally governed virtually all human subjects research conducted by the federal government or in facilities receiving federal funds.

The Common Rule and previous federal regulations addressed a number of vulnerable populations whose ability to give informed consent was compromised, including fetuses, in vitro embryos, and pregnant women (subpart A); prisoners (subpart C); and children (subpart D). Yet in spite of the National Commission's 1979 concerns about the mentally disabled and the 1983 recommendation by the President's Commission that special protections be adopted for this population, serious doubts about the wisdom of such measures remain. The population of those who might be characterized as decisionally impaired is potentially quite large and diverse; many individuals with psychiatric disorders would not fit into such a category. Those who are decisionally impaired or at risk for such an impairment might be stigmatized by this kind of characterization. Psychiatric researchers have also argued that researchers are sensitive to issues of coercion and manipulation in the mentally ill and that psychiatric patients are not as vulnerable as their protectors suggest. Some advocates for the mentally ill argue that special protections are themselves stigmatizing, do not respect patient autonomy, and thus further contribute to the powerlessness and distrust experienced by the mentally ill. Such concerns help account for the fact that the Common Rule does not treat the mentally ill as a vulnerable group in need of special protections. The Common Rule does state that IRBs should be "particularly cognizant" of the needs of all vulnerable subjects, including the mentally disabled, and suggests that IRBs include "additional safeguards" when such populations are included in a study.

The Common Rule controls more human subjects research than any other policy or framework. All federally funded research and all research performed at institutions whose research is subject to a multiple project assurance (MPA) must comply with the Common Rule. An MPA is awarded by the Office for the Protection of Research Risks to institutions that pledge compliance. Thus, the reach of the Common Rule is immense, and we discuss some of its major guidelines in the "Current Issues in Human Subjects Research in Psychiatry" section later in this chapter. At this writing, the National Bioethics Advisory Commission is considering whether current regulations adequately protect the decisionally impaired or whether additional conditions should be imposed on research involving individuals with impaired decision-making capacity. In the next section we discuss some of the reasons for this reconsideration.

Developments Since the Common Rule

Views of patient autonomy and standards of ethical human subjects research have been changing ever since the Common Rule was formulated. A number of court decisions, regulations such as the Patient Self-Determination Act, statements by professional medical societies, and various commission findings have prompted renewed attention to the inadequacies of protections of people in both clinical and research settings.

For example, President Clinton's Advisory Committee on Human Radiation Experiments (1994–1995), which documented thousands of federally funded research projects involving ionizing radiation between 1944 and 1974, also examined the adequacy of consent forms and practices in both radiation and nonradiation research as required under the Common Rule. The committee found that, although there have indeed been "significant advances in the protection of the rights and interests of human subjects" since the 1940s, there is also "evidence of serious deficiencies in some parts of the current system" (Advisory Committee 1995, p. 510).

The deficiencies cited by the committee included inadequate information in research proposal documents about the voluntariness of participation, about risks that are discussed among investigators and IRB members but not in consent forms, and about considerations that enter into the selection of subjects and confusion about the distinction between research and therapy. Of particular importance for psychiatric research, the Advisory Committee on Human Radiation Experiments (1995, p. 510) found that research proposal documents rarely discussed "the implications of diminished capacity for the process of consent and authorization to participate in research, even in studies that appeared to offer no prospect of medical benefit to subjects." The committee also found a high degree of trust in medical research institutions and in the medical research community but warned that unless the problems identified in its studies were addressed, public confidence in medical research might be endangered.

Some states have issued their own regulations about psychiatric research (Delano and Zucker 1994). Several high-profile cases, as well as the efforts of groups such as the National Alliance for the Mentally Ill, have reopened debate over the nature of psychiatric research and the safeguards afforded to the mentally disabled. Newer, more comprehensive regulations may well be the result of these concerns; we discuss that possibility in the following section.

CURRENT ISSUES IN HUMAN SUBJECTS RESEARCH IN PSYCHIATRY

Psychiatric research presents some ethical issues that codes of conduct and federal regulations may not adequately address. Researchers and bioethicists often take opposing positions on these issues, and researchers frequently must use their best judgment to assure the protection of vulnerable subjects in these areas. A review of a few of the more controversial issues may serve to illustrate how much work must still be done to create a standardized set of principles and regulations that will both protect human subjects and allow for the advancement of psychiatric knowledge and therapy. Most of these issues are discussed at greater length in subsequent chapters of this book.

Risk

The Common Rule's framework contemplates three levels of research risk: 1) *minimal risk research,* in which the risks of harm anticipated are not greater, considering probability and magnitude, than those ordinarily encountered in daily life; 2) *greater than minimal risk research that presents the prospect of direct benefit to individual subjects;* and 3) *greater than minimal risk research that does not present the prospect of direct benefit to individual subjects.* Each has its particular protections:

- *Minimal risk research* includes noninvasive procedures, psychometric tests, medical record reviews, venipunctures, medical tests or procedures done in a routine physical examination, diagnosis and treatment of patients, and so forth. According to federal regulations, informed consent requirements may be waived if a study presents minimal risk and meets three other conditions: the waiver or alteration will not adversely affect the rights and welfare of the subjects; the research could not practicably be carried out without the waiver or alteration; and, whenever appropriate, subjects will be provided with additional pertinent information after participation.

- *Greater than minimal risk research that presents the prospect of direct benefit to individual subjects* is often called therapeutic research, although subjects in a study may not receive the potential therapeutic benefit (e.g., they may be assigned to the placebo arm). Patients with decision-making capacity must give informed consent to participate in this kind of research. IRBs must ensure that the research design is methodologically sound and that risks to subjects are reasonable considering the alternatives, including that of no treatment at all.

- *Greater than minimal risk research that does not present the prospect of direct benefit to individual subjects* is sometimes called purely investigational research to distinguish it from research that might present a direct benefit to some subjects. The research must be likely to yield generalizable knowledge about subjects' disorder or condition. Patients with capacity (or the surrogates of incompetent patients) must give informed consent to participate in this kind of research. IRBs must ensure that the research design is methodologically sound and risks to subjects are minimized.

Applying these categories to actual research projects is not simple. For example, there are no firm guidelines to determine minimal risk. Is minimal risk to be interpreted as the average risk a patient might run on a typical day outside of an institution (which may be very high for a homeless person with schizophrenia, for example), some incremental degree of risk above and beyond the risks the person would otherwise face if he or she were participating in a research project, or some universal list of common research procedures or activities that are broadly recognized as relatively safe?

Similarly, *direct benefit to the patient* can be a slippery concept. Any study that involves a routine physical or diagnostic assessment or provides medical supervision that the subject may not otherwise receive can be justified as benefiting the subject. However, such attention usually constitutes the good medical care patients should be receiving (but do not always receive) outside of research protocols, and so the term *benefit* is usually limited to the potential benefit of a drug trial or research directly related to a subject's disorder. Also, IRBs sometimes do not allow surrogate consent on greater than minimal risk research in mentally ill subjects, especially if it promises indirect benefit. In fact, such research is not permitted in some states.

Drug-Free Studies, Washout Studies, and Placebo Research

In May 1994 the Office for the Prevention of Research Risks (OPRR) of the NIH reported on two complaints against schizophrenia researchers at the University of California–Los Angeles (UCLA) from subjects who had participated in studies of Prolixin decanoate, an antipsychotic medication. The study had used a washout strategy, in which the subject is maintained in a drug-free state for a period to establish a baseline level of functioning. The UCLA study's purpose was to identify predictors of successful functioning without antipsychotics. Subjects first underwent a 1-year, fixed-dose study of Prolixin in which they received injections every 2 weeks. Those willing to continue entered a second randomized, double-blind, placebo-controlled study of the same dose of Prolixin. After 12 weeks the two groups crossed over, with subjects who had received active medication now getting placebo and vice versa. After another 12 weeks stable subjects entered a withdrawal protocol, in which medications were stopped and subjects were followed up for at least a year or until they experienced exacerbation or relapse. During this period, one subject experienced a severe relapse and threatened to kill his parents, at one point approaching his mother with a carving knife. One year after leaving the study, a former subject who was drug free but was still being studied by the researchers committed suicide.

Those who complained about the study claimed that the drug withdrawal protocol was unethical because it virtually guaranteed that subjects would relapse; that adequate informed consent was not obtained from the subjects; and that the patients were inadequately monitored by the investigators, who did not restart medication quickly enough when they relapsed. OPRR concluded that the design of the UCLA study was not itself unethical and that monitoring was not deficient but that the informed consent process failed to adequately describe the differences between participating in the study and receiving standard therapy. The agency also concluded that subjects should have been told that their physicians were acting in the role of investigators, not therapists, for this project.

Critics of washout studies maintain that drug-free trials should never be permitted because a basic aim is to induce patient relapse, with all of the suffering relapse entails. The Declaration of Helsinki requires that every subject, including control subjects, be "assured of the best proven diagnostic and therapeutic method" available (Katz 1972, p. 312). Being removed from medication for research purposes may not fulfill this requirement. Advocates of washout studies, on the other hand, argue that all experimentation entails risk, that establishing baseline functioning is critical for determining the efficacy of a new medication, and that with careful monitoring the risk of relapse is no greater than that taken by subjects in other research protocols. Additionally, given the side effects and limitations of current psychotropic medications, determining who can remain drug free and stable could be of great benefit to patients themselves.

Placebo studies are often regarded as the gold standard for investigational drug research. But is it ethical to deny patients known effective treatments in the pursuit of research goals—even laudable ones—when, as in the case of patients with schizophrenia, the results of placebo are likely to be significant discomfort or harm in a percentage of subjects? One way to answer this question is to insist that placebo studies be done only when there is no other way to acquire information of vital importance for subjects with particular ailments and conditions.

Informed Consent

Studies of informed consent tend to show that both experimental patients and control subjects often have a very poor understanding of the risks, benefits, and methods of the protocols to which they consent (Benson et al. 1988; Irwin et al. 1985). Many subgroups of psychiatric patients have even less comprehension, and the clinical terminology used in most informed consent forms further limits understanding (Meisel and Roth 1983). Recently calls have been made for the formulation of more understandable and accessible informed consent procedures for the mentally impaired. Research has shown that improving the quality of information to psychiatric patients increases patient understanding (Benson et al. 1988). Suggested improvements include using videotapes or videodiscs, giving smaller units of information over longer periods of time, encouraging subjects and their families to use audiotaping during the presentation of information about research, appointing an independent patient advocate to answer questions about research, increasing the use of didactic techniques such as repetition and subject summarization, and frequently reinforming patients during the life of the study. Few empirical data exist on the relative usefulness of these innovations, however.

According to the Common Rule, all competent patients must grant informed consent to participate in research, except for those in minimal risk studies, and incompetent patients must be represented by a third party who is charged with safeguarding the subject's welfare. Informed consent must include the following elements:

- A statement that the project involves research, an explanation of the purposes of the research, and a description of the procedures to be followed

- A description of the reasonably foreseeable risks or discomforts to the subject
- A description of any benefits to the subjects or to others that might reasonably be expected
- A disclosure of alternative procedures or courses of treatment
- A statement describing the extent to which the confidentiality of records identifying the subject will be maintained
- For research involving more than minimal risk, an explanation of the availability and nature of any compensation or medical treatment if injury occurs
- Identification of whom to contact for further information about the research and about subjects' rights and whom to contact in the event of a research-related injury
- A statement that participation is voluntary, refusal to participate will involve no penalty or loss of benefits to which the subject is otherwise entitled, and participation may be discontinued at any time without penalty to the subject

The picture is not so simple in psychiatric research or other research involving patients with cognitive or affective deficits. In schizophrenia, for example, psychosis is episodic and cognitive deficits can be subtle; in mood disorders, judgment may be impaired even though the subject seems to clearly understand the facts.

Another challenge facing psychiatric and other researchers is potential conflicts of interest when physicians assume the role of both clinician and researcher. The goals of the clinician and the researcher often differ; the clinician's primary goal is care of the patient, whereas the researcher's is the accumulation of scientific knowledge. These conflicts can be more acute if researchers are given funding to enroll and retain study subjects from their own patient pools. It is difficult for most patients to understand that the physician who has been treating them is now also a researcher using them as experimental subjects. Subjects may fall prey to the *therapeutic misconception,* a belief that the research activity is meant for their direct benefit rather than to help create generalizable knowledge. IRBs need to be aware of potential conflicts of interest and ensure that the informed consent process specifically acknowledges them.

A device suggested by the National Commission, called the consent auditor, could help to ensure patient voluntariness and mitigate the conflict of interest inherent in much research recruitment. The consent auditor is an individual who is not associated with the study and who therefore has no conflict of interest with regard to soliciting subject participation. The auditor's role is to witness the informed consent process and decide whether the subject's apparent consent to participate involves adequate comprehension and judgment and is sufficiently voluntary. If the auditor has any doubts about the subject's voluntariness, he or she can either request an ethics consultation or advise that the subject not be enrolled. The consent auditor is a disinterested party whose involvement adds a further layer of accountability to the process of choosing study participants. However, because using an auditor also adds cost to the research, and may be a time-consuming and cumbersome procedure thought unnecessary or resented by researchers, this process is rarely used.

A further rarely discussed issue that is virtually unique to psychiatric studies is the question of the potential physical harm to subjects' families during a study and the degree to which families might also have a stake in knowing about a member's participation in a research study. In washout studies, relapse of subjects, especially those living at home, may put families at risk for violence as an indirect result of the research protocol. Researchers have a moral duty to warn families who may be at risk, as they do when a clinical patient seriously threatens violence against a family member. Other studies, such as those with persons who are depressed or have eating disorders, may increase families' care and support burden, and therefore researchers should be sensitive to the effect their research may have on subjects' support networks.

Capacity and Competence

The notion of *capacity* is more robust than the more global notion of *competence,* which is a legal term. Capacity is task specific and implies that one may be capable of certain actions or decisions but not others. That an individual has been given a psychiatric disorder diagnosis does not imply that he or she lacks decision-making capacity concerning research, standard medical treatment, or any other life decision. The legal finding that a patient is incompetent for any reason, therefore, requires a further determination, governed by legal requirements of the jurisdiction in which the individual is institutionalized, to determine whether the person lacks the capacity to make medical decisions. Thus, for example, an individual who is incompetent with respect to his or her financial affairs may not lack the capacity to make a decision about how much medication can comfortably be tolerated.

Despite some attempts by scholars in the legal and psychiatric communities to create standardized means to determine capacity (usually for consent to treatment rather than research), judgments of subject capacity are still highly dependent on individual psychiatric assessment. Grisso and Appelbaum (1995), for example, found that the choice of standards used to assess competence affected the identity and proportion of those considered competent; different groups were identified as impaired depending on the measures used, and the proportion increased when multiple or compound measures were employed.

Appelbaum and his colleagues (Appelbaum 1996; Appelbaum and Grisso 1988; Appelbaum and Roth 1982) have created the most cited typology of competence. Noting that competence is a legal concept and can be formally determined only in court, they enumerate the four standards most commonly used by the courts and by those writing about competence:

1. An ability to communicate a choice
2. An ability to understand relevant information
3. An ability to appreciate the nature of the situation and its consequences
4. An ability to manipulate information rationally

Some groups, such as the American College of Physicians (ACP) (1989), have endorsed the idea of preconsent (Ulysses Contracts), whereby a competent patient agrees in advance to consent to research when he or she becomes incapacitated. The ACP mandates a proxy to supervise the subject's participation after becoming incompetent, giving the proxy the responsibility of protecting the subject's welfare and withdrawing the subject from participation if necessary. In the absence of such a contract, surrogates should have the right to consent to participation in research for incompetent subjects consistent with the subjects' best interests.

Surrogacy and Substituted Judgment

Although there are no specific federal regulations concerning research with adults of diminished capacity, the regulations allow an IRB to impose special conditions on research procedures to ensure the ethical participation of this population. In 1986 the Clinical Center (CC) of the NIH voluntarily adopted a set of guidelines for the cognitively impaired in its report entitled "Consent Process in Research Involving Impaired Human Subjects." At this writing, the CC policy is the most fully developed statement of any federal agency and so may serve as a model for broader regulations. The policy recognizes that "consent of impaired subjects is necessary but is not sufficient" for involvement in research. Researchers must also obtain a substituted judgment that the subject would consent to the research if he or she were capable of providing informed consent. The CC policy is summarized in Table 1–1, which describes eight case types representing various combinations of circumstances.

The CC policy presumes that a patient is either capable or, if incapable, has executed a legal document called a durable power of attorney for health care (DPAHC). The DPAHC is not to be confused with a traditional durable power of attorney, which pertains to granting a representative legal authority over

TABLE 1–1.   Typology of impaired subjects according to the Clinical Center
at National Institutes of Health

Eight possible research situations are enumerated in the Clinical Center of the
National Institutes of Health's (NIH's) "Consent Process in Research Involving
Impaired Human Subjects" (1986). Each assumes a different degree of subject
capacity and/or experimental risk and sets forth guidelines for the permissibility
of research under those circumstances.

Case 1: The subject is capable of understanding the durable power of attorney
(DPA), and the research risk is minimal. The DPA is executed, notification is given, and research can proceed. Notification is done by sending copies of the signed and witnessed DPA forms to those designated
on the carbons (Chair, ICRS; Institute Clinical Director; CC bioethicist).

Case 2: The subject is inapable of understanding the DPA, and the research
risk is minimal. The physician shall request an ethics consultation for
the selection of a next-of-kin surrogate. After a positive consultation
report, the substituted proxy consent of the relative can be obtained,
and research can proceed.

Case 3: The subject is incapable of understanding the DPA, and the research
risk is greater than minimal but with a prospect of direct benefit to the
subject. The physician shall request an ethics consultation to assure
that the person appointed by the subject is capable of understanding
the risks and benefits of the study. After the DPA is executed, notification shall occur, and research can proceed.

Case 4: The subject is capable of understanding the DPA, and the research risk
is greater than minimal but with no prospect of benefit to the subject.
The physician shall request an ethics consultation to assure that the
person appointed by the subject is capable of understanding the purpose and risks of the study. After the DPA is executed, notification shall
occur, and research can proceed.

(continued)

certain financial matters, such as signing checks. The DPAHC is a legal device
by which the research subject appoints a surrogate to make decisions for the
subject about his or her participation in research should he or she become
incapacitated. Also, if the subject is incapable of choosing a surrogate through
the DPAHC process, the CC's policy permits a physician to choose a next-of-
kin surrogate, subject to approval through an ethics consultation. Each jurisdiction has special conditions concerning DPAHCs, and not all of them allow
surrogate consent for research rather than standard therapy. Both DPAHC and
next-of-kin surrogacy require consultation with legal counsel to ensure compliance with local law.

TABLE 1–1. Typology of impaired subjects according to the Clinical Center at National Institutes of Health *(continued)*

Case 5: The subject is incapable of understanding the DPA, and the research risk is greater than minimal with a prospect of direct benefit to the subject. No court-appointed guardian exists, but family members desire the patient's participation in the research. The physician shall request an ethics consultation for the family members to assure their understanding of the risks and benefits and also of the CC's policy requiring court appointment of a guardian. Research shall not proceed until family members initiate court proceedings and a court-appointed guardian gives consent for the research.

Case 6: The subject is incapable of understanding the DPA and the research risk is greater than minimal, with no prospect of benefit to the subject. No court-appointed guardian exists, but family members desire the subject's participation in the research. The physician shall request an ethics consultation for the family members to assure their understanding of the risks and lack of benefit in this case. Research shall not proceed until family members initiate court proceedings and a court-appointed guardian gives consent for the research.

Case 7: The subject is incapable of understanding the DPA and the research risk is greater than minimal, with a prospect of direct benefit to the subject. The subject does not have an intact family, i.e., no relatives are alive or able to act as surrogate decision makers. Research can proceed if the situation is a medical emergency, when a physician may give therapy, including experimental therapy, if in the physician's judgment it is necessary to protect the life or health of the patient.

Case 8: The subject is incapable of understanding the DPA and the research risk is greater than minimal, with no benefit to the subject. The subject does not have an intact family or relatives. Research is prohibited in this case.

Subject Selection and Recruitment

The inherently coercive nature of involuntary commitment has led some to suggest that noncoercive experimentation can never be done on this population, because informed consent must be voluntary. However, others argue that consent to participate in research may be a means to empower institutionalized patients. In any case, because such patients routinely participate in decision making about their medical care, there is no reason to judge them absolutely incapable of making decisions in this one area. Still, the power differentials inherent in the locked ward or court-mandated treatment increase the risk that the voluntariness of consent will be compromised (Appelbaum 1995).

There are a number of ways to ensure voluntary consent without denying involuntarily committed populations the opportunity to participate in research. Protocols must be examined for their inherent fairness, and IRBs must be convinced that investigators understand the risks of coercion in such research. Participation in research should not result in additional rewards or privileges that are not available to those who refuse consent (outside of reasonable compensation for expenses and subjects' lost time). Informed consent procedures are best done by someone other than the treating physician, and in some cases consent auditors or patient advocates should participate in the informed consent process.

Ensuring that the burdens and benefits of participation in research are fairly and evenly distributed across eligible populations is important. Poor or uninsured patients should not be relied on as a subject pool to the exclusion of wealthy or insured patients. Likewise, minorities and women should be included as subjects in research, because these populations tend to be underrepresented and may have special needs or circumstances that research confined to only white men does not reveal. Women must know about the risks that new and experimental drugs pose if they are or become pregnant, yet the participation of women in psychiatric research involving drugs should not be neglected out of fears of harm to embryos or fetuses. It is ethical to ask women involved in studies to consent to the use of contraception or to abstain from sexual relations as a condition of study participation.

Direct Benefit Versus Altruism

In 1979 the National Commission allowed mentally disabled subjects to participate in research that did not directly benefit them. Two years earlier, the American Bar Association's Commission on the Mentally Disabled recommended that research using institutionalized persons relate "directly to the etiology, pathogenesis, prevention, diagnosis, or treatment of mental disability," arguing that the mentally disabled are already burdened enough, and so others, free of such burdens, should bear the brunt of research if possible (quoted in Tancredi and Maxfield 1983, p. 25).

Denying the mentally impaired the right to participate in research that benefits others denies them the opportunity to be altruistic and therefore excludes them from a role given to others. If a person is capable of understanding altruism and its risks, there is no prima facie reason to deny that person the right to make a moral choice to participate in research.

CONCLUSION

There is no doubt that researchers are concerned about conducting ethically proper studies and that many persons with mental illness support research that may alleviate their symptoms or even remove the cause of symptoms. It is also true that the history of research with mentally ill patients shows that they have been subjected to abuse and maltreatment. Special vigilance is necessary on the part of those conducting psychiatric research today. Researchers must realize that research is a privilege, not a right. Society can restrict (and has restricted) the right of researchers to undertake studies and inquiries when it has reason to believe that the welfare, health, and dignity of subjects are being compromised. The best rule for a researcher using subjects who are mentally ill is to be absolutely certain that the subject or surrogate fully understands and can appreciate the risk-benefit ratio of the study and that every effort is made to design a study that minimizes risks to subjects to the degree possible. In the end, despite all of the regulations and guidelines, the best protection a subject in research has is the integrity and advocacy of the investigator.

REFERENCES

Advisory Committee on Human Radiation Experiments: Final Report. New York, Oxford University Press, 1995

American College of Physicians: Cognitively impaired subjects. Ann Intern Med 111:843–848, 1989

Appelbaum PS: Consent and coercion: research with involuntarily treated persons with mental illness or substance abuse. Accountability in Research 4:69–79, 1995

Appelbaum PS: Patients' competence to consent to neurobiological research. Accountability in Research 4:241–245, 1996

Appelbaum PS, Grisso T: Assessing patients' capacities to consent to treatment. N Engl J Med 319:1635–1638, 1988

Appelbaum PS, Roth LH: Competency to consent to research. Arch Gen Psychiatry 39:951–958, 1982

Beecher HK: Experimentation in Man. Springfield, IL, Charles C Thomas, 1959

Beecher HK: Ethics and clinical research. N Engl J Med 475:1354–1360, 1966

Benson P, Roth LH, Appelbaum PS, et al: Information disclosure, subject understanding, and informed consent in psychiatric research. Law and Human Behavior 12:455–475, 1988

Clinical Center, National Institutes of Health: Consent Process in Research Involving Impaired Human Subjects. Bethesda, MD, National Institutes of Health, 1986

Delano SJ, Zucker JL: Protecting mental health research subjects without prohibiting progress. Hosp Community Psychiatry 45:601–603, 1994

Department of Health and Human Services: Final Rule, Protection of Human Subjects: Informed Consent. Federal Register 61 (October 2, 1996):51498

Grisso T, Appelbaum PS: Comparison of standards for assessing patients' capacities to make treatment decisions. Am J Psychiatry 152:1033–1037, 1995

Grodin MA, Glantz LH (eds): Children as Research Subjects. New York, Oxford University Press, 1994

Irwin J, Lovitz AA, Marder SR, et al: Psychotic patients' understanding of informed consent. Am J Psychiatry 142:1351–1354, 1985

Katz J (ed): World Medical Association Declaration of Helsinki, in Experimentation With Human Beings. New York, Russel Sage Foundation, 1972, pp 312–313

Levine RJ: Ethics and the Regulation of Clinical Research, 2nd Edition. Baltimore, MD, Urban & Schwarzenberg, 1986

Liberman R: An experimental study of the placebo response under three different situations of pain. J Psychiatr Res 2:233–246, 1964

Meisel A, Roth L: Toward an informed discussion of informed consent: a review and critique of empirical studies. Arizona Law Review 15:265–346, 1983

National Commission for the Protection of Human Subjects of Biomedical and Behavioral Research: The Belmont Report (DHEW Publ No OS-78-0012). Washington, DC, U.S. Government Printing Office, 1978

Shamoo AE, Irving DE: Accountability in research using persons with mental illness. Accountability in Research 3:1–17, 1993

Tancredi LR, Maxfield CT: Regulation of psychiatric research: a socioethical analysis. Int J Law Psychiatry 6:17–38, 1983

Wolpe PR, Merz JF: Hospital ERs on front line of informed-consent debate. Forum for Applied Research and Public Policy 12:127–131, 1997

CHAPTER 2

Issues in Clinical Research Design: Principles, Practices, and Controversies

JEFFREY A. LIEBERMAN, M.D., SCOTT STROUP, M.D.,
EUGENE LASKA, PH.D., JAN VOLAVKA, M.D., PH.D.,
ALAN GELENBERG, M.D., A. JOHN RUSH, M.D.,
KATHERINE SHEAR, M.D., AND WILLIAM CARPENTER, M.D.

I n recent years highly publicized instances of scientific fraud and allegations of abuses of human subjects have led to increased examination of the ethics of biomedical research. Because mental illness is poorly understood by the general public and individuals with mental illness are perceived to be potentially vulnerable to exploitation, the scrutiny has been most intense for psychiatric research. In this chapter we consider the benefits and risks to human subjects of various experimental designs and methods. We focus primarily on experimental designs that involve considerable potential risk to study participants, including medication-free research and studies requiring invasive procedures. Because medical research fundamentally involves the need to balance the goal of scientific discovery with the burden and risks to individual participants, we consider design issues in this context.

We begin this chapter by presenting ethical principles relevant to research design. Second, we review, from the perspective of ethical considerations, some of the statistical design issues that attend the application of a generic clinical trial to psychiatric research. Third, we consider issues related to specific disorders (schizophrenia, bipolar disorder, major depressive disorder, and anxiety disorders). Finally, we consider ethical implications in the design of nontherapeutic research.

It is not our intent to establish definitive standards for research design; society and its policy-making institutions must provide this guidance. Our purpose is to present relevant considerations, ethical principles, and general guidelines for individual investigators as they consider research hypotheses and design studies to test them.

GENERAL CONSIDERATIONS

All research involves important considerations of study design and methods. Because clinical research includes human subjects who may be placed at risk, it also must attend to ethical considerations (Meinert 1996). A clinical study must balance the responsibility of physicians to always act benevolently for their patients with the scientific need to acquire new knowledge for the benefit of future patients (Clayton 1982). These somewhat conflicting obligations present the clinical investigator with vexing dilemmas.

The following guidelines, based on fundamental ethical principles, are generic and should always be applied in study design:

1. A study that cannot be informative is unethical. Any risk is too much in a study without potential benefits.
2. A study should be as informative as possible, within the context of the study's goals.
3. The risks to study participants should be minimized.
4. Individual autonomy must be respected. Participation of subjects must be voluntary.
5. The principles of informed consent must be followed fully. A patient, or his or her legal representative, should consent to participate in a study only after risks and benefits have been effectively communicated.
6. Research is not treatment. Although treatment can be a part of studies, participants should clearly understand that the purpose of research is to produce generalizable information that will benefit science, society, and patients with similar conditions in the future. They should not be led to believe that they are guaranteed to receive any direct benefit other than possible payments.
7. Information learned from a study, whether general or specific to a patient and whether positive or negative, should be made available to the patient and to the medical community in a timely fashion to the extent that such action does not compromise the study.

In the course of considering the initiation of a clinical investigation, a series of questions must be considered:

1. Does the potential benefit of a study exceed its risks?
2. If so, what is the optimal study design to test the research hypothesis?
3. If a therapeutic trial is planned, is an effective treatment already available? If not, a placebo-controlled trial is needed. If an effective treatment exists, is a better and/or safer treatment needed? If existing treatments are not curative or have a low therapeutic index, new therapies are desirable.
4. What are the nature and the severity of the illness being studied? If the illness is life threatening or if irreversible harm will result if treatment is discontinued or withheld, then placebo trials are not acceptable. If the illness is intermittent and spontaneously remitting, placebo trials may help to distinguish therapeutic effects from spontaneous remissions or waxing and waning of symptoms.
5. How can the risks to patients be minimized? The choice of a safe setting and the establishment of criteria for study withdrawal and for the use of rescue medication are important safety measures.

GENERIC ISSUES IN THE DESIGN OF A CLINICAL TRIAL

The elements of a clinical trial are similar to those of all studies, and these generic factors can be used to illustrate important ethical issues. (Ethical and scientific issues, however, must always be considered in the specific context of a study and its subjects.) Clinical studies involve consideration of some or all of the following issues: recruitment of patients, determination of sample size, development of inclusion and exclusion criteria, acquisition of informed consent, choice of treatments and controls, methods for allocating treatments to subjects, use of washout periods, duration of study, duration of treatment after study completion, use of concomitant therapy, blinding of raters and subjects, withdrawal of subjects, termination of study, analysis of statistics, and feedback and dissemination of information. Each of these issues must be weighed in designing a valid, ethical, and cost-effective study. Many of the issues are discussed in other chapters in this volume, but some with particular relevance for design decisions are discussed here.

Motivation and Rationale for the Recruitment and Enrollment of Patients

No study is without risk. Without this risk, there would be no dilemma for researchers or subjects. The justification for research on human subjects is that

society's benefit from the research sufficiently exceeds the risks to study participants. The benefit may be a new and better treatment or therapeutic paradigm
or understanding of disease processes. The investigator has a duty to design a
study that minimizes risks to subjects and ensures that the intended benefits
are obtainable. Potential risks and benefits must be effectively communicated
so that potential subjects can make informed decisions about participation.

Subjects have various motivations for participating in studies. They may
enter studies for genuinely altruistic reasons. Those who have suffered from a
disorder may wish to participate in a study to benefit future patients. Other
participants may expect to derive immediate benefit by receiving better clinical
care. In some circumstances, a subject may hope to benefit by receiving an
otherwise unavailable experimental treatment. If so, it must be clearly understood that individual participants may not be assigned to the experimental treatment group. King (1995, p. 14) emphasizes that physicians and their patients
should engage in "shared decisionmaking" regarding study participation.

Some patients may be invited to enroll in an investigation conducted by
their own physicians, presenting a potential conflict of interest. Because an
investigator's desire to enter and maintain subjects in a trial can conflict with
the physician's fiduciary duty to serve the patient's best clinical interests, subjects
may best be referred to another physician for the duration of a study. When
changing physicians is not possible, an independent clinical consultant must be
readily available.

Payments may influence a potential subject's decision to participate in a study.
Payments may range from travel reimbursements to considerable amounts of
money for time and effort. Depending on the monetary amount and the circumstances of potential subjects, such inducements can be seen as coercive. On
the other hand, there is a legitimate need to compensate participants for their
effort and time.

Sample Size Determinations

In many trials the purpose is to determine whether a difference exists between
two treatments and, if so, to estimate the magnitude of the difference. If two
treatments are equally efficacious, it is possible that the test treatment will be
declared superior to the standard treatment because of random chance. Statistical tests are designed to keep the probability of this Type I error small.

To be ethical, a trial must have a high probability of concluding that there
is a difference between test and standard treatments (if there is one). The probability of finding a difference when indeed there is a difference is called the
power of the test. The power depends on the sample size, the variability of

responses, and the size of the true difference. Of these factors, the only value within the investigator's control is the sample size. The variability of patient responses in similar clinical trials may give an approximate idea of what can be expected in the current trial, but the size of the treatment difference is unknown. How can the investigator pick a sample size that will ensure adequate power? Usually the effect size—a difference between test and standard treatments that is clinically meaningful—is established. Any difference less than the specified amount is considered to be of no consequence. The calculation of the sample size necessary to achieve the desired power, typically .80 or higher, may then be based on this value. If the true difference is larger than the specified effect size, then the trial has a higher probability of finding it. The only drawback is that the trial could have had a smaller sample size to achieve the same testing end. Sample size can also be appraised in terms of the size of a confidence interval for the mean treatment effect.

One method of increasing the probability of detecting a difference between groups is to pick a sample size so large that the chance of an error is extremely small. The obvious drawbacks to this strategy include its costs in terms of the excess patients unnecessarily exposed to risks, the time wasted, and the lost financial resources. Also, physicians and patients are denied information and perhaps even access to the better treatment for the added time it takes to complete the study. Moreover, using a very large sample limits the pool of patients available for participating in other potentially valuable studies. Several authors have tried to establish the optimal sample size to use in terms of the number of patients who will use the new better treatments for the foreseeable future (Armitage 1985; Bather 1985; Colton 1963; Laska and Meisner 1966). To date, such analyses have not led to widely used methods.

Most treatments for mental disorders affect many dimensions, as reflected by the plethora of rating scales typically used in a study. Choosing which variable to use in a power calculation requires ranking the relative importance of the outcome measures. The results for different choices can be quite disparate. For example, an assessment based on a clinical global rating may determine that the sample size needed for .90 power is 30 patients per treatment arm. Yet power analysis to detect differences in the rate of an adverse event of only moderate rarity may determine that for comparable power a sample size of several hundred or more is needed.

In the end, sample size determinations are imprecise and subjective. Neither the true value of the variance nor the value of the difference in the size of the effects of treatments can be known in advance. The power analysis should therefore be viewed as an approximation to help guide the investigator. The sample sizes used in trials of similar agents, in the same institution, and in the literature should all be weighed to arrive at a sensible judgment.

In a *sequential trial,* the sample size is not fixed but depends on the experience of the patients in the trial. As a sequential trial proceeds, the data are analyzed and the summarizing criterion or statistic is compared with pre-specified values. When the value is exceeded, the trial stops and the conclusion follows. There are open and closed schemes. In a closed sequential trial, the sample size is bounded in a way that makes it possible to reach the conclusion that no treatment difference exists. In an open scheme, the trial continues until one or the other treatment is found to be superior. On average the sample size in a sequential trial is smaller than in a comparable fixed sample size study.

Group sequential methods lie between fixed sample size and sequential designs. A fixed number of analyses, perhaps four or five, are planned at the beginning of the study to occur at specified intervals. Because repeated analyses are performed on the accumulating data, the statistical criteria must be adjusted to ensure that if a difference between treatments is declared the claim is valid. Naturally, the statistical hurdle that must be traversed is greater in the early stages than in the later stages when a larger sample gives more confidence in the significance of the outcome.

Sequential trials have been criticized on ethical grounds. Consider the last patient in a sequential trial who is assigned the test treatment. Suppose that the accumulating data show that the chance that this treatment is superior to the standard is nearly zero, but unless another patient participates in the study, the boundary will not be crossed and the probabilities will not be significant (Chalmers 1975; Schafer 1982; Tygstrup et al. 1982). Ware et al. (1985) proposed a partial solution to this concern using a "look ahead" procedure in which the probability that the test treatment is better than the comparison treatment is assessed at every stage. When the data show that this probability (called a futility index) is small, the trial is terminated. Another alternative is a "bet-the-winner" strategy that evaluates early results of a two-arm trial and then increases the likelihood of successive patients being assigned to the initially more successful arm.

Inclusion and Exclusion Criteria

If the study population is too diverse, the ability to find a difference is compromised because of the wide variability in responses to treatment (Shaw and Chalmers 1970; Tygstrup et al. 1982). On the other hand, if the exclusion criteria are too strict and the study population is narrowly constrained, the possibility of generalization is limited. For example, eliminating all women of childbearing age or patients with any history of substance abuse not only limits the sources of subjects but also decreases the generalizability of the results. Moreover, systematic exclusion of segments of the population (e.g., women of childbearing age) may be discriminatory and deprive these groups of the benefits of research on diseases' specific effects on them (Liebenluft 1996). In the United States this issue has been addressed by National Institutes of Health guidelines on the inclusion of women and minorities in research (National Institutes of Health 1994).

Informed Consent

The need to ensure informed consent is part of the bedrock of ethical behavior for those involved in clinical trials. It is important to emphasize, however, that informed consent does not eliminate the need to design ethically sound studies that avoid unnecessary risks and minimize unavoidable ones (Rothman and Michels 1994). Prospective study subjects should be given adequate information about the benefits and risks of the available treatments in the trial and the probability of receiving each of them. They must be competent to understand that information and to make a rational decision, and they must participate voluntarily. Because only competent people can give informed consent, persons deemed incompetent may enter a study only with the consent of a legal guardian, in addition to the assent of the subject.

In longitudinal studies involving multiple phases, investigators should consider a new consent process at each step of the study. Subjects who consent to randomization initially may wish to decline further participation before additional phases begin. Although participants always have the right to drop out of a study, this iterative consent process provides additional safeguards for individual autonomy.

In studies that involve subjects whose judgment may become impaired in the course of the study (e.g., in maintenance treatment studies in which relapse is an outcome), involving significant others in the consent and monitoring process may be important. Appelbaum (1996) has suggested that a durable power of attorney or other substitute decision-making mechanism is desirable if subjects may lose the capacity to act for themselves. In general, even if the research participants are deemed incompetent, they should not be required to participate if they resist unless qualified representatives determine that failure to do so is more harmful than participating. At the same time, issues of confidentiality and autonomy of subjects must be considered and respected. Adult patients who have been independent or have no significant others may have wholly justified yet different points of view from their designated representatives, and their preferences should be considered. In such cases the investigator needs to use judgment analogous to that in clinical situations in which differences in perspective and opinion can occur. Informed consent and the assessment of competence are covered more fully in Chapters 4, 5, and 6.

Choice of Treatments and Controls: When Is a Placebo Warranted?

There is perhaps no more contentious ethical issue than whether to use a placebo in a clinical trial (Addington 1995; Clark and Leaverton 1994; Freedman et al. 1996a, 1996b; Rothman and Michels 1994; Volavka et al. 1996). In a typical clinical trial, patients who complete the placebo washout period are randomly assigned to receive either the experimental treatment (T) or placebo (P) under double-blind conditions. The patients thus form parallel groups (i.e., they are not crossed over from one treatment to another). This double-blind, randomized, placebo-controlled, parallel-group trial has become the gold standard for determining the safety and clinical efficacy of pharmacological treatments (Freedman et al. 1996b; Rothman and Michels 1994).

Proof of efficacy is required by the U.S. Food and Drug Administration (FDA) for any new drug to be marketed in the United States. A placebo comparison is the most straightforward demonstration of efficacy; if a treatment is superior to placebo, the treatment is considered efficacious. Placebo comparisons are thus used to determine (and define) efficacy. However, other proofs of efficacy that meet this FDA requirement are also possible.

Use of a placebo is difficult to justify when the illness is severe and known efficacious therapies are available. However, in some situations there are valid justifications for use of a placebo. For example, if no standard treatment exists, the only way to tell whether a test treatment is effective is to compare it with a placebo. Placebos can also justifiably be used for patients who are refractory to standard treatments, for testing new drugs when the standard treatment has a poor therapeutic index, and for testing unproven augmentation strategies for subjects receiving standard treatments (Freedman et al. 1996a).

A placebo may also be justifiable when an experimental treatment (T) is being compared with a standard treatment (S). Suppose a trial has only two treatments: T and S. If the trial shows that $T > S$ or $T < S$, the results are interpretable. But if a two-armed trial compares S and T and fails to find a difference, the result may mean that neither treatment or both treatments were effective. In many cases this ambiguity is avoidable if a placebo group is used, and therefore many trials introduce a placebo treatment (P). In these studies there are three parallel treatment groups: T, P, and S. With a placebo arm, the possible results are $P < T = S$, $P = T = S$, or (improbably) $P > T = S$. If

P < T = S, both T and S were effective. A placebo arm thus limits the likelihood of inconclusive findings. However, if S = P or S < P, the results of the trial still cannot be interpreted. If the standard treatment is not more effective than placebo, something went wrong in the trial: perhaps the patients were all non-responders, the raters were not adequately trained, or the dose of the standard medication was not appropriate. In any case, the trial had low sensitivity; it failed. An investigator who found that T = S (without knowing that T = S = P) could erroneously conclude that T was effective; after all, T did not differ from the proven S. Thus, a placebo arm is used to establish trial sensitivity. However, trial sensitivity also can be established by using multiple doses (parallel arms) of T and S, assuming that the same dose is either ineffective or less effective than others. It is a matter of current debate whether this design may eliminate or reduce the need for a placebo arm. If one dose is less effective, a larger number of subjects must be exposed to achieve the same power that would be achieved with placebo.

Some argue that the randomized, placebo-controlled clinical trial is the only truly scientifically objective way of answering the question of efficacy (Pledger and Hall 1986). Others, however, advocate the use of historical controls (Dempster et al. 1983; Rothman and Michels 1994), arguing that experience from naturalistic databases and previous studies can supply information about placebo response rates. Nonetheless, historical controls would be regarded by most experts as an unsuitable substitute for placebo control except in very few situations and for studying particular diseases (Carpenter et al. 1997). Prien (1988) has pointed to the variability of placebo responses between trials as a major limitation to the use of historical controls. The value of historical and naturalistic data as a formal or informal control can be enhanced by using techniques such as matching and propensity scores (Rosenbaum 1985; Rosenbaum and Rubin 1984). The results of a clinical trial, however designed, should be compared with existing information to appropriately assess the outcome.

Several strategies have been used to address the dual problems of need for control and need to minimize placebo exposure. One such strategy is unequal randomization. If a sample is large enough and the placebo response rate is fairly well known, a study can be conducted with only a small placebo group. A variation of this approach is the bet-the-winner strategy mentioned earlier, which increases the likelihood of successive patients being assigned to the initially more successful treatment arm. A third strategy is to conduct a discontinuation study rather than use a standard randomized, controlled design. Patients are all initially treated with active medication to a designated improvement level and then randomly chosen to discontinue medication using a double-blind strategy. The rate of symptom recurrence is then measured. Although there is still exposure to placebo in these designs, subject burden is lessened. In unequal randomization and bet-the-winner strategies, fewer subjects are exposed to placebo. In discontinuation designs, relatively well patients, rather than ill ones, are assigned to placebo treatment. Investigators can rapidly reinstitute treatment in a relapsed patient. Discontinuation studies, however, are complicated by the effects of drug withdrawal.

Other alternatives to the use of placebo may be available. If there is a standard treatment for which a dose-response curve exists, then a low dose and a high dose of the treatment serve a function similar to that of a placebo. If the low dose is subtherapeutic and just a substitute for placebo, there has been no ethical gain. However, a low dose on the dose-response curve can be justified if the percentage of patients expected to respond is meaningfully larger than the percentage expected to respond to placebo. Patients who respond to the low dose would be put at a disadvantage were they given the higher dose because of a higher probability of an adverse reaction. Thus, when a dose-response curve exists, multiple-dose standard treatment controls may eliminate the need for a placebo. Yet another design is to add a placebo or experimental drug to a standard drug that patients receive as background therapy. If a therapeutic response is detected, subsequent studies using this design can include a discontinuation phase.

The issue of placebo control is discussed further in the sections on specific psychiatric disorders later in this chapter.

Methods for Allocating Treatments to Patients

Random assignment of subjects to treatment conditions eliminates selection bias in the allocation. This key element of experimental design forms the basis for statistical analysis of the results. Random assignment also facilitates blinding patients, caregivers, and raters and decreases the probability that treatment groups will differ with respect to some underlying characteristic or baseline value likely to affect the outcome. Group differences in these variables can still occur as a result of chance, but adjustments for such differences in the analysis stage, by methods such as analysis of covariance, poststratification, and modeling, are legitimized by randomization. Whenever there are known prognostic variables whose values might affect the outcome, it is wise to take them into account in the allocation procedure. Matching and stratification are commonly used to attempt to control for such variables. A newer method involves keeping track of the numbers of patients assigned to the treatment groups by prognostic variables. The randomization procedure is dynamically adjusted to increase or decrease the probabilities of treatment assignment depending on the direction needed to achieve balance. These methods are called biased coin or urn model randomization schemes (Meinert 1996; Wei 1977; Wei and Lachin 1988).

Placebo Washouts and Drug Discontinuation

If an effective medication is discontinued for long enough to ensure that there is no lingering pharmacological effect, the risks of undertreatment (symptom exacerbation and increased suffering) are present. Nevertheless, a number of reasons have been proposed for including a washout period in a trial: the establishment of a drug-free baseline, improved diagnostic accuracy, allowance for drug elimination to minimize the potential for drug interactions, screening out of placebo responders, possibility of greater treatment response, and assessment of clinical and biological variables without the effects of drug treatment. These factors have been the subject of considerable discussion (Carpenter et al. 1997; Trivedi and Rush 1994; Volavka et al. 1996). The issue of placebo washout is further discussed later in this chapter in the sections on specific psychiatric disorders.

Study Duration

Studies that are too short may fail to find treatment differences that require extended time periods in which to develop. Studies that are too long are associated with subject attrition, which complicates the analysis and interpretation of the results. Other problems with studies that are too long include the fact that potentially useful information is unnecessarily kept from the public and from study participants. Patients who enter the study near the end, as well as those not in the trial who would be helped by the results, may not benefit from the latest information. These considerations argue for scheduled analyses during the course of the study and provisions for early study termination when findings are clear. In clinical trials of medications, optimal study duration is best determined by a phase II trial that provides information about a drug's onset of action.

Poststudy Treatment and Follow-Up of Patients

Following study completion or withdrawal, a mechanism for appropriate follow-up and care of patients should be provided. This aftercare includes ensuring that a careful evaluation is conducted, that recommendations about follow-up treatment are made, and that these recommendations are clearly communicated to the patient and his or her physician.

A difficult question in the case of a clinical trial, particularly a trial involving a drug under development, is whether and how the blind should be broken to determine the best treatment for patients without compromising the study's integrity. Strict fidelity to the scientific goals of the study would militate against breaking the blind until after the entire study has been completed. Any breaking of the blind risks leaking information back to study staff that could influence their attitude toward the study and compromise the blind and thus the study itself. When the blind is strictly maintained until the study is complete, patients are often given the opportunity to undergo the experimental treatment afterward; in this way they are able to try the new treatment without compromising the blind. However, this option is not advantageous for the patient who was randomized to the experimental treatment in the double-blind phase of the study and did not respond. An alternative is to designate a clinician not involved in the study to break the blind and independently determine the best course of action for the patient and ensure that such treatment is administered outside of the study structure.

The National Alliance for the Mentally Ill (1995) has argued that a participant in a clinical trial has the right to know what treatment he or she received during the trial and the investigator's assessment of its value for the individual. Patient advocates have also suggested that if a patient has done well with an experimental treatment, he or she should be able to continue to receive it after study participation is over, even if the treatment has not yet been approved by the regulatory authorities. Systematic implementation of this proposal would require policy changes by the pharmaceutical industry and the FDA.

Early Termination of Subject Participation

A protocol for how to intervene when subjects' conditions worsen during a study must be established. Such a plan entails specification of criteria and procedures for intervention. These criteria should ignore the modest fluctuations that occur in clinical care, instead focusing on sustained worsening. Patients must always be permitted to withdraw from the study at any time should their attitude toward participation or circumstances change in the course of the study. Adequate clinical care must be available for all subjects who leave a study prematurely.

Early Termination of Study

Even in the fixed sample size experiment, as the trial continues and results accrue, interim analyses can lead to the conclusion that the trial should be terminated because of excessive adverse effects or because the evidence favoring one treatment over another is clear. Interim analysis to reach decisions as rapidly as possible is now a firmly established practice (Fleming et al. 1984; Geller and Pocock 1987; O'Brien and Fleming 1979). A data safety monitoring board that examines results according to protocol at predetermined intervals is essential to this process.

Statistical Analysis

In the same way that blind study conditions are used to prevent bias from influencing the observations made in the course of a study, it is necessary to prevent biases from influencing data analyses. Researchers have a natural desire to find significant new results, particularly in support of the a priori hypothesis. Studies that find no differences between treatments or negative results in general are not good news for patients or for the researchers who want to publish their results. Such tendencies can have a profound influence on the way in which data are "cleaned" and prepared for analysis. For example, a questionable or inconsistent data element may need to be revisited, perhaps with the benefit of a review of the case record. To avoid any possibility of bias entering the decision as to the true value of the observation, the review should be conducted without knowing the subject's treatment condition. Some researchers advocate blinding statisticians as well.

Many analytic methods are available to a statistician for a single data set. Different analyses usually yield at least qualitatively the same results. The analysis can be influenced by the selection of which variables are included as covariates, the use of summary or time-specific measures, and the decision to treat a variable as constant or variable. The protocol must be as complete as possible with respect to the analysis and the handling of missing data so that decisions are made before the data are collected and before the blind has been broken to avoid bias or the appearance of bias.

The data collected should be used to the fullest extent possible. If a study takes an extensive time to complete, many scientific questions may arise in the interim; some of these questions may be answered by the data collected. Or the individuals who developed the protocol may not have chosen the optimal statistical analysis, and data may be analyzed beyond the protocol specifications. After a period of time (e.g., 3 years), the data should be made publicly available for further analysis. The answer to those who call these unspecified analyses "fishing expeditions" or "data dredging" is full disclosure. When the results are presented in professional journals, the fact that they are based on analyses not originally specified in the protocol should also be presented. It is then up to the reader to judge the value of the information.

The data on which published articles are based should always be available for scientific inquiry. The issue of what to do with unpublished data is unresolved. Some researchers argue that all data archives should ultimately be open to the public. The pharmaceutical industry is likely to resist this disclosure, however, because it may consider product development information proprietary.

Information Feedback and Dissemination

Investigators, journal editors, and the pharmaceutical industry have a responsibility to make the results of studies available to patients and the public in a timely fashion. If data are suppressed or neglected, participants have put themselves at risk but they and society have received no benefit for their potential loss. An investigator may not wish to publish a failed study for fear that it might tarnish his or her reputation as a clinical researcher or that it might offend a pharmaceutical company or eminent colleague. Furthermore, negative or inconclusive results are difficult to publish in the best scientific journals. Also, with changing circumstances (e.g., change of responsibilities or staff turnover or moves to different institutions), investigators may not have the time to report low-priority data. Nevertheless, even if the study failed to find the expected or positive differences, this information can be useful to the scientific community. For example, in treatment studies adverse event rates and measures of the variability of response can be used by others in planning and interpreting their own studies and those in the literature. Here again, a public data archive may be a partial solution.

CONTROVERSIAL ISSUES IN STUDY DESIGN

We have described a range of issues that must be considered by investigators in designing and implementing studies of psychiatric disorders. In addition to these generic issues, studies of psychiatric disorders that entail greater than minimal risk are currently receiving special scrutiny and warrant additional consideration, particularly for disorders in which patients may have decisional impairment (e.g., dementia, psychosis, and mental retardation). Therefore, the following sections address specific types of high-risk studies as they apply to particular psychiatric disorders. Schizophrenia is used as the model, although the principles also apply to other disorders in which patients are decisionally impaired. Subsequent sections on bipolar disorder, major depressive disorder, and anxiety disorders address issues specific to research in those disorders.

Studies of Schizophrenia

The issue of medication-free research has become particularly vexing in schizophrenia research, partly as a result of highly publicized incidents in which serious harm was alleged to befall subjects in studies involving placebo treatment or drug withdrawal (Appelbaum 1996; Hilts 1995). In addition, a number of investigators have speculated that sustained periods of untreated illness have potentially deleterious effects (Lieberman et al. 1997; Post et al. 1992; Scully et al. 1997; Wyatt 1991). However, the evidence to support or definitively refute this hypothesis is not yet available. Moreover, the concerns raised may not apply to the brief periods of closely monitored medication-free research typically used in contemporary research designs (Waddington et al. 1997; Wyatt 1997).

The issues of drug discontinuation and placebo differ somewhat in short-term and long-term studies. Long-term studies have recently been examined in great depth (Baldessarini and Viguera 1995; Carpenter and Tamminga 1995; Carpenter et al. 1997; Gilbert et al. 1995; Greden and Tandon 1995; Jeste et al. 1995; Meltzer 1995). An extensive body of work has consistently demonstrated the prophylactic efficacy of antipsychotic medication and its lessening of the severity of psychotic relapse. Therefore, it is generally considered undesirable to pursue placebo-controlled maintenance treatment studies in patients with schizophrenia. (An exception may be first-episode patients, for whom the long-term risk-benefit ratio of antipsychotic medications has not yet been clearly determined.) At the same time it should be emphasized that the methods for conducting maintenance treatment studies have evolved in recent years in a way that minimizes the potential risks to patients. To head off relapses and prevent serious disruptions and need for patient hospitalization, the outcomes that trigger rescue interventions in these studies involve not relapse but the appearance of early warning signs of impending relapse (Schooler et al. 1997). Nevertheless, we shall confine the following discussion to short-term trials of acutely exacerbated or persistently symptomatic schizophrenia.

Medication-free periods may be called for in placebo washouts, parallel-arm placebo comparisons, and descriptive research intended to elucidate neurophysiological and psychopharmacological mechanisms. The durations of placebo washout and parallel-arm placebo periods in three recent phase III trials of antipsychotics are displayed in Table 2–1.

Placebo Washout (Lead-In or Run-In)

Most patients with schizophrenia enter acute clinical trials while currently receiving antipsychotic medication (Chouinard et al. 1993; Marder and Meibach 1994; Peuskens 1995). This treatment is typically discontinued before the

TABLE 2–1. Duration of placebo treatments in recent trials of antipsychotics

Study period	Risperidone[a]	Sertindole (study M93–113)[b]	Seroquel[c]
Lead-in placebo washout	3–7 days	4–7 days	3–7 days
Parallel-arm placebo	56 days	56 days	42 days

[a] Marder and Meibach 1994
[b] Schulz et al. 1996
[c] Borison et al. 1996

patients can enter the lead-in period of a clinical trial. Discontinuing treatment has different clinical consequences from delaying treatment (Baldessarini and Viguera 1995). Indeed, combining patients whose treatment is discontinued with those whose treatment is delayed is one of the methodological complexities of the placebo lead-in period.

The purposes of a washout period include the following (Volavka et al. 1996):

1. *To minimize the carryover effects of previous (nonstudy) drugs.* Residual levels of previously administered antipsychotic medication could affect the outcome of the study. More than 1 week may be required for oral antipsychotics to be cleared from the circulating plasma (Hubbard et al. 1987), and considerably more time is required for clearance from the brain (Cohen et al. 1988). Placebo washout for depot neuroleptics is usually 1 month (Volavka et al. 1996), although slow-release injections of antipsychotics can result in measurable plasma levels for up to 8 months (Sampath et al. 1992) and D_2 receptor occupancy levels of 24%–34% as long as 6 months after discontinuation (Nyberg et al. 1996). Thus, the typical placebo washout period may result in variable reduction of the carryover effect, and the washout may be far from complete. At the same time, the relative reduction of medication in patients after the washout period can provide a more realistic (albeit imperfect) baseline from which to view the efficacy and side effects of treatments.

2. *To improve diagnostic accuracy.* Previous use of street drugs by patients entering the study may affect the results because of acute toxic psychosis or a withdrawal syndrome. The differential diagnosis can be clarified during the lead-in placebo period.

3. *To screen out placebo responders.* A small proportion of schizophrenia patients respond to placebo treatment. If a trial design does not include a

placebo condition, a placebo lead-in period may identify patients who would be placebo responders. For example, in one study Volavka et al. (1992) found 3 placebo responders among 176 patients (1.7%) who entered a 1-week placebo lead-in period.

4. *To establish an untreated baseline of psychopathology.* A *true baseline* remains undefined, and whatever definition may be applied, it is unlikely to be met after a mere week taking a placebo. However, psychopathology can increase to a higher level during a placebo washout period, and the therapeutic effect of treatment may be measured using this higher level. The increase of symptoms within a limited time frame cannot, however, be said to reflect a stable baseline level of psychopathology because the symptoms could reflect fluctuations in the context of drug withdrawal. DSM-IV criteria (American Psychiatric Association 1994) stipulate that the signs and symptoms of schizophrenia must be present for a significant portion of time during a 1-month period, and some signs must persist for at least 6 months. Therefore, given the length of most washout periods, only limited enhancement of diagnostic precision may be achieved.

5. *To obtain a greater treatment response.* Because many patients worsen following drug discontinuation, therapeutic response may be greater after a drug washout period than if patients were immediately converted from their prior regimen to the double-blind treatment. However, worsening after drug withdrawal may be a transient phenomenon. The patient's "true" psychopathological state might not be reached until some longer period of drug elimination and physiological adaptation occurs, which may take weeks or months. Thus, only a relative psychopathological baseline may be readily achieved.

In light of these considerations, the stated goals of the lead-in placebo period may be met only partially using the typical 1-week washout model. Yet however desirable longer durations would be for scientific reasons, they are difficult and may not be currently feasible in most clinical research settings in the United States, for both ethical and fiscal reasons.

In patients whose medication is discontinued, symptoms may worsen. In at least one instance, the worsening was statistically significant (Volavka et al. 1992), even though the researchers tried to detect clinical deterioration and shortened the duration of the placebo period when it appeared necessary. The worsening may not be clinically important and may be temporary, and patients may respond promptly when antipsychotic medication is restarted. Nevertheless, the suffering associated with psychosis will be prolonged by the lack of active treatment for a week in patients who are withdrawn from their medication, as well as in those who enter a study unmedicated. However brief this period, it cannot be discounted and must be viewed as a necessary risk for patients to complete the study and for society to gain its benefits. Furthermore, the lead-in placebo period may prolong the time that the patient remains in the hospital and out of his or her normal living circumstances. This situation may affect the patient and his or her family, employer, insurer, and hospital; the sponsor of the drug trial; and any other entity that may bear the cost of longer hospitalization.

In summary, the design advantages of the lead-in placebo washout must be weighed against its potential clinical, ethical, and economic disadvantages (Volavka 1995a). Placebo washouts lessen possible harmful drug interactions and provide a relatively drug-free baseline. Another general purpose of drug withdrawal protocols is to investigate the psychopathology and pathophysiology of disease independent of drug confound and artifact. Many measures employed in the study of psychotic disorders may be confounded by the drugs used in treatment. For example, in a biochemical study testing a dopamine hypothesis, the outcomes will be confounded if the patient is receiving drugs that alter dopamine physiology. Psychological tasks used in research may also be influenced by drug effects. A study of memory function, for example, will be confounded if patients are taking an anticholinergic medication. Therefore, compelling scientific rationales exist for study protocols that require a medication-free period.

Parallel-Arm Placebo Treatment

Determination of efficacy. The general issue of parallel-arm placebo trials to determine efficacy has been discussed previously. In recent studies of schizophrenia, haloperidol has been the typical standard treatment. Haloperidol's antipsychotic efficacy has been demonstrated in many well-controlled trials involving a large number of subjects. It is also well established that haloperidol is not curative and is frequently associated with potentially severe side effects, including extrapyramidal symptoms and tardive dyskinesia. Clearly, better treatments than haloperidol are desirable. The argument that a placebo arm is needed even in some trials using a standard treatment was presented earlier. However, given the availability of an efficacious standard treatment, the severity of psychotic symptoms, and the potential consequences of symptom exacerbation, placebo-arm trials in studies of schizophrenia are very controversial. The advent of atypical antipsychotic drugs that are effective and have fewer side effects than conventional antipsychotic drugs further complicates the argument for using placebo control.

Determination of safety. The principal advantage of the recently tested atypical antipsychotics over haloperidol is their lower propensity to produce extrapyramidal side effects (EPS) (Czobor et al. 1995; Schulz et al. 1996). A recent trial (Czobor et al. 1995), however, has been criticized as "unfair" because multiple-dose regimens of the experimental treatment (T) were contrasted with a single-dose regimen of haloperidol (S), which was perhaps too high a dose. A second trial (Schulz et al. 1996) used three dose regimens of haloperidol, including one as low as 4 mg/day; each of the haloperidol dose regimens produced more EPS than the equally efficacious dose of T. Thus, a possible alternative design to determine the efficacy and safety of antipsychotics is a multiple-dose regimen trial instead of a parallel-arm placebo design (Volavka 1995b).

A parallel-arm placebo design has potential adverse consequences similar to those of the lead-in placebo period. However, because the cumulative duration of placebo treatment in the recent parallel-arm trials of antipsychotics was 49–63 days (Table 2–1), the potential for adverse effects was greater than in a brief washout period. In one trial, placebo was discontinued earlier than intended because of "insufficient response" in 62% of the patients, compared with 17%–46% of patients receiving active treatments (Marder and Meibach 1994). Patients assigned to the placebo arm showed deterioration from baseline on all measures of outcome (Marder and Meibach 1994). To some extent, the high dropout rate in the placebo group reflected conscientious supervision by the researchers, who withdrew patients from the trial and provided timely rescue medication. Nevertheless, the data show that the conditions of the patients taking placebo worsened. This outcome is in agreement with a meta-analysis of antipsychotic drug withdrawal in maintenance groups that demonstrated that the relative likelihood of relapse was highest during the initial 3 months after medication withdrawal (Jeste et al. 1995).

In summary, although clearly an efficient design feature, the placebo arm may not be absolutely necessary for the determination of efficacy and safety of treatments for schizophrenia, and some patients taking placebo may worsen. Other experimental designs, such as multiple-dose regimens, may provide an alternative method to obtain the desired information. Multiple-dose regimens, however, must include a dose that is less effective to serve as an alternative to placebo in establishing efficacy.

Placebo Trials for Adjunctive Treatments

Numerous treatments have been evaluated for their efficacy against specific dimensions of schizophrenic psychopathology (e.g., negative and cognitive symptoms) and complicating or comorbid syndromes (e.g., depression and mania). When there is no standard adjunctive treatment (as with negative symptoms and cognitive deficits), the issue of placebo is less problematic because the study can be conducted while all subjects continue to receive "background" antipsychotic treatment. And because patients are not denied standard treatments and are not at increased risk for psychotic exacerbation, no ethical principle is violated in placebo-controlled trials. Depression and mania, however, have accepted treatments that may make the use of placebo problematic for all of the reasons stated earlier.

Summary

There is substantial evidence that short-term medication discontinuation in the context of research is relatively safe and without long-term adverse consequences. In a meta-analysis of medication discontinuation studies, Gilbert et al. (1995) found patients responsive when medication was reintroduced and little evidence of extensive suffering or long-term harm. A number of prospective studies involving lengthy follow-up of dose reduction have found that the long-term course of schizophrenia is not adversely affected by the brief and controlled medication-free periods associated with typical research designs (Wyatt 1997). An important question is whether the symptom worsening associated with drug withdrawal causes diminished treatment responsiveness or other long-lasting pathological consequences. Although some evidence suggests that the lengthy off-medication periods often encountered in clinical circumstances may have long-term adverse effects, these effects have not been shown for the brief and controlled medication withdrawal periods associated with research. Nevertheless, subjects in drug withdrawal protocols should be closely monitored to ensure that serious events remain extremely rare.

The issue may be put forward in a relatively simple context. Medication withdrawal from patients with psychotic disorders places many at risk for increased psychotic symptoms, with the potential to increase suffering and resource utilization and, in certain circumstances, to cause long-term problems. For example, an employed individual whose symptoms are exacerbated may be vulnerable to job loss, with long-lasting adverse consequences even if the symptom exacerbation is responsive to therapeutic intervention. It must also be recognized, however, that patients with these conditions in nonresearch settings are also at risk for symptom exacerbation and very commonly discontinue medication on their own.

Patients, medicine, and society all have a stake in the acquisition of new information on the pathophysiology and treatment of psychotic illnesses. Existing evidence appears to support the proposition that protocols with drug-free periods can be conducted without long-lasting adverse effects. Development of new prevention strategies and treatments with greater efficacy and safety than current ones depends on the knowledge obtained in such studies (Carpenter et al. 1997). We suggest the following guidelines for study design, patient selection, and therapeutic intervention for the conduct of drug discontinuation studies with psychotic patients:

1. The drug-free period should be as brief as possible given the design and goals of the study.
2. Patients should be selected using guidelines that exclude those at highest risk for significant adverse outcomes (e.g., history of violent or suicidal behavior).
3. Close clinical monitoring, with procedures to ensure early detection of relapse symptoms and early intervention, should be included in the study design.
4. Any increased resource utilization should not come at the expense of the participating subjects.

Studies of Bipolar Disorder

Many of the issues discussed previously in regard to medication-free research with schizophrenia patients also apply to clinical trials of patients with bipolar disorder. Bipolar disorder presents additional complexity in considering research designs and their ethics because it manifests in two acute forms, mania and depression. As better treatments have become available and the research database has increased, discontinuation of active medication and the use of placebo controls have become more problematic ethically. The following section addresses specific issues relevant to trials conducted during acute phases of the illness and issues attendant to research on maintenance therapy.

Drug Discontinuation and Placebo Washout in Acute Bipolar Exacerbations

Mania. Mania and hypomania are severe pathological conditions that subject patients, family members, and their communities to considerable suffering and various risks. Lithium and divalproex have been approved by the FDA as treatments of acute mania. Antipsychotic drugs, carbamazepine, and electroconvulsive therapy (ECT) are also used frequently and have been shown to have clinical efficacy. Benzodiazepines are commonly employed adjunctively. Thus, effective and safe treatments for mania are available (Goodwin and Jamison 1990).

The argument for drug discontinuation in studies of acute mania is the same as for schizophrenia. If discontinuation is necessary, it should be gradual for two reasons. One is that the medication, even though the patient relapsed while taking it because of inadequate efficacy or partial noncompliance, may have been partially effective. The other is that rapidly discontinuing medication can lead to withdrawal symptoms and possibly a state of heightened vulnerability to reemergent psychopathology (Baldessarini et al. 1996). A recommended compromise is to withdraw medication gradually and introduce a new treatment strategy before the previous treatment is totally discontinued (so-called cross-titration). Again, criteria must be clear for withdrawing subjects from the protocol if they show obvious clinical deterioration, and rescue medications should be available.

Availability of adjunctive or rescue medications is a practical necessity in studies of bipolar disorder. Benzodiazepines and antipsychotic drugs should be available for short-term use if psychotic symptoms or excitement becomes excessive. Criteria for using rescue medications should be well defined, enabling the use of these agents to serve as a dependent variable. An increased need for rescue medications presumably demonstrates that a treatment condition (such as placebo) has inferior efficacy.

Similarly, criteria should be well defined for withdrawing a patient from the protocol if his or her clinical condition deteriorates or improvement does not occur within a reasonable period. If these criteria are too liberal, patients may be removed from a protocol prematurely, and an excessive number of premature discontinuations can cripple the design and render an investigation meaningless. At the same time, if the discontinuation criteria are too strict, patients may be exposed to undue suffering and potential harm. Balancing these risks is a crucial research design issue.

Depression. The depressive phase of bipolar disorder remains incompletely understood. Nonetheless, some commonly used treatments are believed to be efficacious. Although mild depression in a bipolar patient may be allowed to go untreated, more severe depression is typically treated with antidepressant drugs or ECT. Because severe depression is associated with considerable suffering and a risk of suicide, failure to provide active treatment for a severely depressed patient is unethical. The use of placebo comparisons may be justified in milder forms of depression when the threshold point at which to use antidepressant drugs is less clear. It is important to determine the threshold of severity beyond which use of placebo is not acceptable.

Rapid cycling and mixed mania. Dysphoric mania and mixed and cycling episodes, which can have worse prognoses than pure mania and depression, are typically more difficult to treat. Anticonvulsant medications may be more efficacious than lithium, and clinicians often use combined antipsychotic and antidepressant treatment. Again, the highly symptomatic nature of these patients and the possible effects of ineffective treatment during the acute phase on the long-term course of the illness make it difficult to justify the use of placebo. In these conditions, a trial including a placebo should provide the safeguards described previously for studies of acute mania.

Drug Discontinuation From Maintenance Treatment in Bipolar Disorder

Studies of maintenance treatment in bipolar disorder present their own problems. If a patient has not been stably maintained on a prior treatment, discontinuing that treatment would be expected to cause few problems. Even so, for the same reasons noted earlier, medication discontinuation should be gradual and subjects should be observed carefully for symptomatic worsening. Cross-titration with a replacement therapy may limit problems. Because subjects in maintenance treatment are often outpatients, investigators must maintain close contact and make emergency services available. Drug discontinuation should perhaps be limited to subjects with supportive family members or other social supports who can serve as an early warning system of any problems.

If a patient has been effectively maintained in a euthymic state without serious side effects on a maintenance regimen, it is difficult to justify withdrawing that treatment. Drug discontinuation exposes the patient to the risk of a recurrent mood episode, and there is no guarantee that a subsequent reinstitution of the same treatment will afford the patient the same degree of mood stability and protection against further recurrences (Post et al. 1992). Placebo use is therefore quite problematic in maintenance studies, except in patients who are treatment resistant.

As noted earlier, it may be justifiable to have a subject "ride out" an episode of subsyndromal depression because of the potential adverse effects of antidepressant treatment and the possibility of spontaneous remission. An episode of hypomania, however, carries a strong risk of leading to a full-blown manic episode (Keller et al. 1992). Subjects whose conditions worsen may need to be dropped from the protocol and treated as indicated clinically. An intermediate position is to specify a protocol for the treatment of hypomania with adjunctive medications such as benzodiazepines or antipsychotic agents. If symptoms are controlled and the patient rapidly returns to euthymia, the adjunctive medications can be withdrawn and the patient maintained in the original study group. The number of such episodes an individual can experience before being dropped from the protocol should be specified. Such dropouts for lack of efficacy can help to demonstrate the inferiority of a treatment.

Studies of Depression

Nearly all of the issues discussed in relation to psychiatric disorders in general, and bipolar and schizophrenic disorders in particular, are relevant to clinical trials in major depressive disorders—especially with severely ill patients. In this section we highlight particular considerations relevant to these nonbipolar mood disorders.

First, a note on the heterogeneity of the depressions: A substantial proportion of patients with major depression are either very severely ill (e.g., with melancholic or psychotic depression), chronically ill (i.e., do not recover fully between episodes or have been symptomatic for years), or both. On the other end of the spectrum, a significant proportion are less symptomatic—although they have reduced function, they are ill for a shorter period, are not psychotic, and are rarely suicidal. The former group poses problems identical to those discussed earlier in regard to schizophrenia or bipolar disorder, whereas the latter group raises less-profound ethical issues in treatment discontinuation or the use of placebo.

A key issue is the range of treatments that may be evaluated (from six visits of counseling to ECT). The dangers are providing a treatment with many side effects when a standard treatment with fewer side effects is available and, conversely, entering patients into a minimal treatment condition when spontaneous remission is unlikely and a more powerful treatment is clinically indicated. To simplify the following discussion, we divide the depressions into psychotic/severe and nonpsychotic/less severe groups.

Matching the population studied to the treatment or treatments to be evaluated is profoundly important in depressed patients. For both ethical and scientific reasons, one would not wish to evaluate ECT in mildly depressed individuals who have received no previous treatment any more than one would want to evaluate six sessions of counseling as the sole treatment for psychotic or severely melancholic inpatients, given the lack of evidence of efficacy of brief psychosocial treatment in severely ill nonpsychotic patients and the availability of effective medications.

Placebo Washout

Nonpsychotic/less severely ill. For mildly to moderately depressed outpatients, a placebo washout is routinely used to decrease the postrandomization placebo response rate. Yet a recent meta-analysis found that among depressed outpatients, the postrandomization placebo response rate was identical for those with and without a pill placebo washout in randomized, controlled efficacy trials (Trivedi and Rush 1994). It is notable, however, that in nearly all of these trials (with and without a placebo washout), two to four outpatient visits were conducted to both provide a reliable diagnosis and evaluate general medical and psychiatric comorbidity. Thus, it would seem that the pill placebo washout can be omitted as long as several prerandomization visits are used for clinical evaluations.

Psychotic/severely ill. Some evidence suggests that the placebo response rate is < 20% in severely ill patients (Nelson et al. 1990). Indeed, a lower placebo response rate is seen with greater chronicity even in less severely ill outpatients with major depression (Fairchild et al. 1986; Khan et al. 1991). Thus, the scientific need for a placebo washout (or an extended pretreatment evaluation period) is weaker for the more severely ill. As its scientific relevance drops, the ethics of using this method become more questionable—especially given the danger of suicide or subject attrition.

Parallel-Arm Placebo Treatment

Nonpsychotic/less severely ill. In published reports of medication trials, the usual placebo response rates (not remission rates) in outpatients with non-psychotic major depression are 25%–35% versus 50%–55% for antidepressant medications (Depression Guideline Panel 1993). However, many unpublished studies have found no drug-placebo difference. Many investigators believe that the major reason for this lack of difference is that there is a high placebo response rate in acute-phase treatment studies. The danger of not including a placebo group in the evaluation of a new treatment is that without a placebo control, efficacy may be incorrectly inferred if the new treatment and a standard treatment are found to be equally efficacious. Here the scientist faces another ethical dilemma—namely, incorrectly declaring efficacy when none may exist versus asking individual patients to take a placebo when standard treatment would be more beneficial for them. Nevertheless, because of the high placebo response rates in the nonpsychotic/less severely ill depressed patient group, a pill placebo cannot be avoided in trials attempting to determine the efficacy of new medications.

Psychotic/severely ill. For the psychotic/severely ill patient group, particularly because of the risk of suicide, a pill placebo has serious disadvantages—just as in schizophrenia. Here one may prefer a placebo for scientific rigor, but alternatives such as a multiple-dose strategy, a bet-the-winner strategy, or both can usefully reduce the individual's disadvantage.

Discontinuation Trials

Nonpsychotic/less severely ill. There is strong evidence from a variety of maintenance-phase randomized clinical trials that longer (as opposed to shorter) durations of active treatment are associated with lower relapse and recurrence rates in those with recurrent depression (see Depression Guideline Panel 1993, pp. 109–118, for a review). Because many patients with recurrent depression have recurrences years after remission from their prior episode, there is only a modest disadvantage for many patients in such trials. However, for some individuals another disabling depressive episode may exact tremendous personal cost (e.g., loss of marriage, job). Thus, for placebo-controlled discontinuation studies, careful and frequent monitoring is called for to detect a recurrence at the earliest time possible and minimize costs to the individual.

Psychotic/severely ill. The same ethical issues are found for psychotic/severely ill patients as for those with schizophrenia and bipolar disorder. For this group, either a multiple-dose or a bet-the-winner strategy is preferable. However, neither approach reduces the need for intensive and frequent monitoring of clinical status throughout the duration of the discontinuation study.

Placebo for Psychotherapy

Nonpsychotic/less severely ill. The issue of an "adequate placebo" for nonpsychotic/less severely ill patients remains controversial. Historically, a waiting list control has been used, but this contrast is nearly certain to define any reasonable treatment as efficacious. It contains no obvious (or only very minimal) therapeutic elements (e.g., the patients know they will receive treatment sometime soon). It also contains countertherapeutic import (e.g., the patients feel bad but cannot get treatment now). In this case different doses of the same therapy (e.g., once- versus twice-weekly sessions) or different formats for delivery—in that some (but not all) of the same elements are found in the experimental treatment (e.g., bibliotherapy versus individual therapy)—may be preferable. Such approaches deliver treatment of some form to all patients and reduce the likelihood of differential attrition from the two treatment cells. However, because the specific therapeutic ingredient in psychotherapy cannot be delineated, a strict placebo in the medication sense (i.e., everything but the potentially active ingredient) is not forthcoming. Furthermore, an active medication contrast may not be sufficient because therapy may work for some for whom medication is ineffective or vice versa. Thus, the population or case mix in a particular study may dictate whether medication or psychotherapy is more or less effective.

Psychotherapy Run-In

Nonpsychotic/less severely ill. It is logical, although rare, to use psychotherapy as a run-in condition before randomization to pill placebo or medication. Only 50% of moderately ill depressed outpatients respond to time-limited, depression-targeted psychotherapies. One would expect that the pill placebo response rates in patients who have not responded to formal psychotherapy would also be quite low. The issue for this group is whether a pill placebo is ethical. Perhaps a high- versus low-dose medication strategy would be more useful and more ethical, as long as the lower dose involved some degree of efficacy. Alternatively, patients who fail to respond or cannot tolerate a medication might be a highly informative population in which to compare the efficacy of an alternative medication and formal psychotherapy. This design, which mirrors routine clinical practice for many patients, has not been used yet is highly ethical and scientifically rigorous.

Studies of Anxiety Disorders

Anxiety disorders are chronic, potentially debilitating conditions that have been recognized for only a few decades as distinct psychopathological entities. Over this period, specific treatments have been identified for these disorders. Proven efficacious pharmacological and cognitive-behavioral treatments (CBT) exist for each anxiety disorder. Nevertheless, there is a continued need to improve these treatments. The availability of two distinct types of effective therapy, medication and CBT, affords unique opportunities as well as difficulties in designing clinical studies. We review here ethical considerations in treatment studies as they relate to anxiety disorders.

Anxiety is associated with considerable suffering. A persistent or recurrent high level of anxiety is painful and distressing. Anxiety disorders are also associated with substantial impairment in daily life, increased morbidity from physical illness, increased mortality from suicide and possibly from physical illness, and sometimes aggression toward others. Further, anxiety is a risk factor for onset of depression. These findings suggest that the course of anxiety disorders is not benign and raise the possibility of significant and perhaps permanent deleterious effects of complications from untreated illness. Thus, research designs that withhold treatment present risks.

On the other hand, there is little evidence for persistent deleterious effects of a sustained period of untreated anxiety disorders, although much more information is needed before this hypothesis can be confirmed. Treatment studies document that some patients with long-term anxiety disorders improve substantially or even recover completely when provided with an efficacious treatment. This finding suggests that the problem of leaving patients untreated may be less pressing for patients with anxiety disorders than for patients with disorders that might progress or become relatively refractory during periods without treatment.

The proven effectiveness of psychological treatment alone for patients with anxiety disorders is an important issue. In some cases CBT may even be superior to medication. More studies that compare medication and psychotherapy, as well as combination treatment studies, are needed. However, such studies present difficult design questions. Given the high efficacy and safety of CBT, there may be ethical questions about withholding this treatment to conduct a straightforward pharmacological treatment trial.

Placebo Washout and Drug Discontinuation

Many patients with anxiety disorders are prescribed benzodiazepines, often in doses too low to adequately treat their illness. These patients are taking medication when recruited for research, creating a difficult problem. Medication discontinuation is desirable for an ideal study design, but discontinuation affects the generalizability of results and adds the factor of withdrawal symptoms. Researchers have managed this problem in different ways. Pharmacotherapy studies of anxiety disorders most often include a placebo washout phase. However, CBT studies typically have not done so; instead, these studies have required that medication dosages be stable (e.g., not increased over a specified period before study entry) and that a symptom severity criterion be met while taking medication.

Although there is good reason for continuing low-dose medication, the addition of psychotherapy to ongoing pharmacotherapy is a different intervention from psychotherapy alone. Moreover, in at least one pharmacotherapy study, combination benzodiazepine and tricyclic medication resulted in poorer outcomes than tricyclic medication alone. Because continuation of medication is thus a potentially serious design problem, it is essential to conduct studies with patients who have been withdrawn from psychotropic medication. A further important issue is the relationship between neurophysiological or neuropsychological processes and treatment outcome in patients with anxiety disorders. To be sure of assessing disease-related phenomena without potentially confounding treatment effects, baseline data should be obtained from patients in a drug-free state. However, in some populations (e.g., the elderly) benzodiazepine withdrawal may be difficult or even impossible until another treatment is substituted. Moreover, because of the widespread use of chronic benzodiazepine treatment for anxiety, studies need to be conducted with symptomatic patients who, at least initially, continue to take medication. Study conditions will then resemble usual clinical practice. Studies in which subjects meet standard inclusion criteria but are maintained on low doses of medication may produce results that are more generalizable than those in which a washout is required.

Withdrawal symptoms that occur when benzodiazepines and other anxiolytics are discontinued pose a second problem for anxiety studies. Withdrawal symptoms include anxiety, which can be difficult or impossible to distinguish from reemergence of the illness. Rapid benzodiazepine withdrawal also brings a risk of withdrawal seizures. Furthermore, rebound anxiety can occur in which anxiety reaches a level higher than baseline. Theoretically, discontinuation symptoms can be managed by allowing sufficient time after withdrawal for these to subside, but patients may be unable or unwilling to tolerate this phase without some help. Moreover, the precise time required to ensure that remaining symptoms are true anxiety is unclear. Further, discontinuation requirements may bias a study against more severely ill patients, because subjects clearly must be informed of the likelihood of developing withdrawal symptoms.

The usefulness of a placebo washout to establish baseline psychopathology is also unclear. Hypothetically, several weeks of a single-blind placebo should improve the precision of baseline symptom definition. In panic disorder studies, there is consensus that a minimum of 2 weeks of panic monitoring is needed to establish an adequate baseline for measurement of panic symptoms. The baseline can be established using a placebo lead-in or a no-treatment baseline. Some anxiety patients, particularly those who are wary of medication, find a no-treatment baseline reassuring. For panic disorder patients, self-monitoring has been shown to be an active intervention. Because such monitoring is standard during treatment, it is important that it be instituted during baseline to control for its effects.

Placebo lead-in is used to identify placebo responders and eliminate them from the study. Placebo response is uncommon in patients with obsessive-compulsive disorder and social phobia but occurs frequently in those with panic and generalized anxiety disorder. However, although some patients appear to improve during a placebo lead-in period, anxiety studies that use this procedure to screen out responders have not succeeded in lowering the placebo response rate. This result may be partly due to the natural variability of anxiety symptoms. In many patients, anxiety levels vary from week to week, and an apparent placebo response may simply represent a waning phase.

The use of medication-free periods in subjects with anxiety disorders must be considered in the context of a study's objectives. For studies focusing on mechanisms of action, patients should be in as "pure" a state as possible. Obtaining this state may require lengthy pretreatment management and careful monitoring to ensure safe and effective discontinuation of benzodiazepines after long-term use, which is common in anxiety patients. A long period of baseline monitoring also helps to ensure a stable pretreatment baseline. On the other hand, studies focusing primarily on identifying active interventions for highly comorbid, multiproblem patients such as those typically seen in treatment settings may be best done in a more naturalistic manner, allowing patients to continue taking medication as long as sufficient symptoms are present to meet standard inclusion criteria.

Parallel-Arm Placebo Designs

The various anxiety disorders are associated with different response rates to placebo. As noted previously, obsessive-compulsive disorder generally has a very low placebo response rate, whereas generalized anxiety disorder has a high placebo response rate. The use of a placebo control is especially important for patient groups known to have high placebo response rates. These studies also require "calibration" to ensure that the particular study group is not one with a high placebo response rate. In such a situation, without a placebo group, the new treatment could be erroneously believed to be efficacious. Placebo controls thus help to establish the validity of a study's findings and to decrease the ambiguity of results. Placebo comparisons are also important for accurate identification of side effects.

On the other hand, the use of a placebo treatment arm carries risks similar to those of the placebo lead-in described earlier. If patients are too symptomatic to tolerate a placebo treatment, they will drop out of the study, and high attrition rates threaten study integrity.

Placebo and Psychotherapy

Efficacious CBTs that have few known side effects are available for all of the anxiety disorders. Thus, these treatments are effective and safe. To test the hypothesis that the primary goal of medication should be to enhance psychotherapy, studies could be designed comparing CBT plus placebo with CBT plus active medication. If there is no medication-placebo difference in this kind of study, researchers could conclude that patients should receive CBT alone.

Several types of psychotherapy other than CBT are now under study. These forms of therapy show some promise of efficacy but may be less effective than CBT. These treatments could be used to establish the efficacy of medication compared with placebo in the context of supportive psychotherapy, such as might be done currently by many practitioners.

Drug-Psychotherapy Comparison Studies

Given the high response rate of anxiety disorder patients to CBT, studies are needed to compare the relative effectiveness of medications and psychotherapy and to clarify their advantages and disadvantages. It remains unclear whether there are indications for choosing one type of treatment over the other. It is also unclear whether medication and psychotherapy work through the same or different mechanisms. Little information is available on the possible benefits of combined treatment.

Comorbidity and Outcome Measurement

Persons with anxiety disorders frequently have other Axis I diagnoses. Comorbidity with other anxiety disorders, substance abuse, and/or depression is common with patients with panic disorder, generalized anxiety disorder, and social phobia. The presence of comorbidities in patients who enter a study for a specific diagnostic group creates potential clinical and ethical problems. The objective of a treatment study is to determine whether a given treatment performs better than a comparison control treatment. To accomplish this goal, treatment targets a single symptom or set of closely related symptoms. A patient with comorbidity has symptoms that are not targeted by the study treatment and are not expected to respond to the test treatment. In contrast, a treating clinician takes into consideration the patient's full range of problems and symptoms in an effort to achieve the best possible results for that patient. Further, the desired outcomes for patients in research are predetermined and constant for all patients in the study. In clinical settings, outcomes are individualized, and the patient may even decide which outcomes are most important to him or her. Thus, from an individual patient's perspective, research and clinical goals are only partially overlapping.

In summary, clinical research has documented the efficacy of specific interventions for particular sets of anxiety symptoms. Yet there is a pressing need for such investigations to continue. Perhaps paradoxically, the better the research results, the more complicated it becomes to design ethical studies.

NONTHERAPEUTIC RESEARCH

Descriptive research that does not directly test treatments but seeks to elucidate neurobiological processes frequently employs procedures that expose subjects to more than minimal risks, including pain, discomfort, or the activation of symptoms. These procedures have been used to great advantage throughout biomedical research. Examples of invasive procedures used in nontherapeutic research include provocative (or challenge) tests, lumbar punctures, and neuroimaging assessments. Provocative tests involve the potential transient induction or exacerbation of the symptoms of a specific disorder. Lumbar punctures involve insertion of a needle into the vertebral column, a potentially painful procedure with rare neurological consequences. Neuroimaging procedures can be noninvasive, as in magnetic resonance imaging, or they may involve catheter insertion into a peripheral artery or vein and injection of a radioactive tracer as in positron-emission tomography scans. All of these procedures are complex and may involve some level of discomfort, but they bring a very low risk of enduring consequences or life-threatening complications. Many of these techniques are used as standard diagnostic procedures in other clinical disciplines (e.g., neurology, cardiology, and endocrinology).

Provocative tests have been particularly controversial because they cause transient activation of symptoms (although not the induction of relapses or new episodes of illness). Examples of such tests include, in schizophrenia, tests with dopamine agonists (amphetamine, L-dopa, and methylphenidate) (Lieberman et al. 1987) and more recently N-methyl-D-aspartate (NMDA) receptor antagonists (ketamine) (Krystal et al. 1994); in dementia, tests with cholinomimetic and anticholinergic agents (Mohs et al. 1985); in depression, the use of cholinomimetic agents (Janowsky and Overstreet 1995) and tryptophan depletion procedures (Delgado et al. 1990); in anxiety disorders, tests with sodium lactate (Gorman et al. 1987), carbon dioxide (Gorman et al. 1987), and pentagastrin (Abelson et al. 1994); and in obsessive-compulsive disorder, tests with m-chlorophenylpiperazine (Zohar et al. 1987). Proponents of this type of research note that provocative tests are commonly used in clinical medicine, ranging from exercise electrocardiogram stress testing for coronary artery disease to the use of glucose tolerance tests for diabetes and tensilon (acetyl cholinesterase inhibitor) tests for myasthenia gravis (Lieberman 1996). They argue that the information gained from this research is unique and highly valuable and obtained with acceptable levels of risk.

Neuroimaging studies have provided an enormous amount of information about disease pathophysiology and a means of exploring mechanisms of action of psychotropic drugs in a variety of ways. Technological advances now provide a relatively noninvasive window into the brain. Magnetic resonance imaging poses no known risks, and the radioactive tracers required in other neuroimaging studies employed in research protocols are commonly used in diagnostic studies and involve only modest risk.

Nevertheless, it must be recognized that descriptive research is inherently different from therapeutic research. Opponents of nontherapeutic research focus on the risks and benefits to individual subjects. In descriptive neurobiological research individual subjects receive no direct benefits other than possible modest payments. The justification for engaging in such studies and exposing patients to these procedures can only be that this research can and will produce scientific and societal benefits. If the requirement that individual benefits exceed individual risks is the standard, nontherapeutic studies involving any risk would not be feasible and their potential scientific benefits would be lost (Lieberman 1996). Proponents of nontherapeutic research agree that individual risks must be minimized and undertaken with informed consent but argue that risks must be judged against the potential societal benefits to be gained from the study.

Studies involving invasive procedures must adhere faithfully to the general guidelines for research design described earlier in this chapter. Risks to subjects must be minimized and fully disclosed to potential study participants. For example, because provocative testing can transiently activate or worsen symptoms, the potential for the patient to do something untoward during this period (e.g., self-injury or violence toward others) must be considered and appropriate precautions taken. Sample criteria that exclude patients with histories of dangerous behavior should be adopted, and extensive safeguards should be implemented. In challenge studies, the minimum dose of the test agent needed to achieve the study goals should be utilized; the investigator must thus determine the requisite dose range from the literature or from preliminary work.

For imaging studies involving ionizing radiation, standard limits of exposure must be applied. Similarly, for lumbar punctures or venipunctures, standard methods of sterile technique and limits on volumes of fluid and blood should be required. As always, the design and methods of the study must be adequate to ensure that study hypotheses can be rigorously tested.

CONCLUSION

Based on the principles we have outlined in this chapter, how should clinical investigators view research involving drug withdrawal, placebo control, and invasive procedures? Questions about the short- and long-term consequences of psychiatric symptoms remain unresolved. Because these questions have not been answered definitively and because of the scientific importance of such research designs, it is premature to prohibit the use of drug withdrawal and placebo controls in patients with serious psychiatric disorders. At the same time, we must continue to investigate systematically the potential hazards of untreated symptoms. Subsequent elucidation of these issues will resolve some of the current design controversies. Current evidence is inadequate to prove that temporary drug-free periods or other procedures that may lead to short-term symptoms or transient illness exacerbation have enduring or irreversible consequences. If and when new evidence emerges that confirms the risks of repeated symptomatic episodes of any duration, it may become necessary to eliminate study designs that include a significant risk of symptom exacerbation or prolongation.

The research designs and procedures discussed in this chapter are commonly used throughout clinical biomedical research. To limit their use in psychiatric research without valid justification would be unfair and discriminatory to patients who could benefit from the results of the research. Although regulations and safeguards focus on protecting research participants with severe mental disorders, it should not be forgotten that current and future patients are the ultimate beneficiaries of this research. Investigators conduct research because of concern for these patients and the desire to prevent future patients' suffering. It might be easier to include in studies only mildly ill patients (for whom issues of competence and need for substituted judgment are less problematic), but to do so would not serve the interests of society and its most seriously afflicted. It is the most seriously affected patients who stand to gain the most from research. Nevertheless, clinical investigators must design and conduct studies that are consistent with current ethical standards. Subjects must be enrolled in studies voluntarily and with informed consent. Any risks to subjects must be reasonable in relation to the significance of the knowledge reasonably expected to result from the investigation. The health and rights of research subjects must be protected, but they must be balanced with the need for more knowledge of the causes of and better treatments for psychiatric disorders (Appelbaum 1997).

REFERENCES

Abelson JL, Nesse RM, Vinik AI: Pentagastrin infusions in patients with panic disorder, II: neuroendocrinology. Biol Psychiatry 36:84–96, 1994

Addington D: The use of placebos in clinical trials for acute schizophrenia. Can J Psychiatry 40:171–176, 1995

American Psychiatric Association: Diagnostic and Statistical Manual of Mental Disorders, 4th Edition. Washington, DC, American Psychiatric Association, 1994

Appelbaum PS: Drug-free research in schizophrenia: an overview of the controversy. IRB: A Review of Human Subjects Research 18:1–5, 1996

Appelbaum PS: Rethinking the conduct of psychiatric research. Arch Gen Psychiatry 54:117–120, 1997

Armitage P: The search for optimality in clinical trials. International Statistical Review 53:15–24, 1985

Baldessarini RJ, Viguera AC: Neuroleptic withdrawal in schizophrenic patients. Arch Gen Psychiatry 52:189–192, 1995

Baldessarini RJ, Tondo L, Faedda GL, et al: Effects of the rate of discontinuing lithium maintenance treatment in bipolar disorders. J Clin Psychiatry 57:441–448, 1996

Bather JA: On the allocation of treatments in sequential medical trials. International Statistical Review 53:1–13, 1985

Borison RL, Arvanitis LA, Miller BG: A comparison of five fixed doses of "seroquel" (ICI 204,636) with haloperidol and placebo in patients with schizophrenia (abstract). Schizophr Res 18:132, 1996

Carpenter WT Jr, Tamminga CA: Why neuroleptic withdrawal in schizophrenia? Arch Gen Psychiatry 52:192–193, 1995

Carpenter WT Jr, Schooler NR, Kane JM: The rationale and ethics of medication-free research in schizophrenia. Arch Gen Psychiatry 54:401–407, 1997

Chalmers T: Ethical aspects of clinical trials. Am J Ophthalmol 79:753–758, 1975

Chouinard G, Jones B, Remington G, et al: A Canadian multicenter placebo-controlled study of fixed doses of risperidone and haloperidol in the treatment of chronic schizophrenic patients. J Clin Psychopharmacol 13:25–40, 1993

Clark PI, Leaverton PE: Scientific and ethical issues in the use of placebo controls in clinical trials. Annu Rev Public Health 15:19–38, 1994

Clayton D: Ethically optimized designs. Br J Clin Pharmacol 13:469–480, 1982

Cohen BM, Babb S, Campbell A, et al: Persistence of haloperidol in the brain. Arch Gen Psychiatry 45:879–880, 1988

Colton T: A model for selecting one of two medical treatments. Journal of the American Statistical Association 58:388–400, 1963

Czobor P, Volavka J, Meibach RC: Effect of risperidone on hostility in schizophrenia. J Clin Psychopharmacol 15:243–249, 1995

Delgado PL, Charney DS, Price LH, et al: Serotonin function and the mechanism of antidepressant action: reversal of antidepressant-induced remission by rapid depletion of plasma tryptophan. Arch Gen Psychiatry 47:411–418, 1990

Dempster AP, Selwyn MR, Weeks BJ: Combining historical and randomized controls for assessing trends in proportions. Journal of the American Statistical Association 78:221–227, 1983

Depression Guideline Panel (Rush AJ, Chair): Clinical Practice Guideline, No 5. Depression in Primary Care, Vol 2: Treatment of Major Depression (AHCPR Publ No 93-0551). Rockville, MD, U.S. Department of Health and Human Services, Public Health Service, Agency for Health Care Policy and Research, 1993

Fairchild CJ, Rush AJ, Vasavada N, et al: Which depressions respond to placebo? Psychiatry Res 18:217–226, 1986

Fleming TR, Harrington DP, O'Brien PC: Designs for group sequential tests. Control Clin Trials 5:348–361, 1984

Freedman B, Weijer C, Glass KC: Placebo orthodoxy in clinical research, I: empirical and methodological myths. Journal of Law, Medicine, and Ethics 24:243–251, 1996a

Freedman B, Glass KC, Weijer C: Placebo orthodoxy in clinical research, II: ethical, legal, and regulatory myths. Journal of Law, Medicine, and Ethics 24:252–259, 1996b

Geller NL, Pocock SJ: Interim analyses in randomized clinical trials: ramifications and guidelines for practitioners. Biometrics 43:213–223, 1987

Gilbert PL, Harris MJ, McAdams LA, et al: Neuroleptic withdrawal in schizophrenic patients: a review of the literature. Arch Gen Psychiatry 52:173–188, 1995

Goodwin FK, Jamison KR: Manic-Depressive Illness. New York, Oxford University Press, 1990

Gorman JM, Liebowitz MR, Dillon D, et al: Antipanic drug effects during lactate infusion in lactate-refractory panic patients. Psychiatry Res 21:205–212, 1987

Greden JF, Tandon R: Long-term treatment for lifetime disorders? Arch Gen Psychiatry 52:197–200, 1995

Hilts P: Agency faults a UCLA study for suffering of mental patients. New York Times, March 10, 1994, pp A1, A11

Hubbard JW, Ganes D, Midha KK: Prolonged pharmacologic activity of neuroleptic drugs (letter). Arch Gen Psychiatry 44:99–100, 1987

Janowsky DS, Overstreet DH: The role of acetylcholine mechanisms in the affective disorders, in Psychopharmacology: The Fourth Generation of Progress. Edited by Bloom FE, Kupfer DJ. New York, Raven, 1995, pp 945–956

Jeste DV, Gilbert PL, McAdams LA, et al: Considering neuroleptic maintenance and taper on a continuum: need for individual rather than dogmatic approach. Arch Gen Psychiatry 52:209–212, 1995

Keller MB, Lavori PW, Kane JM, et al: Subsyndromal symptoms in bipolar disorder: a comparison of standard and low serum levels of lithium. Arch Gen Psychiatry 49:371–376, 1992

Khan A, Dager SR, Cohen S, et al: Chronicity of depressive episode in relation to anti-depressant-placebo response. Neuropsychopharmacology 4:125–130, 1991

King NMP: Experimental treatment: oxymoron or aspiration? Hastings Cent Rep 25:6–15, 1995

Krystal JH, Karper LP, Seibyl JP, et al: Subanesthetic effects of the noncompetitive NMDA antagonist, ketamine, in humans: psychotomimetic, perceptual, cognitive, and neuroendocrine responses. Arch Gen Psychiatry 51:199–214, 1994

Laska E, Meisner M: A decision theory procedure for a binomial population with a beta prior distribution. New York Statistician 18:7–8, 1966

Liebenluft E: Women with bipolar illness: clinical and research issues. Am J Psychiatry 153:163–173, 1996

Lieberman JA: Ethical dilemmas in clinical research with human subjects: an investigator's perspective. Psychopharmacol Bull 32:19–25, 1996

Lieberman JA, Sheitman B, Kinon BJ: Neurochemical sensitization in the pathophysiology of schizophrenia: deficits and dysfunction in neuronal regulation and plasticity. Neuropsychopharmacology 17:205–229, 1997

Marder SR, Meibach RC: Risperidone in the treatment of schizophrenia. Am J Psychiatry 151:825–835, 1994

Meinert CL: Clinical Trials Dictionary: Terminology and Usage Recommendations. Baltimore, MD, Johns Hopkins Center for Clinical Trials, 1996

Meltzer HY: Neuroleptic withdrawal in schizophrenic patients: an idea whose time has come. Arch Gen Psychiatry 52:200–202, 1995

Mohs RC, Davis BM, Greenwald BS, et al: Clinical studies of the cholinergic deficit in Alzheimer's disease, II: psychopharmacologic studies. J Am Geriatr Soc 33:749–757, 1985

National Alliance for the Mentally Ill: Policies on Strengthened Standards for Protection of Individuals With Severe Mental Illnesses in Research. Arlington, VA, National Alliance for the Mentally Ill, 1995

National Institutes of Health: NIH Guidelines on the Inclusion of Women and Minorities as Subjects in Clinical Research. Federal Register 59 (March 28, 1994):14508–14513

Nelson JC, Mazure CM, Jatlow PI: Does melancholia predict outcome in major depression? J Affect Disord 18:157–165, 1990

Nyberg S, Farde L, Halldin C: Longtime persistence of D_2 dopamine receptor occupancy after discontinuation of haloperidol decanoate (abstract). Schizophr Res 18:199–200, 1996

O'Brien PC, Fleming TR: A multiple testing procedure for clinical trials. Biometrics 35:549–556, 1979

Peuskens J: Risperidone in the treatment of patients with chronic schizophrenia: a multinational, multi-centre, double-blind, parallel-group study versus haloperidol. Br J Psychiatry 166:712–726, 1995

Pledger GW, Hall D: Active control trials: do they address the efficacy issue? (with discussion). Proceedings of the Biopharmaceutical Section, American Statistical Association, Alexandria, VA, 1986, pp 1–10

Post RM, Leverich GS, Altshuler L, et al: Lithium-discontinuation-induced refractoriness: preliminary observations. Am J Psychiatry 149:1727–1729, 1992

Prien RF: Methods and models for placebo use in pharmacotherapeutic trials. Psychopharmacol Bull 24:4–8, 1988

Rosenbaum PR: Observational Studies. New York, Springer-Verlag, 1985

Rosenbaum PR, Rubin DB: Reducing bias in observational studies using subclassification on the propensity score. Journal of the American Statistical Association 79:516–524, 1984

Rothman KJ, Michels KB: The continuing unethical use of placebo controls. N Engl J Med 331:394–398, 1994

Sampath G, Shah A, Krska J, et al: Neuroleptic discontinuation in the very stable schizophrenic patient: relapse rates and serum neuroleptic levels. Human Psychopharmacology 7:255–264, 1992

Schafer A: The ethics of the randomized clinical trial. N Engl J Med 307:722–723, 1982

Schooler NR, Keith SJ, Severe JB, et al: Relapse and rehospitalization during maintenance treatment of schizophrenia: the effects of dose reduction and family treatment. Arch Gen Psychiatry 54:453–463, 1997

Schulz SC, Mack R, Zborowski J, et al: Efficacy, safety, and dose response of three doses of sertindole and three doses of Haldol in schizophrenic patients (abstract). Schizophr Res 18:133–134, 1996

Scully PJ, Coakley G, Kinsella A, et al: Psychopathology, executive (frontal) and general cognitive impairment in relation to duration of initially untreated and subsequently treated psychosis in chronic schizophrenia. Psychol Med 27:1303–1310, 1997

Shaw LW, Chalmers TC: Ethics in cooperative clinical trials. Ann N Y Acad Sci 169:487–489, 1970

Trivedi MH, Rush AJ: Does a placebo washout or a placebo treatment cell affect the efficacy of antidepressant medications? Neuropsychopharmacology 11:33–43, 1994

Tygstrup N, Lachin JM, Juhl E (eds): The Randomized Clinical Trial and Therapeutic Decisions. New York, Marcel Dekker, 1982

Volavka J: Lead-in placebo washout period (letter). Br J Psychiatry 167:694, 1995a

Volavka J: Placebo reconsidered (letter). Can J Psychiatry 40:426–427, 1995b

Volavka J, Cooper T, Czobor P, et al: Haloperidol blood levels and clinical effects. Arch Gen Psychiatry 49:354–361, 1992

Volavka J, Cooper TB, Laska EM, et al: Placebo washout in trials of antipsychotic drugs. Schizophr Bull 22:567–575, 1996

Waddington JL, Scully PJ, Youssef HA: Developmental trajectory and disease progression in schizophrenia: the conundrum, and insights from a 12-year prospective study in the Monaghan 101. Schizophr Res 23:107–118, 1997

Ware JH, Muller JE, Braunwald E: The futility index: an approach to the cost-effective termination of randomized clinical trials. Am J Med 78:635–643, 1985

Wei LJ: A class of designs for sequential clinical trials. Journal of the American Statistical Association 72:382–386, 1977

Wei LJ, Lachin JM: Properties of the urn randomization in clinical trials. Control Clin Trials 9:345–364, 1988

Wyatt RJ: Neuroleptics and the natural course of schizophrenia. Schizophr Bull 17:325–351, 1991

Wyatt RJ: Research in schizophrenia and the discontinuation of antipsychotic medications. Schizophr Bull 23:3–9, 1997

Zohar J, Mueller EA, Insel TR, et al: Serotonergic responsivity in obsessive-compulsive disorder: comparison of patients and healthy controls. Arch Gen Psychiatry 44:946–951, 1987

CHAPTER 3

Providing Quality Care in the Context of Clinical Research

Nina R. Schooler, Ph.D., and Robert W. Baker, M.D.

I n this chapter we provide information to help investigators ensure that high-quality clinical care is provided in conjunction with high-quality clinical research. Several characteristics of clinical research present opportunities and challenges for clinical care, both during the implementation of a protocol and after a subject's participation has ended. First, it is extremely rare for a research protocol to specify all parameters of treatment for research subjects; protocols generally leave some aspects of treatment to ad hoc accommodation. Second, protocols may include elements that offset potential problems or complications. Third, because all research protocols are time limited, questions of clinical care can be addressed once a subject has completed participation in the research.

Altruism is not the only motivation for researchers to provide high-quality clinical care. High-quality care can also make subjects more likely to consent to study participation and make oversight bodies more likely to accept a protocol. All psychiatric research in the United States supported by federal sources or the pharmaceutical industry must have the approval of institutional review boards (IRBs). And virtually all other research must meet this requirement because the agencies in which the research is conducted mandate IRB review. A major tenet of IRBs is that subjects or their agents must provide informed consent before

We thank the reviewers whose critical analysis of the chapter allowed us to consider changes, some of which we made. Those we can identify by name include William T. Carpenter Jr., Steven Kenny Hoge, and Donald F. Klein. In addition, we thank our colleagues with whom we share our clinical research efforts at Mayview State Hospital: Joan Bezner, Roy Chengappa, and Joyce Bell Delaney. At Western Psychiatric Institute and Clinic the conjunction of research and clinical concerns is shared with Lois DiFrank, Matcheri S. Keshavan, and Nancy Miller McLaughlin. Finally, we gratefully acknowledge the participation of the many patients who agreed to be the subjects of our research and the families who supported their decision.

participating in a research protocol. If the protocol involves a randomized comparison of treatments with two different medications or a novel psychosocial treatment and "usual care," the research subject has chosen to forgo treatment selection on the basis of a clinician's judgment of what is best. However, all nonprotocol-specified aspects of care allow and indeed require the application of clinical judgment, making the consideration of quality of care in the research setting critical.

Because the clinician's judgment of what is best may not be perfect and some of the treatments under study may offer advantages beyond those clinically available, individuals who elect to participate in a research study may gain some advantages simply from participation. Further, it is our contention that research participants should be provided with the highest-quality clinical care that a treatment setting can provide. All elements of the care not dictated by the research protocol should reflect the clinician's best judgment of the appropriate treatment for the individual subject-patient.

In the sections that follow we first discuss the tension between research and clinical care and identify several models, with their attendant advantages and disadvantages. We then discuss issues in clinical management during protocol participation, distinguishing four broad categories of protocols: protocols that manipulate pharmacological treatment, protocols that manipulate psychosocial treatment, protocols that entail assessment but do not alter clinical care, and protocols that involve pharmacological probes or other biological procedures that may be invasive. In the next section we discuss "wraparound care," or clinical care following research protocol participation. In the final section we discuss relationships with both family members and the community and hospital.

RESEARCH-CLINICAL TENSION

Ideally a clinician providing psychiatric care can access a body of knowledge about treatments and tailor it to the needs of individual patients. Unfortunately, this body of knowledge is not complete; many treatment questions have no definitive answers, and even apparently definitive answers change. Many treatments have fallen in and out of favor over time. Further, no individual physician is likely to possess all of the available knowledge. Nevertheless, using the available knowledge and the history of an individual patient, the doctor and patient embark on a treatment plan and adjust that plan over time in response to the patient's course, availability of resources, willingness to continue in treatment, and any number of other factors. Research protocols that specify treatment elements limit this adjustment process to a greater or lesser extent, depending on the specific protocol. These restrictions are not necessarily adverse to treatment and may even enhance it, but they define the boundaries of clinical care during research participation.

Research strives to generate information that may benefit individuals other than the research subject. When this goal requires protocol-dictated treatment that differs from routine clinical judgment, considerable tension and strain may be generated for both clinicians and researchers. In the following sections, we consider three paradigms under which this relationship may express itself: the clinician and researcher are the same individual, the clinician and researcher are different individuals, or an outside monitor oversees the clinician-researcher or clinician and researcher.

Clinician-Researcher

In the clinician-researcher model, the individual who is responsible for a patient's clinical care is also responsible for the research protocol. The research may be conducted in the clinical facility in which the patient is being treated, such as a research ward. Or by agreeing to be a subject, the patient may be transferred to the care of the clinician-researcher, such as in a research clinic in which all patients participate in research protocols. One advantage of this model is that the clinician-researcher may be very experienced in meeting the challenges of clinical care in the context of research. A second benefit is that the clinical setting can be organized to optimize tailoring of nonresearch-specified elements to clinical needs. For example, a research clinic in which pharmacological treatment is studied may have a higher staff-to-patient ratio than a routine clinical setting and may offer more flexible appointment scheduling and an enriched psychosocial milieu. A clinic in which psychological therapies are studied may incorporate a sophisticated pharmacological approach. A research ward in which medication is discontinued for periods of time may offer advanced diagnostic procedures or subsequent access to psychopharmacological expertise.

The disadvantages of the clinician-researcher model reflect the tension between research and clinical care. The clinician-researcher may be perceived by others as concentrating on research goals at the expense of optimizing treatment for individual patients. When the research protocol specifies a course that is less than optimal for a particular subject, the clinician-researcher may also have concerns. (See the section "Clinical Management During Protocol

Participation" for strategies to protect the interest of the individual subject while maintaining the research protocol.)

Separate Roles for Clinician and Researcher

In the separate roles model, clinicians who are not directly associated with the research protocol provide treatment. Clinicians participate in the research endeavor by agreeing to limit the full exercise of clinical judgment in treatment or by agreeing to the participation of subjects in assessments that are not of direct benefit to the patient. The clinician may serve as a gatekeeper to research participation at the beginning: patients will not be approached for participation without the consent of the treating clinician. Further, during a study the clinician relates to and observes individual patients independent of the research. The advantage of this model is that an independent voice represents clinical care. The disadvantage is that the patients referred for research may not be representative of the clinical population under study. Furthermore, the clinical setting may not be optimal for research, the clinician may not have full knowledge of the research interventions or procedures of which the subject is a part, and the researcher-subject relationship may be diminished.

Oversight

In the oversight model, the individual who has clinical responsibility for patient care may or may not also have responsibility for the research protocol. In either case, outside individuals oversee the protocol to ensure that research goals are not being furthered at the expense of subjects' clinical needs. An oversight model may be used in situations that entail considerable risks for subjects. Oversight may include a range of activities, including guaranteeing that potential subjects are clear about the risks and benefits of the research before they consent to participate, monitoring patients' clinical course to ensure that subjects are discontinued from a protocol when appropriate, and reviewing the early results of a study and requiring that it be discontinued if these early findings suggest that continuation would place subjects at undue risk. This model is expensive and can diminish research productivity if the researcher-overseer working relationship is strained. It may also diminish the personal relationship between researcher and subject.

The use of safety committees in large multicenter trials represents another oversight option. These committees provide guidance in regard to study design and regularly review both efficacy data and adverse events to facilitate early trial discontinuation if the results clearly favor one treatment arm.

CLINICAL MANAGEMENT DURING PROTOCOL PARTICIPATION

Insofar as a protocol affects diagnosis or treatment or poses risk to the subject-patient, the study has a clinical component. Quality care in such studies requires clear communication and mutual understanding among the researcher, clinician, and subject. If the same individual serves as the researcher and clinician, the number of individuals involved in this communication process is smaller, but the issues remain important.

Artful clinical management during research requires skillful and timely manipulation of nonprotocol-mandated aspects of treatment and, at times, recognition of a clinical imperative to terminate the research participation of a given subject. One bit of the art is achieving these clinical objectives without undermining the project's capacity to adequately test its hypothesis. If a study involves randomized treatments that differ, the difference can be overwhelmed by disproportionate application of supplemental, nonprotocol-specified therapy to the subjects in one treatment arm.

In the sections that follow we address issues, tensions, and techniques that are relevant across research areas and then turn to special problems associated with particular types of research. We begin by emphasizing the value of maintaining study participation despite clinical obstacles to that goal.

The Benefit of Completing Trials

Dropout rates of half or more are reported in even relatively brief clinical trials. The issue of termination of subject participation has drawn attention because dropouts reduce the credibility of the findings of these studies and also reflect the operation of clinical priorities in research settings. Just like patients in routine clinical care, research subjects experience treatment side effects and treatment-refractory symptoms. Subjects are often withdrawn from studies because of clinical issues such as unsatisfactory improvement of their target symptoms or adverse physical events. Even terminations that are not ascribed to adverse events may in fact be driven by clinical factors. For example, in our schizophrenia treatment studies most subjects who have withdrawn consent have done so because of discomfort or paranoia incompatible with continued participation; that is, withdrawal of consent might have been averted had the subjects' responses to treatment been better.

In our experience, most decisions to terminate a given subject's participation reflect informal, case-by-case reanalyses of the risk-benefit ratio. At the time of informed consent, weighing of risks and adverse outcomes hinges on potential harm or discomfort; during the study, after clinical deterioration or adverse physical events have ensued, this discomfort is actual and the risk-benefit ratio is less favorable to continued study participation. Similarly, lack of improvement in the target symptoms within a given interval may lower the expectation of benefit to be gained by the experimental treatment and also tilt the risk-benefit ratio against continued participation. In these situations, subjects, clinicians, and clinician-researchers tend to vote with their feet, breaking blinds and withdrawing subjects from the study.

We do not dispute the ethical imperative of terminating study participation for an individual when increasing risk or decreasing benefit is apparent. However, one common mistake is failure to consider the full range of potential benefits. We suggest that there is both individual and global benefit to remaining in a protocol long enough for the individual's outcome to inform the study results. Put another way, the overall value (benefit) of a study hinges on its ability to test its hypothesis; failing this, participation for any subject does not outweigh even small risk. This issue is handled during study design by power calculations that anticipate likely dropouts. During protocol execution, the need to usher subjects through the protocol makes quality clinical care a research imperative. Therefore, although many of the themes we elaborate on later relate to patient safety and comfort, they also have the goal of sustaining protocol participation despite clinical problems. We discuss several approaches to maintaining participation: preparation of staff and subjects, anticipation of problems in the protocol itself, consideration of requests by subjects to change the terms of study participation, and consideration of the natural history of illnesses and side effects. The challenge to clinical investigators is to use these and similar approaches to balance the priority of completing the study with the obligation of acting in patients' best interests.

Educating Subjects and Clinicians About Common Pitfalls

When it comes to health, ambiguity is especially uncomfortable. Experimental protocols can concern everyone involved, doubly so if interventions are blind or of uncertain safety or efficacy. In this environment, any unpleasant surprise may provoke precipitous study termination. Thus, there is real clinical utility in carefully preparing subjects and other interested parties about likely experiences, particularly unfavorable ones. Common adverse experiences should be anticipated and predicted, including their likely time course, management, and consequences. Staff or subjects may view experimental treatment as a failure if more testing or closer confinement becomes necessary because of clinical deterioration or side effects. However, these events are less likely to disrupt the protocol or provoke emotional distress when viewed by participants as expected, normal, or manageable. Careful attention to such possibilities during the in-formed consent process can be most beneficial to research completion.

Anticipating Clinical Problems During Protocol Design

In designing protocols, researchers can build in mechanisms for dealing with likely clinical problems. For example, a planned ability to shorten placebo wash-out periods in the face of symptom exacerbation can provide an alternative to protocol termination or tolerating the subject's worsening. Available adjunctive medications can ameliorate emerging behavioral symptoms such as anxiety, insomnia, agitation, or aggression. These drugs can jeopardize clean assessment of the effects of experimental probes or treatment, but they are an invaluable tool for clinical management. Nonmedical interventions may or may not be carefully codified, but they can offset temporarily inadequate treatment. Some protocols specify a priori numerical (rating-instrument-based) criteria for using adjunctive treatment or changing treatment status. These criteria tend to en-hance the uniformity of interventions, yet reliance on rating-scale changes may or may not match sound clinical judgment. For example, a change that demands clinical intervention but is captured by only one or two rating items (e.g., sui-cidality) may fail to raise a total psychopathology score to the threshold required to intervene. If such requirements postpone or prevent supplemental clinical measures, they may increase the likelihood of dropout or adverse outcome. Conversely, mandatory dropout due to "worsening" on a particular scale may sacrifice subjects who appropriately could persevere in the research protocol. We suggest allowing clinical judgment to override such rating-scale mandates.

When the Subject Wants to Alter the Terms of Study Participation

How should investigators deal with their subjects' requests to change or quit their protocol? Clearly the answer depends on the situation. When it appears medically best to stop the study, the investigator must quickly honor the request; indeed, if this is the case the investigator should have moved toward terminating participation before the subject requested it. On the other hand, subjects may want to withdraw for reasons other than what appears to be in their best medical interest. Although the guiding principle is that subjects have the absolute right to decline study participation, appropriate responses to requests for study ter-mination vary.

Often subjects' dissatisfaction can be dealt with by less dramatic measures than study termination, such as prescription of a medication to treat insomnia or permission to visit home despite a protocol policy of remaining in the hos-pital throughout a placebo period. The request may be nonverbal, such as consuming alcohol despite prohibition by the experiment. Our best success in these situations has come from approaching them as we might any clinical matter: individually, with the maximal allowable flexibility and pragmatism. It is helpful if researchers anticipate these situations, because the allowable flexibility and pragmatism depend on the rigidity of the protocol and what has been promised to the sponsor and the IRB.

Are attempts to persuade withdrawing subjects to remain in a study ethical? Good care requires close monitoring of the subjective experience of study participants throughout their participation, which is especially important when the subject is dissatisfied. Both research and clinical practice seem to demand inquiry about why a subject would like to drop out; if this inquiry reveals problems that can be addressed, it seems appropriate to address them and then reevaluate the participant's willingness to proceed. For example, if a volunteer wants to quit blind treatment for hypertension because of light-headedness, application of support stockings may relieve the light-headedness and materially affect his or her willingness to remain in the trial. Similarly, if a subject objects that appointments for research evaluations interfere with working, rescheduling these appointments to evenings and renegotiating study participation may salvage the subject's participation and are as ethical as immediate study termination. Not uncommonly, a narrow component of the protocol may be the noxious precipitant to a request for termination. For example, large multicenter trials of antibiotic treatment for infection may recruit a subsample for determination of the pharmacokinetics of the study drug. One subject in the subsample may withdraw consent after experiencing discomfort from repeated phlebotomy or venous catheterization. In this case, it may be scientifically beneficial and ethically sound to allow a subject to discontinue participation in the objectionable pharmacokinetics study while maintaining participation in the parent double-blind study of antibiotic treatment.

Subjects with impaired mentation may require special consideration in addressing their requests to stop study participation. Informed consent is more a process than an event. Patients with delusions, thought disorder, ambivalence, or impulsiveness may nevertheless retain an ability to understand medical or research treatment and make informed decisions about treatment. These subjects deserve very clear information about their options and probably repeated assessment over time of their competence and willingness to consent. Similarly, time and care should be taken in assessing their requests to withdraw. Although an active treatment component should never be administered over a subject's objection (i.e., the research pills should not be administered if a subject does not want them), delay of irrevocable study termination can be appropriate. For example, an impulsive subject may respond with irritation when awakened for a morning intervention: "I don't want to be involved in this research anymore";

if this subject is likely to competently choose to continue the study when wide awake a few hours later, it would seem a mistake to immediately terminate study participation (though, of course, it is necessary to withhold whichever intervention provoked objection that morning). Similarly, when in the course of schizophrenia trials objections seem delusional ("Those capsules contain feces"), it is appropriate to assess and address the objections for a day or so before final termination of participation.

In contrast to the preceding examples, in some situations we have ended double-blind treatment over the objection of the participating subject. In all cases these were patients in clinical trials of antipsychotic drugs with improved subjective well-being but decline in reality testing or judgment to a point that ongoing research treatment seemed imprudent. This situation illustrates a responsibility of the investigator to exercise medical care in protecting subjects from the risks of experiments even when they do not themselves recognize the need for protection.

Considering the Natural Course of Illness, Recovery, and Adverse Events

Sound knowledge of the natural course of the illness under study and rational expectations for speed of improvement and occurrence of side effects may assist management of an unsatisfactory clinical course.

To illustrate, antidepressant and antipsychotic drugs often ameliorate symptoms over weeks rather than days. Therefore, it seems wise to resist urges to terminate a placebo-controlled trial after a week or so because of inadequate change in the target symptoms. This time factor is an important issue in study design, especially if the trial takes place in a setting subject to pressures for quick change, such as a hospital unit monitored by impatient third-party payers. Such protocols are difficult to accomplish unless they include reasonable methods to relieve symptoms while awaiting the onset of action of the experimental treatment. The experience and comfort of the clinical research staff affect how the situation is approached as well; resourceful, experienced clinicians are better able to handle clinical problems by using interventions compatible with the study.

Symptoms fluctuate spontaneously in most psychiatric illnesses. Research can control for this fluctuation by employing parallel treatment groups. In managing individual subjects, it is worthwhile to keep this natural variability in mind. That is, not every change is due to the experimental treatment, and not every worsening requires prompt cancellation of the treatment.

Adverse event–related choices also benefit by considering the expected effects of each of the treatments under study. Life-threatening or other very serious adverse events generally require immediate intervention. With less serious problems, investigators can move less precipitously. Recognizing that placebo-treated groups typically have a high incidence of some adverse events (e.g., headache or insomnia), clinical researchers may resist overascribing such complaints to an experimental drug and encourage subjects to persist a bit in the protocol. Some side effects are common and transitory, such as nausea during the initial weeks of serotonin reuptake inhibitor treatment or temperature elevation during clozapine titration. In these cases it is appropriate and potentially beneficial to reassure the subject that his or her discomfort is common and probably temporary. On the other hand, however, extreme prolongation of the corrected Q-T interval on the cardiograms of subjects in clinical trials of quinidine-like psychotropic or cardiovascular drugs may herald sudden death; the investigator may thus need to intervene quickly even if the subject is asymptomatic.

Concerns in Particular Types of Psychiatric Research

As indicated earlier, we divide clinical research into four rough categories: treatment trials studying a pharmacological intervention, treatment trials studying a psychosocial or nonpharmacological intervention, studies entailing assessment but not altering clinical care, and studies involving pharmacological probes or other procedures that may be invasive. Some studies, such as those in which a pharmacological probe serves as the baseline for a clinical trial comparing medications or (rarely) those that involve manipulation of both medication and psychosocial treatment, may raise concerns from more than one of these categories.

Psychopharmacological Studies

Psychopharmacological treatment studies may be open, single-blind, or double-blind trials. Although many issues are common to these designs, the discussion that follows focuses on double-blind studies. In their use of treatments of uncertain identity, double-blind trials differ notably from routine clinical practice and consequently represent the greatest challenge to clinical investigators. We discuss an approach to coping with the ambiguity present in double-blind studies.

Applying parallel clinical reasoning. Clinical research protocols codify many but not all aspects of treatment. In working with subjects in double-blind protocols, clinicians typically encounter two classes of problems: 1) management of situations for which the protocol does not supply guidelines and 2) management of situations in which the protocol's guidelines seem clinically unwise or inadequate.

During double-blind protocols at least one key aspect of the clinical puzzle is missing. For example, how can one respond to a subject's physical complaints without knowing what medication is prescribed and therefore which side effects are common? A useful strategy for addressing the problem involves considering each treatment arm in the study design as a separate question. An intervention or course of action can be chosen by evaluating each possible scenario separately: "If the treatment is A, I should do B; if the treatment is X, then Y is the best intervention," and so on. Ideally, at the conclusion of this exercise the researcher can choose a strategy that includes each intervention that would be appropriate for a given arm of the blinded treatment. However, if management that is appropriate if the subject is in one arm of the study would be inappropriate or dangerous if he or she were in one of the other arms, it may be necessary to drop the subject from the protocol and possibly to unblind that individual's treatment. This approach may be clarified by the examples that follow.

Consider a subject who complains of light-headedness during a double-blind comparison of three treatments for depression: imipramine, phenelzine, and placebo. It is easiest to approach this situation as three different problems. The first is how to understand and manage light-headedness in a placebo-treated patient. Could the light-headedness be somehow related to withdrawal from whatever treatment preceded the double-blind trial? Is it a somatic manifestation of anxiety due to the subject's fears about research or perhaps inadequate biological treatment of depression and associated anxiety? Could it represent a physical condition unrelated to depression or placebo treatment? Might simple reassurance ameliorate the light-headedness? In short, the investigator should review the "normal" evaluation and management of light-headedness in depressed patients taking no medication and for the most part evaluate and manage the research subject in the same way (except as forbidden by the research protocol or contradicted by the steps listed in the following). The second problem is how to understand and manage light-headedness in a patient treated with phenelzine. Most of the considerations in a placebo-treated patient would still apply here, but the biological effects of phenelzine also need consideration. Does light-headedness reflect postural hypotension? At this stage, the researcher should measure the subject's lying and standing pulse and blood pressure. If postural hypotension is present, worthwhile clinical interventions are evident— counseling the patient to sit or stand slowly, prescribing support stockings and perhaps more liberal salt intake, and, the protocol permitting, slowing the study drug titration or reducing the dose. The third issue is how to approach light-headedness in a patient treated with tricyclics. In addition to the previous considerations, prudent clinicians may want to exclude cardiac disturbance by obtaining an electrocardiogram (ECG). Prolonged intracardiac conduction might necessitate medical intervention and protocol termination; on the other hand, a normal ECG result would be reassuring. At the conclusion of this exercise, taking into account all possibilities, the clinical researcher might find it best to reassure the subject, check the orthostatic vital signs, and order an ECG.

As another example, consider a subject who becomes pregnant during a placebo-controlled trial of a drug for acne. Most management decisions will hinge on whether the subject has been taking the active drug. Must the treatment be stopped immediately? The researcher might first consider the known effects of the active drug in pregnancy. If the study drug is known to be safe, double-blind continuation might be entertained. On the other hand, if the medication is early in development or recently marketed, its effects in pregnancy may be relatively unknown and the decision must be made to terminate double-blind treatment. Parallel reasoning should be applied to the question: should the subject be dropped from the protocol and have her treatment assignment be unblinded? An appropriate question might be that, assuming the subject received the active drug, what is the best prenatal management? If that management poses negligible risk or discomfort, or does not differ from routine prenatal care, the pressure for immediate unblinding diminishes.

Sometimes physical problems during a protocol require consultation with nonpsychiatric physicians. In this case, good communication between the consultant and researcher is critical. The consultant may need to apply parallel clinical reasoning similar to that described earlier. The researcher is responsible for explaining to the consultant why this approach is preferable to simply dropping the subject from the protocol.

Psychosocial Treatment Studies

Unlike pharmacological treatment studies, studies of psychosocial treatments are never fully blinded. Many of the issues we have considered for research generally and for pharmacological studies specifically are also applicable to psychosocial treatment studies. However, two issues are particularly important in psychosocial treatment studies. The first is the possibility of differential added care or attention to patients in a control group. The psychosocial treatment researcher who allows pharmacological treatment to "run free" may find substantial differences between groups that represent wide variations in clinical care and can compromise the validity of the research. Psychosocial treatment protocols vary in their requirements for standardization of treatment beyond those specified by the research. A phrase frequently found in research reports is that "pharmacological treatment was optimal." From the vantage point of both research and clinical care, efforts should be made to ensure that *optimal* applies equally to all subjects who participate in a study.

The second issue is the question of wraparound care following study participation. In a subsequent section we describe several options for further care that are particularly applicable to pharmacological trials: referral to other clinical systems, provision of medication for a fixed period, or treatment until a specified clinical milestone is reached. The problem for psychosocial treatment studies is somewhat more complicated because the options may be more limited. The psychosocial treatments under study are likely not available through other clinical systems, and the provision of "open label" psychotherapy may not be feasible. Consequently, the treatment the subject has received as part of protocol participation may represent the limit of clinical care that the research is able to provide. Of course, a referral to another clinical setting is mandatory, but it may not include all (or even any) of the treatments that were part of the research protocol.

Assessment and Diagnosis

Because psychiatric assessment and diagnosis are based mostly on history and mental status examination, they carry less risk, less potential for inconvenience, and a much lower likelihood of long-term impact than treatment studies do. Consequently, quality-of-care considerations are generally indirect, but the study may have an impact on ongoing clinical care. We highlight two examples in the following.

Time considerations. Research participants are precious, and protocols can mushroom to take full advantage of them, adding multidimensional assessments and proliferating secondary questions. Multidimensional assessments are perhaps more likely in multi-investigator collaborations: More questions require more assessments to be performed. Such a situation can be detrimental to the subjects' comfort, but from the viewpoint of this chapter the biggest concern is for the subject to retain enough time and energy to effectively pursue clinical management of his or her problems. The subject may not reliably protect his or her time and energy, and a surrogate or ombudsman may be necessary, especially in large-scale assessment studies. Practically speaking, those responsible for clinical care are most likely to speak up when that care is compromised.

Communication to the clinician. When diagnostic and assessment studies uncover information not previously available to the treating clinician, handling of that information may not be straightforward. The subject-investigator relationship obviously affects the accuracy and completeness of data provided by the subject. That is, openness in providing information may reflect the trust placed in the investigator, which in turn reflects the expectation for what is to be done with that information. Clinical care may be enhanced by new information, especially pressing data such as new suicidal ideation or evidence that some third party is in danger. On the other hand, feeding these data back to the clinician may betray an assumed confidentiality; knowledge that confidentiality is lacking may undermine the candor of the subject in providing data. If the study is tracking a naturalistic course, the provision of data to clinical personnel may influence that course and undermine the study's intent.

A related issue is what to do when the research diagnosis or assessment does not agree with that of the responsible clinician. This can be a delicate situation, because a referring source may be upset by contradiction of his or her conclusions. On the other hand, passing on this information may inform and thereby improve the patient's care. Also potentially vexing is what to say to the subject-patient if the investigator disagrees with the clinical diagnosis or management. No fully satisfying answer may exist, but basing the solution on an a priori agreement rather than an ad hoc decision may be the best approach when a potential disagreement arises.

The best solution to potential communication problems is to discuss procedures when a study is initiated, to include the issue of communication in the process of obtaining informed consent, and to be certain that all parties, including subjects, clinicians, and researchers, have a common understanding. Quality of care is likely to profit from open communication, and therefore the bias should be toward communicating new data to the responsible clinician. For example, if a researcher knows that a subject is hiding suicidal intent from the treating clinician, the researcher should not maintain passive silence. The subject must of course be told that the information is being provided to the treating clinician. Strong justification, such as safeguarding subject confidentiality, is required for the shielding of information, but it must always be clear to all involved that information that places the subject or another individual at risk must be revealed. We have used the following language in some situations: "If I agree, information from clinical interviews may be shared with my treatment team. . . . [I]f in the course of this research, information relevant to my protection or the protection of others is learned, it will be released."

Biological Procedures

Biological procedures include pharmacological probes, imaging studies, and bodily fluid collection. Although these procedures may not require modification of clinical care per se, they may influence the clinical care patients receive. For example, medication administration may need to be delayed to permit blood to be drawn to obtain trough concentrations of medication, anticholinergic medication may be held before an imaging procedure, or a patient may be asked to stay on the ward rather than go to a scheduled activity because of a research procedure. Further, if adverse clinical events present after a patient has been a subject in a biological study, there may be questions about whether the event is attributable to earlier research participation. Commonly, the clinician and researcher are not the same individual, making communication between the clinician and researcher crucial. The researcher should inform the clinician about the procedures that his or her patient will undergo and any potential clinical consequences of the research.

In general, these procedures may have a negative impact on clinical care if they delay treatment, have direct adverse consequences, or are associated with long-term adverse events. On the other hand, patients may benefit if the information obtained in the research can be subsequently communicated to the clinician. For instance, information regarding the relationship of plasma concentration and dose may be informative. Data from research imaging studies may have treatment implications if they include clinically significant findings, such as a previously unsuspected mass or lesion.

Minimizing clinical risk and enhancing benefit require vigilance and communication both during the course of the study and for subsequent follow-up. Researchers know the importance of maintaining good relationships with the clinicians who are responsible for patients who enter protocols as well as nursing and other clinical staff who carry out the protocol. Here we emphasize the two-way nature of those interactions: information that may be useful to the clinical group should be provided on an ongoing basis, and, as noted earlier, information regarding study findings, even if not relevant to an individual patient, may be relevant to future clinical work.

WRAPAROUND CARE

What should we do when the study is over? An important question in provision of care to patients who have participated in studies is the extent of the responsibility of the researcher following research participation. There is always some responsibility. When the protocol has involved treatment manipulation or a procedure that could change clinical course, the responsibility appears to us to be greater than when the research involves only assessment and observation. Several options are available for wraparound care, and which one is most appropriate depends on the particular clinical setting, the resources the research protocol makes available, and the clinical needs of the individual patient. Aside from being ethically appropriate behavior on the part of the researcher, attention to wraparound care is politically prudent in terms of relationships to the hospital and community with which researchers need to interact. (See the later section on relationships to the community and hospital for further comments on this aspect of the topic.)

The minimum requirement in our view is attempting to leave the patient at his or her baseline condition or better and to provide an appropriate referral for further clinical care if the patient desires. Ensuring that a patient involved in a research protocol is no worse than when he or she started may require either little or much time depending on both the nature of the study and the person's response to it. Sometimes, despite the best efforts of the clinical researcher, a subject cannot be improved to the baseline state, especially if the subject has a deteriorating illness such as Alzheimer's disease. In some situations the level of clinical care provided in the research setting cannot be matched in a community referral, but the investigator has a clear obligation to provide a referral. The referral should include information about the patient's course and as much information as possible regarding the patient's treatment. If treatment has been blinded so that some treatment information cannot be provided at the time of initial referral, the investigator should provide that information as soon as it becomes available. From the perspective of the relationship to the patient, it is important to prepare for this transition and to avoid rushing the transition. From the point of view of the research, it is valuable to avoid contaminating outcome in the clinical study by raising questions of study termination. Thus, both scientific rigor and clinical concern suggest that the process of termination from clinical care be divorced from the end of a protocol and patients be followed up for a period after a protocol ends even when the goal is transfer to other clinical care.

Some research protocols, particularly studies of investigational drugs, offer subjects the opportunity to receive the investigational medication for some period following participation in double-blind trials. The chance to try a new and hopefully improved treatment can be a powerful motive for research participation. In industry-sponsored trials, restrictions limiting access may include exclusion of subjects whose participation is discontinued because of an adverse effect or before completing the full trial. In our opinion, restricting access only to subjects who complete the full trial period, regardless of the reason for discontinuation, is unfortunate. If the trial includes placebo arms or dosages that may prove less effective, then the subjects who are randomized to treatments that are later determined to be less effective are doubly disadvantaged. First, if they receive a treatment that requires them to be withdrawn from the study early, then the treatment has not been satisfactory. Second, if they withdraw from the study, they are barred from the opportunity to receive a novel and potentially beneficial medication. We recommend that all patients who have contributed to research by participation in such a clinical trial have equal access to postprotocol treatment with the experimental drug.

In the absence of access to an open label trial of medication in conjunction with a research protocol or if that trial is not clinically useful, a further option may be considered: the provision of clinical care using best available treatment according to the clinician-researcher's best judgment until some time-defined or outcome-based endpoint. Examples of outcome-based endpoints include discharge for hospitalized patients or the end of the episode for outpatients. Examples of time-dependent outcomes are a period equal to or longer than the trial duration. Some investigators report that they continue to treat some patients virtually indefinitely following trial participation; we do not recommend this default strategy because the researcher will accrue clinical obligations that are difficult to manage. Rather, a clear endpoint should be defined, negotiated with the patient, and adhered to. We also believe that the sponsors of psychiatric research should recognize a financial obligation to support some elements of care following research participation. The extent of such support depends on the level of risk that the subject incurs in participation.

Another aspect of wraparound care is the application of knowledge gained in an assessment or treatment study to future clinical management. Communication with clinical staff is addressed under the earlier section "Assessment and Diagnosis," but virtually all research produces information of potential value to a patient, including how he or she fared with the experimental or control treatment. This information may not be immediately available when a given subject completes participation. For example, in some treatment studies, the blind is maintained until all data are collected. Given this constraint, the treatment identity should be unblinded at the earliest feasible moment and communicated as a priority to the subject and the involved clinician.

RELATIONSHIPS TO OTHERS

Family Members

If patients who are participating in research agree, it is appropriate and helpful to contact family members to inform them that their relative is participating in research. Family members often become staunch allies in research, recognizing the importance of participation and providing support in adherence to protocol requirements. If the research participant lives or is in frequent contact with the family, relatives may be the first to notice changes in behavior that are important for clinical monitoring and management.

Relating to family members can place the clinician-researcher on the horns of a dilemma that also exists in usual clinical care but is particularly difficult in research. What should we do when the patient refuses permission to contact his or her family? Patients who are competent to provide informed consent have the right to refuse permission to contact their family members. On the other hand, the National Alliance for the Mentally Ill, a family organization, has taken the position that family members have a right to know when a mentally ill family member is participating in research. They argue that if adverse consequences result, family members will likely be the ones who have to cope with problems and that they should have advance notification. It is our view that we cannot violate a patient's right to refuse permission for us to contact his or her family. In our own research with schizophrenia patients, we generally raise the question of contacting family members early in the process of obtaining informed consent. If the patient is adamant about our not contacting the family and protocol participation entails substantial risk, we take this refusal into account in our own judgment regarding the advisability of including the patient as a research subject.

The Community and Hospital

Fostering a successful working relationship with the clinical facilities from which patients are recruited as research subjects is an important aspect of providing clinical care for patients participating in research. Clinicians who refer patients need to be confident that patients will receive appropriate care and that when they return to the clinical facility they may have benefited from research participation or at least have not been harmed.

Providing educational in-service programs in hospitals and other facilities for clinical staff ensures that they are aware of research protocols for which subjects are being recruited. Equally important, parallel presentations after a study is completed should provide feedback regarding the outcome of the study. During a study it may be hard to recognize progress or see any direct benefit. It is therefore very encouraging to learn the outcome—regardless of whether the tested hypothesis was confirmed or rejected. One point to stress is that benefit does not necessarily mean that the study confirmed the tested hypotheses. Learning that a treatment is not useful or that a procedure does not successfully predict outcome is a valuable contribution to clinical science. Providing this information to clinical colleagues represents a benefit to clinicians and therefore indirectly to the patients they serve.

In an earlier section we noted that the treatment of patients after study participation can affect the relations of the research program to the clinical facilities that serve as referral or treatment sites for potential subjects. If researchers are seen as "using" patients and then returning them to the hospital or clinic without benefiting them, clinicians are less likely to be enthusiastic about referring future potential research subjects. The strategies discussed previously for wraparound care are the reflection on a case-by-case basis of the structural relationship to clinical facilities or clinicians.

CONCLUSION

Clinical research generally moves some aspect of care from the realm of clinician's best judgment to a protocol-mandated prescription. This situation may produce tension between research and clinical care. We have described several models for managing this tension and a few approaches to balancing the research agenda with the priority of quality clinical care. The suggestions are derived primarily from our own clinical research experience and emphasize the need for close communication among subjects, research personnel, clinical personnel, and other interested parties before, during, and after protocol execution.

SUGGESTED READINGS

This chapter represents our opinions and suggested strategies for successfully managing clinical care in the context of research. We found it difficult to provide citations for specific points that are made throughout the chapter. Rather, we list here a number of articles, some old and some quite recent, that we have read and that have influenced our thinking. We include articles by both authors with whom we agree and others whose perspectives do not accord with our own. Obviously, none of the authors should be taken to task for the use, understanding, or misunderstanding that we have of their views.

Beecher HK: Some guiding principles for clinical investigation. JAMA 195:1135–1136, 1966

Brody BA: Ethical Issues in Drug Testing, Approval, and Pricing: The Clot-Dissolving Drugs. New York, Oxford University Press, 1995

Carpenter WT Jr, Schooler NR, Kane JM: The rationale and ethics of medication-free research in schizophrenia. Arch Gen Psychiatry 54:401–407, 1997

de Groot JM, Kennedy SH: Integrating clinical and research psychiatry. J Psychiatry Neurosci 20:150–154, 1995

Freedman B: Equipoise and the ethics of clinical research. N Engl J Med 317:141–145, 1987

Gallant D, Krinsky SL: Ethical and legal considerations in drug trials, in Clinical Evaluation of Psychotropic Drugs: Principles and Guidelines. Edited by Prien RF, Robinson DS. New York, Raven, 1994, pp 261–280

Garfinkel PE, Goldbloom DS, Kaplan AS, et al: The clinician-investigator interface in psychiatry, I: values and problems. Can J Psychiatry 34:361–363, 1989

Garfinkel PE, Kennedy SH, Kaplan AS, et al: The clinician-investigator interface in psychiatry, II: the role of the clinical investigation unit. Can J Psychiatry 34:364–368, 1989

Huth EJ: Conflicts of interest in industry-sponsored clinical research, in Conflicts of Interest in Clinical Practice and Research. Edited by Spece RG Jr, Shimm DS, Buchanan AE. New York, Oxford University Press, 1996, pp 389–406

Lieberman JA: Ethical dilemmas in clinical research with human subjects: an investigator's perspective. Psychopharmacol Bull 32:19–25, 1996

Rothman DJ: Ethics and human experimentation. Henry Beecher revisited. N Engl J Med 317:1195–1199, 1987

Shimm DS, Spece RG Jr, DiGregorio MB: Conflicts of interest in relationships between physicians and the pharmaceutical industry, in Conflicts of Interest in Clinical Practice and Research. Edited by Spece RG Jr, Shimm DS, Buchanan AE. New York, Oxford University Press, 1996, pp 321–357

Taylor KM, Kellner M: Interpreting physician participation in randomized clinical trials: the physician orientation profile. J Health Soc Behav 28:389–400, 1987

CHAPTER 4

Subjects' Capacity to Consent to Neurobiological Research

Jessica Wilen Berg, J.D., and Paul S. Appelbaum, M.D.

Persons' capacity to make health care decisions has become a popular topic of discussion among physicians, lawyers, philosophers, and researchers. The increased interest in capacity was prompted by changes in informed consent law over the last 40 years. Historically, physicians rarely sought informed consent from patients and frequently disclosed to patients neither the nature of their disorder nor the intended course of treatment. Thus patients' capacity to make health care decisions was usually unimportant. In fact, the previously common decision-making model stemmed from the idea that all patients were per se incompetent to make medical decisions (because they lacked medical training) and therefore such choices should be left to experts (i.e., medical professionals).

One of the first American cases to speak of a consent requirement rejected the notion that patients should not be allowed control over their medical care and noted that "every human being of adult years and sound mind has a right to determine what shall be done with his body" (*Schloendorff v. Society of New York Hospital* 1914). The case emphasized the concept of voluntary consent; that is, the patient must freely give permission for a specific procedure to occur. Although a person not of "sound mind" was presumed unable to consent, most cases during this period focused simply on whether the patient did or did not consent, regardless of the competence of that consent. The current view of informed consent in this country began with a trio of cases in the late 1950s and early 1960s. The first of these, *Salgo v. Leland Stanford Junior University Board of Trustees* (1957), coined the term *informed consent* and held not only that patients must freely consent but also that they must be fully informed by practitioners about treatment options. It was this information requirement that prompted increased scrutiny of patient capacity—if a patient is not able to understand the information disclosed, he or she should not be considered competent to consent.

Today valid informed consent requires that a patient be given sufficient relevant facts; be free from coercion, undue influence, and unfair manipulation; and be competent to make a decision. *Competence* is used here to mean that individuals have sufficient cognitive capacities to reach decisions in a rational fashion.[1] This element of a valid consent derives from the view that some minimal degree of rationality in decision making is required if individual interests are to be protected; otherwise, decisions with regard to the interests of the person essentially will be random. Thus competence, like the other informed consent requirements, is linked to autonomy—a competent person is one who is able to make decisions autonomously, or in accordance with his or her preferences (Morreim 1991). This element of informed consent is our focus.

About the same time as the legal doctrine of informed consent to medical treatment was evolving, the doctrine of informed consent to research (prompted by the Nuremberg Code) gained attention. Historical abuses in medical experimentation (e.g., Nazi experiments during World War II, the Tuskegee syphilis experiments, and the Willowbrook hepatitis experiments) resulted in the promulgation of a series of ethical codes constraining biomedical research. Inspired by concern that human subjects not be misused, federal regulations and common law have combined to ensure that informed consent requirements are fully applicable to research (Appelbaum et al. 1987a; Department of Health and Human Services 1991; National Commission 1978). According to the current guidelines of the Department of Health and Human Services, "no investigator may involve a human being as a subject in research . . . unless the investigator has obtained the legally effective consent of the subject or the subject's legally authorized representative" (§46.116). Although the regulations set forth specific disclosure requirements, as well as additional protections for vulnerable populations to ensure voluntary consent, they do not address the requirements for subject capacity. Moreover, cases and statutes that articulate standards of decision-making competence (all of them in the treatment arena) often lack sufficient explanation of both the terms used (such as *rationality*) and the mechanisms for applying the standards (Berg et al. 1996). As a result, investigators have had little guidance in regard to assessments of the decision-making competence of potential research subjects (Appelbaum 1997).

In this chapter we set forth a framework for thinking about the capacities

---

[1]It is important to note that *competence* is a legal construct—in most jurisdictions only a court can decide whether a person is incompetent. Assessments of *capacity,* on the other hand, are left in the hands of medical or mental health professionals. We use the terms interchangeably, and unless otherwise specified, we are referring to clinical assessments of capacity, not legal determinations of competence.

involved in medical decision making, including decisions about research participation. Using this framework, we then examine empirical studies relating to the capacity of subjects to consent to neurobiological research and the implications of these studies for policy-related questions. Finally, we provide practical guidance for investigators engaged in research that involves cognitively impaired subjects.

CAPACITY TO CONSENT TO RESEARCH

Issues related to competence present particular problems for neurobiological researchers (Shamoo and Irving 1993). Many of the target subjects of such research have disorders that impair the very cognitive faculties on which they must rely to decide whether to participate in research. Concerns about capacity thus arise in several subject populations, including persons with mental illness (Elliott 1997); AIDS patients (Marks et al. 1992); elderly persons (Cassel 1988), especially those with dementia such as Alzheimer's disease (High et al. 1994); people with organic brain damage; and people with substance abuse problems. The National Institute of Mental Health's Epidemiologic Catchment Area (ECA) study estimates that during the course of 1 year 2.7% of the adult population (or 4,293,000 people) has severe cognitive impairments (Regier et al. 1993). These disorders may render some proportion of potential subjects incompetent to consent to research, requiring that they not be entered into studies (even if they appear to be agreeing to participate) or that alternative mechanisms for authorizing their participation be developed (Berg 1996). To evaluate the capacity of these and other potential subjects to consent to research, standards of competence must be established.

The following discussion draws on standards of competence articulated in legal, medical, psychological, and ethical literature related to patient capacity to make treatment decisions. Several reasons are cited for applying the standards developed for competence to consent to treatment to decision making related to research. First, many research projects involve administration of treatment; in such cases, the tasks of deciding about treatment acceptance and research participation are intertwined. Second, the legal standards elaborated for competence to consent to treatment are closely related to standards for other decision-making tasks, such as making contracts (White and Denise 1991), writing wills, giving gifts, and even making decisions related to criminal defense (Bonnie 1993). Third, when we turn from the legal literature to medical, psychological, and bioethical writings, we find a similar approach: commentators do not distinguish between competence to consent to treatment and competence to consent to research (Appelbaum and Roth 1982). Although the types of information that the physician and the investigator must disclose may differ, and different procedures may be necessary to avoid infringing on persons' voluntary choice, the capacities needed to make a meaningful decision are much the same.

Standards for Determining Decision-Making Competence

Drawing on earlier work by Roth et al. (1977; Appelbaum and Roth 1982), Drs. Paul Appelbaum and Thomas Grisso have developed a framework of four standards that can stand alone or serve as components of an overall standard of competence: 1) ability to communicate a choice, 2) ability to understand relevant information, 3) ability to appreciate the nature of the situation and its likely consequences, and 4) ability to manipulate information rationally (Appelbaum and Grisso 1988). These standards are reflected in, and in fact drawn from, the law (Berg et al. 1996). Moreover, many commentators evince general agreement about the standards, although they may disagree about which standard should be applied in a specific situation (Berg et al. 1996). Each of the four elements is discussed in more detail in the following section.

Ability to communicate a choice is the least stringent standard applied by courts and legislatures. Potential subjects fail this test because of inability to either reach a decision (i.e., a patient simply cannot make up his or her mind or vacillates to such a degree that it is impossible to implement a choice) or effectively make known their wishes regarding research. Many courts use this standard as a threshold determination of competence, on the assumption that a person who cannot reach a decision or make that decision known to the outside world ought not to be afforded the power to guide his or her own affairs. Although ability to communicate a choice may be a necessary component of competence, it is not in itself sufficient: a person who can communicate a choice does not necessarily have the capacity to make a choice autonomously. Thus, many courts and commentators combine this standard with one or more of the others. Comatose, mute catatonic, or severely depressed persons, individuals with manic or catatonic excitements, and persons with severe psychotic thought disorders or severe dementia fall into this category.

> Ms. A has chronic undifferentiated schizophrenia. When she initially is approached regarding participation in a new protocol designed to test the effect of her present medication on eating habits, she is enthusiastic. She appears to understand all of the implications of the study and consents to participation. Later that day, when the research assistant approaches Ms. A, she refuses to participate. Over the course of the next few days Ms. A repeatedly alternates

between agreeing and refusing to participate. Because Ms. A is unable to make up her mind for a period of time long enough to allow the research to proceed, she should not be included in the study.

Mr. B has been admitted to a hospital for an acute psychotic episode. Unfortunately, the level of medication necessary to control his symptoms leaves him almost completely sedated. If the dose of medication is lowered, however, he rapidly reverts to a severe state of psychotic disorganization and disorientation. In neither his unmedicated psychotic nor his sedated state is Mr. B able to interact with people. Because he cannot communicate, he does not have the capacity to consent to research participation at this time.

The second and most common standard—*ability to understand relevant information*—focuses on the patient's comprehension of information related to the decision at hand. *Understanding,* in this sense, is defined simply as the ability to comprehend the concepts involved in the informed consent disclosure; it does not necessarily include the ability to relate that information to the situation at hand. Thus a person may understand the information, but unless he or she can retain the information long enough for a decision to be made, he or she is not competent to consent. Impairments of intelligence, attention, and memory, whether due to organic or functional disorders, can affect this ability.

Mr. C has Wernicke-Korsakoff syndrome. Although he is able to take care of his daily needs, his short-term memory is almost nonexistent. When approached by a research assistant regarding participation in a long-term protocol, Mr. C appears to understand and is at first eager to help. However, after the research assistant has completed the informed consent disclosure, Mr. C has no recollection of anything that has been explained to him. A few minutes later, he does not even remember meeting the research assistant. Mr. C does not have the capacity to consent.

Ms. D is severely mentally retarded and lives in an institution. She can communicate with her caretaker on a rudimentary level but is unable to engage in higher-level discourse. When asked to do something that she does not like, she becomes agitated and resistant. Ms. D is approached by a graduate student at the institution and asked to participate in a study of behavioral reinforcements that would involve restricting her usual access to food. She indicates her understanding of the graduate student's instructions by her compliance with them. When the student attempts to assess her understanding of the experiment, however, Ms. D demonstrates no comprehension of the research. Thus, despite her compliance with the graduate student's instructions, Ms. D does not have the capacity to consent.

Ms. E is in the midst of an acute manic episode. She is constantly active, and her attention span usually lasts no more than a minute. A research assistant has tried a number of times to explain what is involved in a particular protocol. Each time, Ms. E interrupts any explanation within a couple of minutes, saying that she is willing to do whatever the doctor wants and then immediately launches into a monologue on a different subject. Ms. E does not have the capacity to consent.

The third standard, *ability to appreciate the nature of the situation and its likely consequences,* requires that the subject be able to apply abstractly understood information to his or her own situation. Therefore, this standard is often combined with an understanding requirement. Persons who understand that their physician believes they are ill but in the face of evidence that would persuade a reasonable person deny that this is so would not meet this standard. Denial (often called "lack of insight"), delusions, and psychotic levels of distortion can impair appreciation of the nature of the situation.

Mr. F has paranoid schizophrenia. He is college educated, well-read, and extremely intelligent. When approached by a research assistant regarding participation in a protocol, he is able to comprehend all of the information regarding the study, including the scientific basis for the experiment. He explains to the assistant that he knows that the physicians in the hospital are planning to kill him and that the research assistant is a covert agent sent to secret him away under cover of the research. Mr. F does not have the capacity to consent.

The fourth and final standard is the *ability to manipulate information rationally.* It focuses on reasoning capacity and addresses a person's ability to employ logical thought processes to compare the risks and benefits of treatment options. This standard does not look at the outcome of a decision but, like the understanding and appreciation elements, is concerned with the decision-making process. Thus, a person who can understand, appreciate, and communicate a decision may still be impaired if he or she is unable to process information logically, in accordance with his or her preferences. Conversely, a person may employ logical thought processes but base them on impaired understanding or appreciation.

Ms. G is 84 years old and has multi-infarct dementia. She is asked to participate in a drug trial for a new medication that may slow the progress of her disease. She is told that the study has a small chance (20%) of benefiting her personally, but given the advanced state of her vascular disease it probably will not increase her predicted life span. She tells the research assistant that she is very excited about this protocol because the 20% potential for benefit is much better than the 80% probability of no benefit that was explained to her with respect to a previous drug protocol. When the assistant questions this reasoning, he discovers that Ms. G lacks the ability to compare the risks and benefits of different alternatives. Because of this deficit in probabilistic reasoning skills, Ms. G may not have the capacity to consent. Efforts will now be made to teach her about relative risks, after which her reasoning ability will be retested.

Mr. H, who has AIDS-related dementia, is approached by a research assistant regarding participation in a drug trial. The protocol involves almost no chance of direct therapeutic benefit and a moderate degree of risk, and it requires the subject to remain at the study site for the duration of the experiment (6 weeks). Mr. H has made it clear throughout his illness that he would like to move to a home care situation. Moreover, he has stated more than once that he has accepted that there is nothing that can be done to cure his illness and thus he would rather spend what time he has left with his family. When he consents to participate in the study, his primary care physician is concerned that the reasoning behind his choice is not consistent with his expressed desire to go home. Further inquiry is required regarding the basis for his choice and his ability to consent to research participation.

Empirical Studies of Decision-Making Capacity

Several empirical studies have examined how well persons perform on these standards of decision-making competence. Most of the findings on decision-making performance are from studies of consent to treatment, not consent to research (Appelbaum and Grisso 1995). However, these findings have important implications for research decision making. For example, the recent MacArthur Treatment Competence Study compared the capacity to make treatment decisions of newly hospitalized patients with schizophrenia, major depression, and angina pectoris with the capacity of community control subjects matched for age, gender, race, education, and occupation (Appelbaum and Grisso 1995; Grisso and Appelbaum 1995; Grisso et al. 1995). Because the study looked at both patients hospitalized with mental illness and patients hospitalized with medical illness,[2] it enabled the investigators to examine the effect of mental illness per se (as opposed to the undifferentiated effects of hospitalization) on decision-making abilities. Moreover, the researchers were able to draw conclusions about the decision-making capacity of medically ill persons, and this

---

[2] Mental illnesses are medical illnesses, but for clarification we separate the two here.

information can be used as a standard against which to examine decision making by impaired populations. If subjects who have illnesses that commonly result in cognitive impairments do no worse on measures of decision-making capacity than medically ill subjects, there is less need for investigators to implement special precautions when engaging in research with these groups. This finding does not, of course, mean that no protections should be instituted. If subjects in general (regardless of type of illness) show impairments of decision-making capacity, a prudent researcher should take steps to ensure that competent decision making occurs.

Neurobiological researchers are likely to be most concerned about the abilities of subjects who have disorders that make them candidates for research participation but whose illnesses often result in cognitive impairment. It is these groups—for example, persons with mental illness and elderly persons (especially those with some form of dementia)—on whom we focus here. Although researchers have undertaken numerous studies on the neuropsychological performance of substance abusers, and on the effects of alcohol-induced impairment, we could find no empirical studies of the capacity of substance abusers to consent to research participation or to make treatment decisions. Nevertheless, a recent paper by the College on Problems of Drug Dependence (1995) expressed concern about the capacity of substance abusers to assess objectively the risks inherent in research. Similarly, Kleber (1989) noted that drug use can affect subject comprehension and lead individuals to overestimate their ability to deal with the experimental procedure; Kleber concluded that informed consent should therefore be acquired only when the investigator is certain that the subject is no longer intoxicated. Because of the lack of empirical studies involving this population, we focus primarily on data from elderly and psychiatric populations, bearing in mind that substance abusers probably present many of the same issues. Indeed, the high incidence of HIV and mental illness in this population may result in an even greater percentage of cognitively impaired subjects than in elderly and psychiatric populations.

Individuals who fail to meet the first standard (communication) are the least problematic from the perspective of neurobiological researchers: potential subjects' inability to offer consent will be evident and consent will be sought elsewhere or subjects will be excluded from the study. Thus, here we address only potential subjects' ability to understand, appreciate, and reason.

Understanding

Although a number of studies have explored psychiatric subjects' ability to consent to research, many of the early investigations neglected to ascertain whether the appropriate information had been communicated to subjects (Riecken and Ravich 1982). Thus, it is difficult to know whether poor performance was a result of cognitive deficits or inadequate disclosure. Not all studies have suffered from this flaw, however, and those that examined understanding after controlled information disclosure found that significant numbers of individuals with cognitive impairments had substantial difficulty understanding disclosed information. For example, the MacArthur study examined hospitalized angina patients' understanding of 1) the nature of the disorder, 2) the nature of the treatment being recommended, 3) the probable benefits of the treatment, 4) the probable risks and discomforts of the treatment, and 5) the relevant benefits and risks of an alternative treatment; researchers then compared angina patients' understanding with that of schizophrenia patients and community control subjects. Subjects with schizophrenia did significantly worse than subjects with angina or community control subjects when tested on a measure of understanding: 28% fell in the impaired range compared with 7.4% of angina patients and 2.4% of control subjects. (Impaired subjects were defined as those who, after comparison with everyone else, scored in the bottom 5% of the distribution of scores for the total study sample.) Depressed subjects, on the other hand, performed no differently than medically ill subjects or non-ill control subjects (5.4% scored in the impaired range).

Two studies by Loren Roth and his colleagues in the early 1980s examined psychiatric patients' decision making in the research rather than treatment context. In the first study, 41 patients with affective disorders (of whom only 5 were psychotic) were asked to participate in a study of their electroencephalogram patterns during sleep (Roth et al. 1982). Approximately one-quarter of the subjects understood half or less of the disclosed information, and a mere 5% understood 87% or more of the information. Of the 19 subjects whose consent discussions were videotaped, 4 were rated as probably incompetent by independent judges. The second study (Benson et al. 1988) examined the understanding of 88 psychiatric patients recruited to participate in four research projects. Data analysis revealed that

> while prospective research subjects generally demonstrated good understanding of the purpose of the written consent form and their right to refuse or withdraw from the study . . . they frequently did not understand the psychiatric research project's purpose, or why they had been asked to participate in it. Subjects also often demonstrated poor understanding of important methodological aspects of the study, including the randomized and double-blind treatment assignment. (p. 469)

These findings suggest that how well we rate the ability of psychiatric patients to understand information in research settings depends on what types of information we consider it important for them to comprehend. The Roth et al. study also found that patients with schizophrenia and those with high levels of psychopathology (measured by the Brief Psychiatric Rating Scale [Overall and Gorham 1962]) performed more poorly than patients with borderline personality disorder and subjects who were generally less impaired.

Studies of elderly subjects have shown similar difficulties in understanding. Fitten and Waite's 1990 study of decision-making capacity in elderly persons found that while healthy elderly individuals showed little or no impairment of understanding ability, hospitalized medically ill patients (who were neurologically and psychiatrically intact) "failed to substantially understand key issues in treatment despite language and form simplification of consent documents" (p. 1720). Stanley and colleagues (1984) used a series of hypothetical research studies to assess the capacity of medical patients to consent to research. They found that elderly patients demonstrated poorer comprehension of consent information than younger patients. These findings are consistent with studies of understanding in treatment settings in which elderly patients were less able to remember information and less able to understand consent forms (Stanley et al. 1988).

These deficiencies in understanding, however, may be remedied. For example, a study testing the effect of different disclosure formats on the understanding and reasoning capacity of elderly residents in a long-term care facility found that comprehension was significantly better when the information was presented in a simplified or storybook format (Tymchuk et al. 1988). A more serious problem is the high incidence of dementia in this subject population, which may result in permanent impairment of decision-making capacity (Speer 1990). One estimate suggests that approximately 6% of individuals over age 65 have severe dementia, and an additional 10%–15% have mild to moderate cognitive impairment (Cummings and Benson 1992). Another study has estimated that the incidence of Alzheimer's disease in persons over age 65 is 10% (Evans et al. 1989).

A study by Sachs et al. (1994) examined the willingness of persons with dementia to participate in four hypothetical research protocols. Interviewers judged subject capacity based on subjective evaluation of the consistency and quality of responses related to why subjects would or would not participate. They found that persons with dementia were less able than the well elderly to give cogent reasons for their decisions and were less able to identify specific risks and benefits. Preliminary results in another study of treatment decision making by patients with Alzheimer's disease showed that elderly control subjects without Alzheimer's disease performed significantly better than both mild and moderate Alzheimer's disease patients on measures of understanding (Marson et al. 1994). Moreover, the mildly ill patients performed significantly better than the moderately ill group, providing support for the notion that greater severity of illness leads to greater impairment in decision-making capacity.

Appreciation

The ability to appreciate the nature of a situation and its likely consequences has been the subject of extensive exploration in psychiatric populations because of its close connection to core symptoms of mental disorders. Diminished ability to appreciate that one is ill has been found to be the key diagnostic feature of schizophrenia in two multinational studies (Carpenter et al. 1976; Wilson et al. 1986). In addition, patients with schizophrenia or severe depression may be impaired in their ability to appreciate the potential value of treatment. The MacArthur Treatment Competence Study found that subjects with schizophrenia were more likely to deny completely the presence of illness than were depressed patients (35% versus 4%), although similar proportions of both groups denied the potential for effective treatment (13% versus 14%). On a composite measure of appreciation of the presence of illness and the potential for treatment, a total of 22.6% of subjects with schizophrenia scored in the impaired decision-making range compared with 11.9% of depressed subjects and 4.8% of angina subjects. (This measure was not administered to non-ill control subjects.)

Appreciation problems have been clearly demonstrated in connection with consent to research. Potential subjects with psychiatric disorders often fail to appreciate the nature of the research and its potential impact on their treatment. One recurring problem is the prevalence of therapeutic misconception (Appelbaum et al. 1987b). A study of psychiatric patients found that many of them misconstrued the nature of the research they were involved in and erroneously believed that they would be receiving the treatment their doctors thought was best for their condition (Appelbaum et al. 1982). More specifically, the study found that schizophrenic and depressed subjects involved in a double-blind experiment were unaware that they would be assigned randomly to different drug regimens and that the researchers would not know which drug they were taking. Therapeutic misconception is not limited to psychiatric patients, however. A study of patients undergoing randomized clinical trials for the treatment of cancer found that a significant number had difficulty distinguishing between the treatment and research components of the protocol and more than half failed to understand an explicit explanation of randomization (Simes et al. 1986).

Sachs et al. (1994) noted that the inability of most dementia patients to recognize that they have a memory problem provides one explanation for why such individuals fail most competence standards. The Marson et al. study (1994, p. 13) that examined treatment decision making of Alzheimer's disease patients specifically looked at patients' "capacity to 'appreciate' the emotional and cognitive consequences of a choice." Consistent with the study by Sachs et al., this study found that patients with mild Alzheimer's disease performed significantly better than patients with moderate Alzheimer's disease, and control subjects without Alzheimer's disease performed better than both groups of ill patients.

Reasoning

Few studies of persons' ability to manipulate information rationally have been undertaken, and they often rely on paradigms that bear little resemblance to decision making in clinical or research contexts. For example, one study employed a gambling paradigm to measure the ability of patients with schizophrenia to weigh risks, benefits, and probabilities in an internally consistent manner (Rosenfeld et al. 1992). The study found that involuntarily committed inpatients with chronic schizophrenia were significantly less able to consistently weigh risks, benefits, and probabilities than chronic schizophrenia outpatients and nonpatient family control subjects.

The MacArthur Treatment Competence Study examined the degree to which subjects demonstrated an ability to 1) seek information, 2) consider the consequences of treatment alternatives, 3) compare two treatment alternatives, 4) consider a number of treatment alternatives at one time, 5) generate potential real-life consequences of the disclosed risks or discomforts of the treatment, 6) consistently apply personal preferences, 7) make logical inferences about ordinal relationships (i.e., A > B, B > C, choose the largest), and 8) distinguish correctly the relative values of numerical probabilities. The study found that subjects with schizophrenia or severe depression performed significantly worse than angina subjects and community control subjects. In percentage terms, 24% of schizophrenic subjects, 7.6% of depressed subjects, 0% of angina subjects, and 2% of control subjects fell into the impaired range. Impaired performance by schizophrenia patients on this and other measures of capacity (understanding and appreciation) was positively correlated with conceptual disorganization, unusual or delusional thought content, and, to a lesser extent, hallucinations.

If one takes decision outcome as a proxy for rationality of decision process, three studies of research decision making by Barbara Stanley and colleagues also are relevant here. Looking at a group of psychiatric patients with mixed diagnoses who were asked whether they would participate in hypothetical research projects, Stanley et al. (1982) found that 40% of acutely hospitalized patients said they would agree to take part in high-risk/low-benefit projects, whereas up to 32% refused low-risk/high-benefit participation. Although this finding suggests poor performance in the weighing of risks and benefits, a similar study that compared psychiatric and medical inpatients found no difference between the groups in willingness to participate in studies of either high or low risk (Stanley et al. 1981). Decision outcome is thus probably not a very good proxy for reasoning ability. Stanley et al. (1984) also found that although a significantly greater proportion of elderly than younger patients agreed to participate in a high-risk/low-benefit study, there was no overall difference in the quality of reasoning of elderly and younger medical patients. Although their age may not pose a problem per se, elderly patients who have dementia may demonstrate greater impairment of reasoning ability. For example, Marson et al. (1994) found that subjects with either mild or moderate Alzheimer's disease performed significantly worse than non-ill control subjects on a test of rational thinking (with the mild group performing better than the moderate group).

GUIDANCE FOR POLICY MAKERS

What are the implications of these findings for research involving subjects with cognitive impairments? First, although specific concerns can be identified, broad generalizations should be avoided. It cannot reasonably be maintained that psychiatric patients or elderly patients as a class are incompetent to offer (or refuse) their informed consent for participation in research. Many of these people, perhaps most, retain decision-making abilities indistinguishable from those found in the general population. However, it cannot be argued that decisional incompetence is simply not a problem among these populations. On the contrary, substantial impairment is not uncommon. Thus, researchers need to be especially sensitive to the possible difficulties in obtaining informed consent from people with severe mental illness, elderly persons (especially those with some form of dementia), and people with substance abuse problems.

Second, because cognitive impairment varies in degree, problems may range from mild difficulties in understanding consent documents to severe incapacity rendering the subject incompetent to make any research decision. Although diagnosis cannot generally be used as a means of classifying incompetent subjects, different groups of cognitively impaired subjects may present different issues for investigators. Many people with mental illness (and substance abusers), for example, have intermittent periods of increased capacity. As a result, although certain types of experimentation may be impermissible at one time, they may be possible at another, either when the individual is competent to give his or her own consent or through the use of advance directives or instructions to a proxy in anticipation of later relapse. Other people, such as those with Alzheimer's disease or AIDS, are likely to become more impaired as the research progresses. Therefore, it is important to discuss all aspects of the research (including future involvement) with the subject during the early stages of the illness.

> Mr. I is a long-time substance abuser. He has been drug free for 2 months. However, in the past he has failed to remain drug free for long periods of time. He has recently started using phencyclidine (PCP) again when he is approached by a research assistant, who is unaware that Mr. I is no longer drug free. Although Mr. I consents to participate in the research, over the next few days the assistant notices that the subject's behavior becomes increasingly erratic and that he has developed delusions about the research project. Mr. I no longer has the capacity to consent and should not be included in the protocol. A few weeks later, at the urging of his wife, Mr. I is back in treatment and again drug free. At this time he may be asked again to consent to research participation.

> Ms. J has recently discovered that she has Alzheimer's disease. Except for minor lapses in memory, she has not yet begun to show signs of the illness. Her physician asks her whether she would be interested in taking part in a long-term research protocol studying the progression of her illness. She indicates her willingness and includes her newly appointed proxy decision maker in the discussions regarding research participation. She makes it clear that the proxy is authorized to consent to her continued participation in the protocol even after she becomes incapacitated.

How, then, should policy makers react to the current concern that incompetent patients may be consenting to research participation in violation of the principles of informed consent and to their personal detriment? Whatever action is taken should be sensitive to the balance of interests involved. Protection of the rights and well-being of potential subjects is of great importance. So, too, however, is the advancement of knowledge of disorders affecting the brain. As we guard patients' rights and interests, the burden of additional protections on the conduct of research must also be taken into account. The real issue is not whether we can add enough safeguards (because another safeguard can usually be added) but rather whether the additional protection it provides is worth the potential negative impact on the advance of knowledge. In the end, we seek to achieve a balance between the need for new scientific knowledge to advance medical treatment and the protection of individual autonomy (Candilis et al. 1993).

With this issue in mind, we need to address problems related to competence to consent to research in these areas. First, we need a more precise formulation of the degree of capacity required for competent consent to research. Second, we need a means of identifying persons who may lack the requisite capacities. Third, we must develop approaches to compensate for decision-making impairment among potential research subjects, including mechanisms for more easily obtaining substituted consent when appropriate. Each of these problems is considered in the following sections.

Capacities Necessary

A standard for competence to make research decisions should result in the optimum proportions of people being correctly identified as competent and incompetent. That is, we should be as concerned about incorrectly labeling autonomous agents as incompetent as we are about labeling nonautonomous agents as competent. We must take into account a number of aspects of formulating a standard. Initially, the choice of components is important, because different standards may result in different people and different numbers of people being identified as impaired. Assuming, for our purposes, that all four components described previously (communication, understanding, appreciation, and reasoning) should be included in a standard of competence (Berg et al. 1996), the question remains where the cutoff points should be. That is, below what level of performance should we say that a person is not competent to give or withhold consent? This consideration breaks down into two issues. First, in addition to deciding to apply an understanding standard, we must also establish how much understanding is necessary in a quantitative sense: Is it sufficient if a subject manifests understanding of only 50% of the disclosed information, or must a subject understand 95% of what he or she is told? Second, the necessary aspects of performance must be identified. For example, a subject may understand that the research in question will involve a comparison between people who actually get the experimental medium and control subjects who will get a placebo but fail to grasp that assignment to a group is random. Is understanding of both pieces of information necessary?

Demanding total comprehension and appreciation, along with high-level reasoning abilities, from subjects with cognitive impairments is unrealistic because most members of the general population would fail such tests. Comparisons with nonpatient groups, suitably matched, might provide a statistical basis for identifying levels of performance that fall so far below the general norm as to justify calling a person incompetent, but this approach, too, is likely to be unsatisfactory. A rigid cutoff of this sort fails to take into account the possibility, for example, that different levels of capacity may be required depending on the nature of the research project to which consent is being sought. Thus, instead of using a fixed level of competence, a sliding scale could be applied (Drane 1984; President's Commission 1982). This scale would allow competence determinations to take into account the features of the subject's situation, which many commentators believe is desirable. For example, a subject would be required to demonstrate both understanding and appreciation for all treatment decisions, but the level of understanding or appreciation required might vary depending on the specific context. A subject who showed minor impairments on the competence measures might be competent to make simple research decisions, but those same impairments would be of greater concern if the research decision involved more complex elements. Relevant factors to consider might include the complexity of the research protocol, the amount of risk entailed, and the potential for direct therapeutic benefit. For minimal risk research, unless substantial direct therapeutic benefit is possible, it may be reasonable to allow persons to make their own decisions, even in the face of considerable impairment, knowing that adverse consequences are unlikely to ensue whichever way they decide. As the risks of either participating or not participating rise, however, more demanding levels of capacity may be required (Berg 1996).

Mr. K is in his mid-50s and has mild dementia following a stroke. He is asked to participate in a study of lifestyle changes of early-onset stroke victims. After explaining how the study will be run and indicating that it involves little or no risk and has no potential for direct therapeutic benefit, the research assistant asks Mr. K whether he has any questions. Mr. K demonstrates comprehension of most of the information imparted (approximately 70%) and indicates that he is aware that he will derive no direct therapeutic benefit from the study. He is unclear, however, about why researchers would want to include him because he did not have a stroke. Nevertheless, he is willing to participate because he feels that medical research is important. Although Mr. K demonstrates somewhat impaired appreciation (he does not deny the symptoms of his dementia—including loss of memory and increased difficulty in understanding—just their origin), he probably has the capacity to participate in this low-risk study.

A few weeks later another investigator, hearing about Mr. K's willingness to participate in research, approaches him to ask whether he would be willing to participate in a drug trial. This protocol involves a significant degree of risk but also has a potential for direct therapeutic benefit. Mr. K's failure of appreciation may be of more concern here. If he cannot appreciate the potential therapeutic benefit (because he denies the stroke), he may lack the capacity to consent (because he cannot weigh the risks and benefits of participation). Moreover, Mr. K's difficulties in understanding are also a problem because this protocol involves higher risk.

As noted previously, reliance on quantitative data alone (e.g., how much the subject understands) to determine who lacks competence may be inappropriate, because certain aspects of understanding, appreciation, and rational manipulation may be so crucial to competent consent that we would not feel comfortable allowing a person to make a decision in their absence. A patient who scores above the cutoff point for impairment on a given measure (because he or she does not score in the lower range of the score distribution when compared with the rest of the population) arguably still should be considered incompetent if he or she is incapable of demonstrating a particular capacity that is essential for competent decision making. For example, a subject who is asked to enter a research protocol and understands the procedure in which he or she is asked to participate but fails to understand the distinction between ordinary treatment and research probably should be considered incompetent to consent to participate in the experiment.

To date, resolution of these issues has been left to the decentralized mechanisms we have developed for overseeing research. Institutional review boards (IRBs) may ask investigators to provide assurance that incompetent subjects will be excluded from participation, but they rarely (if ever) have specified how to define that population. Moreover, investigators themselves may be untutored in the nuances of assessing competence, and they usually leave recruitment of subjects in the hands of research assistants. As a result, practices vary widely across research projects. Our inability to say definitively what level of capacity is required in any project makes it difficult to supervise investigators and unfair to criticize them for not following standards that may be formulated only after the fact. Were general standards developed, they would have to be flexible enough to allow application to a wide variety of research projects with very different patient populations. Although difficult, the task should not be impossible. Important considerations include which of the four components (communication, understanding, appreciation, or reasoning) should be made part of a standard of competence, what level of ability a subject must demonstrate to meet the standard, and to what the standard should be applied.

Identifying Impairments

Once clear criteria exist for determining whether potential subjects are competent to consent to research, it is necessary to develop means to identify persons who may lack the requisite capacities. The creation of generally agreed-upon criteria would permit the development of screening mechanisms to identify subjects at risk for incompetence. These screening methods might be based on clinical judgment, measures of psychopathology or dementia correlated with significant impairment (Berg et al. 1996; Schachter et al. 1994; Stanley et al.

1985), or tests aimed at consent-related abilities per se. For example, Appelbaum and Grisso are testing a condensed version of the MacArthur competence assessment instruments for possible use in a research setting. Once reliable indicators of capacity are identified or developed, special training in the use of assessment instruments may be required for those engaged in subject recruitment. In some cases the assessment may be done by research assistants or clinicians, who are ordinarily involved in obtaining informed consent. In other cases, consent specialists who are trained to screen and obtain consent in different settings may be needed. Given the economic and time constraints of many protocols, a screening mechanism for research participation ideally should be easily administered (e.g., by research assistants) and adaptable to a number of different research projects.

Whether a screening mechanism should be used routinely to assess subjects' decision-making capacities depends on the cost of applying the procedure to the target population balanced against the benefit of identifying incompetent decision makers (assuming the screening mechanism is effective—that is, it appropriately identifies impaired or incompetent subjects). Three factors are crucial here: first, the cost of the screening depends on the method used; second, the degree of benefit depends on the prevalence of incapacity in the population, or the base rate; and third, benefits also depend on the extent of harm avoided.

For the general population, competence screening is probably unwarranted because the incidence of incapacity is relatively low. Thus, the likelihood that an incompetent person will be allowed to make a decision is correspondingly low. This likelihood is much higher, however, in populations with schizophrenia or Alzheimer's disease. Even for these groups, competence screening may not be economically feasible except for more severely ill people. Consequently, a maximally efficient screening process would focus only on subjects who are clearly thought disordered, delusional, or otherwise severely cognitively impaired. As the risk inherent in a decision increases, however (e.g., a high-risk research project involving subjects with schizophrenia or a study with an uncertain risk-benefit ratio involving subjects with Alzheimer's disease), so does the justification for routine screening.

The Role of IRBs

Although developing standards and screening mechanisms is basically a task for national policy makers, local IRBs could take a more active role in ensuring appropriate consent. For example, IRBs could specify what standard of competence should be used for a particular protocol and when a capacity screening mechanism is warranted. Furthermore, as part of the initial protocol approval process, IRBs could require investigators to provide information on the use of screening mechanisms. Alternatively, IRBs could actively oversee the consent process or perhaps view a random sample of consent interactions. In addition, IRBs could provide information on appropriate consent mechanisms for subjects who are found to lack decision-making capacity. For example, an IRB might draft a basic document explaining what is meant by *substituted judgment* or *best interests* and give examples of how substitute decision makers should apply the standards in specific cases. The IRB could also specify the level of certainty needed to make a decision: Is it sufficient if the proxy believes that the subject more than likely would have consented if he or she had been competent (>50% likelihood), or should a higher degree of certainty be required (such as 75% or even 90%)? The level of certainty needed may vary depending on the decision in question—less certainty is needed for lower-risk studies and more certainty is needed for higher-risk studies (Berg 1996). In cases in which there is a concern that either subjects or proxies will not understand the experiment because of the complicated nature of the research, and there are high risks involved, the IRB might require that the investigators take additional steps to ensure comprehension, such as employing a neutral third-party educator. The extent of the protections required depend on the case, but IRBs can clearly take a more active role in this context (Berg 1996; Bonnie 1997; Keyserlingk et al. 1995).

PRACTICAL GUIDANCE FOR RESEARCHERS

Though we lack definitive answers to the questions outlined previously (i.e., where to draw the line for incompetence and how to reliably identify incompetent subjects), the following suggestions may provide investigators with techniques for dealing with these uncertainties. First, investigators need to be aware that there will be some percentage of incompetent individuals in most populations with severe mental illness or dementia. Protocols submitted to IRBs should openly acknowledge this possibility, and practical means for dealing with such subjects should be designed.

Second, investigators need to specify for their project what constitutes an acceptable level of capacity. Because there is not a clear legal standard of competence to apply in research situations, investigators should develop one for their specific research protocols. The standard should identify the key information that must be understood by a subject before allowing participation and the disabling impairments (such as failure to appreciate the difference between research and treatment or inability to demonstrate internally consistent reasoning supporting participation) that will bar subject involvement. Because the levels of understanding, appreciation, and reasoning abilities required may vary with the degree of study risk, researchers need to specify these levels beforehand.

> Dr. L is an investigator at a large university. He is seeking approval to recruit subjects for a new protocol that he has developed. The study targets subjects with severe depression, entails a moderate degree of risk, and has a high potential for direct therapeutic benefit. Assignment to groups will be random, and a crossover design will be used. Given the subject population, the moderate degree of risk, and the high potential for benefit, Dr. L reasons that subjects should be able to demonstrate understanding of at least 80% of the information they are told; be able to appreciate the risks, benefits, and consequences of participation; and engage in at least low-level reasoning. He instructs his assistants that all subjects must understand that 1) the protocol will involve 10 visits to the hospital, each lasting 1 hour; 2) blood will be drawn on each of these visits; 3) initial assignment to groups is random, but each group will be given the experimental medium at some point; and 4) the primary risk is agitation as a side effect of the medication.

Third, the consent process itself needs to be structured to allow assessment of subject capacity. The staff in charge of recruitment must be informed of the standards that have been decided on and instructed how to apply them. Moreover, a process of assessment, either formal or informal, should be specified. At present, an informal process (i.e., the research assistant judges the relevant capacities during individual interactions) is permissible because no validated tools for formal assessment exist. However, if effective screening tools are developed in the future, they may take the place of less formal approaches. Furthermore, research staff should be monitored for adherence to the competence assessment protocol. Because implementation of such a protocol may conflict with the aim of recruiting as many subjects as possible, targets can be employed to establish reasonable percentages of subjects who should be excused from the consent process because of incompetence. For example, for a given subject population, an investigator may be aware that a certain percentage of individuals (e.g., 10%) are likely to be incompetent. This percentage should be used to guide the research assistant who is recruiting subjects. That is, the rates of potential subjects from whom consent was not solicited (in this example, 10%) should reflect the probable incidence of incompetence in the subject population. Research assistants need to be encouraged to exclude such subjects from the sample.

> Dr. L's study has been approved, and subject recruitment has begun. In reviewing the initial subjects recruited, Dr. L notices that one research assistant has a 100% inclusion rate, whereas the other has a 90% inclusion rate. Because they

are both drawing from the same population, Dr. L reviews recruitment procedures with his assistants. He makes it clear that he expects that a certain number of potential subjects approached will not have the capacity to consent and should not be included. He asks both assistants to carefully review the subjects they have included thus far and make sure they meet all of the requirements. When recruitment is complete, approximately 9% of all potential subjects approached are excluded because of incapacity. This figure is what Dr. L initially expected, and he notes this information in his subsequent write-up.

Finally, investigators need to make efforts to compensate for impairments detected. When impaired subjects are identified, they should not be excluded automatically from a study. Decision-making abilities are not fixed but highly context dependent. Investigators can take a number of steps to both compensate for decision-making impairment and safeguard impaired subjects who are enrolled in a protocol.

Many studies now suggest that modifications of disclosure methods can significantly improve potential subjects' understanding (Benson et al. 1988; Cournos 1993; Grisso et al. 1995; Tymchuk et al. 1988). For example, the temporal dimension for obtaining consent may be important. Severely disordered patients may need repetitive disclosures (Munetz et al. 1982). Even subjects who are not cognitively impaired have a tendency to forget information and do not always understand when something is explained to them for the first time (Jaffe 1986). Using long consent forms or giving too much information at one time can be confusing (Grisso and Appelbaum 1995; Silva and Sorrell 1988). It is particularly important that the investigator ask questions at different points during the disclosure to assess the subject's understanding so that corrective steps can be taken if necessary. In addition, a number of aids to increase understanding can be employed, such as videotaped disclosures to augment discussion with researchers and employment of independent educators whose sole job is to teach subjects about the studies to which they are being asked to consent (Benson et al. 1988). Investigators may also attempt to convey pertinent information with the aid of other persons such as the subject's family. Subjects should be given information to take home, read, think about, and discuss with others and then have an opportunity to return to have their questions answered.

In addition to previously mentioned aids to understanding, more severely impaired subjects may need supplemental safeguards. It is important to acknowledge that some important research questions may never be answerable without involving subjects with severe and irremediable decision-making impairments. For example, studies aimed at discovering treatments for schizophrenia or Alzheimer's disease necessitate inclusion of subjects with those disorders, many of whom are impaired. We need creative approaches to authorizing surrogate decision makers to act for subjects in a manner protective of their interests (American College of Physicians 1989; Berg 1996; Keyserlingk et al. 1995). One example is the present National Institutes of Health (NIH) Clinical Center policy of using the durable power of attorney prospectively to authorize research with incompetent Alzheimer's patients (Fletcher et al. 1985). Another is the use of a Ulysses Contract, or self-binding psychiatric advance directive authorizing research participation (DeRenzo 1994a). A definitive resolution of this problem will be difficult because many of the issues involved are subject to state laws that vary widely (DeRenzo 1994b). Even so, various solutions are possible, and mechanisms can be adapted for implementation in different jurisdictions.

CONCLUSION

Subject capacity to consent to research has become a focal point for heated discussions among investigators, subject populations, and families. The judiciary, too, has been drawn into the fray, as evidenced by recent cases in New York and Texas (T.D. v. New York State Office of Mental Health 1997; Flynn 1995). Clearly, biomedical research is necessary if we are to find treatments and possibly cures for some of the most devastating illnesses that exist in our society (e.g., schizophrenia and AIDS). Investigators should be permitted to conduct such research, and individuals who are interested should be allowed, and perhaps even encouraged, to participate. Yet the populations involved in such research are among the most vulnerable in our society. Although we are interested in allowing these individuals the same freedom to make choices as other members of our society, we are concerned about protecting persons whose capacity to make decisions autonomously is impaired. The suggestions in this chapter will not resolve all of the difficult issues (e.g., should incompetent subjects be permitted to participate in high-risk/low-direct-benefit protocols?); they will, however, aid in our understanding of subject capacity in the context of biomedical research. Moreover, they should help us to identify impaired subjects and to develop mechanisms designed to deal with those impairments.

REFERENCES

American College of Physicians: Cognitively impaired subjects. Ann Intern Med 111:843–848, 1989

Appelbaum PS: Rethinking the conduct of psychiatric research. Arch Gen Psychiatry 54:117–120, 1997

Appelbaum PS, Grisso T: Assessing patients' capacities to consent to treatment. N Engl J Med 319:1635–1638, 1988

Appelbaum PS, Grisso T: The MacArthur Treatment Competence Study, I: mental illness and competence to consent to treatment. Law and Human Behavior 19:105–126, 1995

Appelbaum PS, Roth LH: Competency to consent to research: a psychiatric overview. Arch Gen Psychiatry 39:951–958, 1982

Appelbaum PS, Roth LH, Lidz CW: The therapeutic misconception: informed consent in psychiatric research. Int J Law Psychiatry 5:319–329, 1982

Appelbaum PS, Lidz CW, Meisel A: Informed Consent: Legal Theory and Clinical Practice. New York, Oxford University Press, 1987a

Appelbaum PS, Roth LH, Lidz CW, et al: False hopes and best data: consent to research and the therapeutic misconception. Hastings Cent Rep 17:20–24, 1987b

Benson PR, Roth LH, Appelbaum PS, et al: Information disclosure, subject understanding, and informed consent in psychiatric research. Law and Human Behavior 12:455–476, 1988

Berg JW: The legal and ethical complexities of consent with cognitively impaired research subjects: proposed guidelines. Journal of Law, Medicine, and Ethics 24:18–35, 1996

Berg JW, Appelbaum PS, Grisso T: Constructing competence: formulating standards of legal competence to make medical decisions. Rutgers Law Review 48:345–396, 1996

Bonnie RJ: The competence of criminal defendants: beyond Dusky and Drope. University of Miami Law Review 47:539–601, 1993

Bonnie RJ: Research with cognitively impaired subjects: unfinished business in the regulation of human research. Arch Gen Psychiatry 54:105–111, 1997

Candilis PJ, Wesley RW, Wichman A: A survey of researchers using a consent policy for cognitively impaired human research subjects. IRB: Review of Human Subjects Research 15:1–4, 1993

Carpenter WT, Bartko JJ, Carpenter CL, et al: Another view of schizophrenia subtypes: a report from the international pilot study of schizophrenia. Arch Gen Psychiatry 33:508–516, 1976

Cassel C: Ethical issues in the conduct of research in long term care. Gerontologist 28:90–96, 1988

College on Problems of Drug Dependence: Human subject issues in drug abuse research. Drug Alcohol Depend 37:167–175, 1995

Cournos F: Do psychiatric patients need greater protection than medical patients when they consent to treatment? Psychiatr Q 64:319–329, 1993

Cummings J, Benson DF: Dementia: A Clinical Approach. Boston, MA, Butterworth-Heinemann, 1992

Department of Health and Human Services: Rules and Regulations for the Protection of Human Research Subjects, 45 Code of Federal Regulations §§46.101–46.409 (1991)

DeRenzo EG: The ethics of involving psychiatrically impaired persons in research. IRB: Review of Human Subjects Research 16:7–9, 11, 1994a

DeRenzo E: Surrogate decision making for severely cognitively impaired research subjects: the continuing debate. Camb Q Healthc Ethics 3:539–548, 1994b

Drane JF: Competency to give an informed consent: a model for making clinical assessments. JAMA 252:925–927, 1984

Elliott C: Caring about risks: are severely depressed patients competent to consent to research? Arch Gen Psychiatry 54:113–116, 1997

Evans DA, Funkenstein HH, Albert MS, et al: Prevalence of Alzheimer's disease in a community population of older persons. JAMA 262:2551–2556, 1989

Fitten LJ, Waite MS: Impact of medical hospitalization on treatment decision-making capacity in the elderly. Arch Intern Med 150:1717–1721, 1990

Fletcher JC, Dommel FW, Cowell DD: A trial policy for the intramural programs of the National Institutes of Health: consent to research with impaired human subjects. IRB: Review of Human Subjects Research 7:1–6, 1985

Flynn G: Suit challenges involuntary use of mental patients. Houston Chronicle, August 22, 1995, p A12

Grisso T, Appelbaum PS: The MacArthur Treatment Competence Study, III: abilities of patients to consent to psychiatric and medical treatments. Law and Human Behavior 19:149–174, 1995

Grisso T, Appelbaum PS, Mulvey E, et al: The MacArthur Treatment Competence Study, II: measures of abilities related to competence to consent to treatment. Law and Human Behavior 19:127–148, 1995

High D, Whitehouse PJ, Post SG, et al: Guidelines for addressing ethical and legal issues in Alzheimer disease research: a position paper. Alzheimer Dis Assoc Disord 8:66–74, 1994

Jaffe R: Problems of long-term informed consent. Bull Am Acad Psychiatry Law 14:163–169, 1986

Keyserlingk EW, Glass K, Kogan S, et al: Proposed guidelines for the participation of persons with dementia as research subjects. Perspect Biol Med 38:319–362, 1995

Kleber HD: Drug abuse liability testing: human subject issues, in Testing for Abuse Liability of Drugs in Humans (NIDA Research Monograph Series No 92). Edited by Fichman MW, Mello NK. Washington, DC, National Institute on Drug Abuse, 1989, pp 341–356

Marks ES, Derderian SS, Wray HL: Guidelines for conducting HIV research with human subjects at a U.S. military medical center. IRB: Review of Human Subjects Research 14:7–10, 1992

Marson DC, Schmitt FA, Ingram KK, et al: Determining the competency of Alzheimer patients to consent to treatment and research. Alzheimer Dis Assoc Disord 8(suppl 4):5–18, 1994

Morreim EH: Competence: at the intersection of law, medicine, and philosophy, in Competency: A Study of Informal Competency Determinations in Primary Care. Edited by Cutter MAG, Shelp EE. Dordrecht, Kluwer, 1991, pp 93–125

Munetz MR, Roth LH, Cornes CL: Tardive dyskinesia and informed consent: myths and realities. Bull Am Acad Psychiatry Law 10:77–88, 1982

National Commission for the Protection of Human Subjects of Biomedical and Behavioral Research: The Belmont Report: ethical principles and guidelines for the protection of human subjects of research (DHEW Publ No OS-78-0012). Washington, DC, U.S. Government Printing Office, 1978

Overall JE, Gorham DR: The Brief Psychiatric Rating Scale. Psychol Rep 10:799–812, 1962

President's Commission for the Study of Ethical Problems in Medicine and Biomedical and Behavioral Research: Making Health Care Decisions: A Report on the Ethical and Legal Implications of Informed Consent in the Patient-Practitioner Relationship, Vol 1: Report. Washington, DC, Superintendent of Documents, October 1982

Regier DA, Narrow WE, Rae DS, et al: The de facto US mental and addictive disorders service system: epidemiologic catchment area prospective 1-year prevalence rates of disorders and services. Arch Gen Psychiatry 50:85–94, 1993

Riecken HW, Ravich R: Informed consent to biomedical research in Veterans Administration hospitals. JAMA 248:344–348, 1982

Rosenfeld B, Turkheimer E, Gardner W: Decision making in a schizophrenic population. Law and Human Behavior 16:651–662, 1992

Roth LH, Meisel A, Lidz CW: Tests of competency to consent to treatment. Am J Psychiatry 134:279–280, 1977

Roth LH, Lidz CW, Meisel A, et al: Competency to decide about treatment or research: an overview of some empirical data. Int J Law Psychiatry 5:29–50, 1982

Sachs GA, Stocking CB, Stern R, et al: Ethical aspects of dementia research: informed consent and proxy consent. Clinical Research 42:403–412, 1994

Salgo v Leland Stanford Junior University Board of Trustees, 317 P2d 170, 181 (1957)

Schachter D, Kleinman I, Prendergast P, et al: The effect of psychopathology and the ability of schizophrenic patients to give informed consent. J Nerv Ment Dis 182:360–362, 1994

Schloendorff v Society of New York Hospital, 105 NE 92, NY (1914)

Shamoo AE, Irving DN: Accountability in research using persons with mental illness. Accountability in Research 3:1–17, 1993

Silva MC, Sorrell JM: Enhancing comprehension of information for informed consent: a review of empirical research. IRB: Review of Human Subjects Research 10:1–5, 1988

Simes RJ, Tattersall MH, Coates AS, et al: Randomized comparison of procedures for obtaining informed consent in clinical trials of treatment for cancer. BMJ 293:1065–1068, 1986

Speer DC: Comorbid mental and substance disorders among the elderly: conceptual issues and propositions. Behavior, Health, and Aging 1:163–171, 1990

Stanley B, Stanley M, Lautin A, et al: Preliminary findings on psychiatric patients as research participants: a population at risk? Am J Psychiatry 138:669–671, 1981

Stanley B, Stanley M, Peselow E, et al: The effects of psychotropic drugs on informed consent. Psychopharmacology 18:102–104, 1982

Stanley B, Guido J, Stanley M, et al: The elderly patient and informed consent. JAMA 252:1302–1306, 1984

Stanley B, Stanley M, Stein J, et al: Psychopharmacologic treatment and informed consent: empirical research. Psychopharmacol Bull 21:110–113, 1985

Stanley B, Stanley M, Guido J, et al: The functional competency of elderly at risk. Gerontologist 28:53–58, 1988

T.D. v New York State Office of Mental Health, 690 N.E. 2d 1259 (N.Y. 1997)

Tymchuk AJ, Ouslander JG, Rahbar B, et al: Medical decision-making among elderly people in long-term care. Gerontologist 28(suppl):59–63, 1988

White PD, Denise SH: Medical treatment decisions and competency in the eyes of the law: a brief survey, in Competency: A Study of Informal Competency Determinations in Primary Care. Edited by Cutter MAG, Shelp EE. Dordrecht, Kluwer, 1991, pp 149–166

Wilson WH, Ban TA, Guy W: Flexible system criteria in chronic schizophrenia. Compr Psychiatry 27:259–265, 1986

CHAPTER 5

Surrogate Decision Making and Advance Directives With Cognitively Impaired Research Subjects

TREY SUNDERLAND, M.D., AND RUTH DUKOFF, M.D.

O btaining informed consent for research is difficult enough when potential subjects have full cognitive capacities. When subjects are cognitively impaired, the complexities increase markedly (High 1992). Nonetheless, an orderly system for the consent process is required both to protect cognitively impaired patients who do not want to participate in research and to allow those who do want to participate in research to do so. As noted by the President's Commission for the Study of Ethical Problems in Medicine and Biomedical and Behavioral Research (1983, pp. 132–133), "Important studies on problems such as senile dementia of the Alzheimer type might not be conducted because of the absence of Federal guidance on ethical issues." Despite more than a decade of progress since the commission's report, the system for informed consent for cognitively impaired subjects is still very much in the developmental stage (DeRenzo 1994; Keyserlingk 1995).

Currently, there are two major mechanisms for including or excluding cognitively impaired individuals in research: advance directives (ADs) and surrogate decision making. Each has its own advantages and disadvantages. In this chapter, we discuss these mechanisms and note how they might apply to research with subjects whose independent informed consent is threatened by cognitive impairment. Before describing the actual process of obtaining informed consent from cognitively impaired subjects, however, we must first define three key terms: *cognitive impairment, surrogate decision making,* and *advance directives.*

COGNITIVE IMPAIRMENT

Although the courts are the final arbiters of competence in times of legal dispute, the clinical determination of cognitive impairment is usually made in a medical setting. The evidence of impairment may come from self-report, family reports, and/or the direct observations of a medical team. Generally, cognitive impairments are heralded by indications of trouble learning new information or recalling recently learned information (memory impairment). In addition, individuals may have difficulty recognizing or identifying objects despite intact sensory function (agnosia); they may experience language difficulties (aphasia); or they may demonstrate disturbances in planning, sequencing, or organizing procedures (executive ability dysfunction) (American Psychiatric Association 1994).

These cognitive symptoms may be seen alone or in combination with dementia of varying degrees of severity, depending on the underlying cause of the cognitive impairment and the stage of the illness. However, not all memory impairments or language difficulties preclude an individual from giving informed consent for a research protocol. The patient must be medically evaluated, paying particular attention to neuropsychological testing and the subject's ability to make independent decisions. The evaluation of individuals' capacity to consent is described in Chapter 4.

Unfortunately, although guidelines exist, measures for assessing cognitive impairment are not exact. Furthermore, because no absolute gold standard exists for the measurement of cognitive impairment, there is much room for interpretation of competence and the cognitive threshold at which it is lost, especially in discussing the issue of transferring the responsibility for consent to another person. When cognitive impairments are severe, there is no debate about the capacity to give informed consent or choose a surrogate, and research is not possible in the absence of an AD. The difficult decisions come in the early or mild stages of cognitive impairment when the capacities for informed consent are more intact and the individual is eager to proceed with research. It is here, at the crossroads of individual capacity for consent and alternative approaches to informed consent, that acceptable guidelines and coordinated efforts by the medical-ethical-legal team are needed. Unfortunately, no national statute governs alternative approaches to informed consent for research with cognitively impaired individuals. Even state law is silent on this issue; yet research with these subjects continues under the supervision of institutional review boards (IRBs) throughout the country. For this discussion, we cite approaches used in Maryland at the National Institute of Mental Health (NIMH); however, these options should be viewed as examples only. Individual researchers should modify their own research designs to fit whatever regulations exist in their jurisdiction.

SURROGATE DECISION MAKING

The Maryland Health Care Decisions Act (1984, p. 112) established standards for surrogate decision making by stipulating that the surrogate base "decisions on the wishes of the patient, and if the wishes of the patient are unknown or unclear, on the patient's best interest." To determine the patient's best interests, the act identifies the following issues for the surrogate to consider:

1. Current diagnosis
2. Expressed preferences
3. Relevant religious, moral, and personal values
4. Behavior, attitude, and past conduct of the individual
5. Reaction to the withholding or withdrawal of treatment of others
6. Expressed concern about the decision's effect on family and friends

Various principles have emerged to help the assigned surrogate make decisions for the patient, but the most widely cited standard is known as the "substituted judgment" standard, which was recommended for use by the President's Commission for the Study of Ethical Problems in Medicine and Biomedical and Behavioral Research (1983). Simply put, this standard directs the surrogate to make the decision covering medical treatment that the patient him- or herself would have made had he or she been fully competent to consider the options. Although this approach is not endorsed without question by the medical-bioethics community (Baergen 1995a, 1995b; Gutheil and Appelbaum 1985), and there is evidence of imperfections in the process of substituted judgment (Seckler et al. 1991), substituted judgment is still the most widely accepted standard in the difficult arena of medical decision making for cognitively incapacitated patients (Smith and Nunn 1995).

The surrogate decision-making procedure codified by Maryland's Health Care Decisions Act is designed to deal with deliberate health care decisions. However, the act is silent on the issue of entering into a research project for emergency procedures and on the issue of more prospective research involvement without direct clinical benefit. For emergency research procedures, a consensus statement concerning informed consent has recently been published by representatives of the Society for Academic Emergency Medicine and the American

Heart Association (Biros et al. 1995). According to this statement, patients "with sudden catastrophic illness receiving emergency or critical care and acute resuscitation should be identified as a new class of vulnerable patients for whom some additional safeguards must be defined." The statement calls for new federal regulations to explicitly address informed consent in this vulnerable population such that they are protected from "research risks without excluding them from research benefits" (Biros et al. 1995, pp. 1205, 1206).

Although the population served by emergency medicine staff may well be cognitively impaired during the immediate emergency period, it is quite possible, depending on the patient's underlying medical condition, that the impairment is reversible and temporary. In that situation, the need for surrogate decision making is also temporary, and the process of informed consent reverts back to the routine procedure once the cognitive impairment is resolved. Therefore, these emergency guidelines are not applicable to those with slowly progressive cognitive impairment. In this chapter we focus on the surrogate decision-making process for nonemergency research, in which the likelihood of continued or progressive cognitive impairment is greater. The expectation for a speedy return to autonomous informed consent is minimal, and protections must be in place if subjects are to participate in research.

One form of progressive cognitive impairment is found in the dementia of Alzheimer's disease. Given the limitations of current medical treatments, it is generally expected that Alzheimer's disease patients with mild cognitive impairment will progress to a more impaired state over time. However, early in their illness they may be quite competent to give informed consent for research according to the standards outlined in Chapter 4, and they may express a clear wish to continue in research beyond the reach of their capacity to give informed consent. It is here that a surrogate may be of benefit to the individual losing his or her autonomy of choice. And, indeed, at this point individuals may still be capable of freely selecting another person from their family, friends, or the community at large who can represent their best interests in the future. It is important to note, however, that the act of appointing a surrogate for research decisions is not a license for continuing research involvement. Rather, the surrogate takes on the responsibility of assessing all aspects of a research procedure and protecting the individual from future unnecessary risks.

ADVANCE DIRECTIVES

Simply put, ADs are the written or oral preferences of individuals in regard to future medical treatments. Presumably initiated at a time of intact cognitive abilities, ADs are intended to provide "clear and convincing" evidence of patients' wishes when they are no longer able to state those wishes (*Cruzan v. Director, Missouri Department of Health* 1990). The law now requires hospitals and most nursing homes to provide patients with written information about ADs. Although acceptance of the AD process has expanded tremendously (Emanuel and Emanuel 1989; Emanuel et al. 1991; President's Commission 1983), there is still much debate about how strictly the directives should be followed (Sehgal et al. 1992) and how they are applicable to individuals who already have some cognitive impairment (Finucane et al. 1993; Grisso and Appelbaum 1995). This latter issue is of particular interest for our discussion because ADs have generally been employed in end-of-life decisions (i.e., withdrawal of life supports), not in the context of research.

ADs are usually targeted at specific issues that can be predicted ahead of time, and relatively little flexibility exists in the documents that establish ADs. In a world of rapidly changing medical practice, tightly worded ADs can quickly become antiquated, thereby undermining the intentions of individuals when they were cognitively intact and established the AD (Sehgal et al. 1992). This rigidity of ADs has led to a search for other approaches to informed consent with cognitively impaired subjects.

Proxy Decision Making for Research: Durable Power of Attorney

One of the most widely used mechanisms for the transfer of personal authority is a power of attorney. Generally, powers of attorney are employed for short periods of time, often for financial matters, but they can be extended to become more long lasting. Faced with the difficult task of getting informed consent from patients experiencing progressive decline, the National Institutes of Health (NIH) Clinical Center established the model of a durable power of attorney (DPA) for research in its 1987 policy on the use of ADs (see Appendix 5–1).

The DPA mechanism was designed to provide a surrogate decision maker in situations in which progressive cognitive impairment was likely and the patient demonstrated an obvious interest in participating in research over time (Fletcher and Wichman 1987; Wichman and Sandler 1995). By definition, therefore, the DPA designee is a surrogate or proxy decision maker of the patient's own choosing (i.e., an agent) who takes on increasing responsibility in the research setting as the patient's cognitive impairment increases. The DPA designee decides on the patient's behalf about participation in future research protocols based on the expressed wishes or substituted judgment of his or her best interest. (The concept of *substituted judgment* is used here rather than *best interests* because of the previous relationship the DPA designee has had with the patient before taking on the responsibility of making research decisions.) Often, the specific issues addressed in a research protocol were not anticipated exactly by any preexisting AD. For this reason, the NIH Clinical Center has decided that ADs should not be considered replacements for DPAs but rather should be reviewed as a complementary process in health care decision making (see Appendix 5–2).

One of the major procedural questions in use of a DPA is how a cognitively impaired subject can choose a surrogate in the first place. If the level of cognitive impairment is clearly moderate at the time of DPA assignment, we handle this decision process at the NIMH with the help of a bioethics consultation or formally with the courts through a legally appointed guardian (see cases 2–6, Appendix 5–2). Obviously, bioethicists are not available as consultants in most medical settings. Other unbiased arbiters might include members of the local IRB or pastoral counselors, and the courts can be used as the final arbiters if necessary. More commonly, the cognitive impairment is mild at the time of DPA assignment, and the patient's own abilities are still mostly intact. At this stage, informed consent for research is usually still achievable with the patient alone, although the surrogate decision maker (i.e., DPA designee) may well participate in the decision-making process to gain experience with the individual's style and personal wishes about research. The DPA designee will presumably be well informed about the individual's wishes when progressive cognitive impairments later blur the patient's ability to fully execute informed consent: the DPA designee must be a full and willing partner in the ongoing consent process (see Table 5–1).

The purpose of the DPA is to allow research to proceed beyond the individual's capacity for informed consent. The intention is to project one's wishes into the future of cognitive impairment, when one's choices are otherwise severely limited in conventional research settings. So long as the DPA designee acts with the expressed wishes and best interests of the individual in mind, the mechanism allows for continued autonomy, even if that autonomy includes

TABLE 5–1. Essential criteria to establish a durable power of attorney (DPA) for research with potentially cognitively impaired subjects

1. Subject understands the meaning of DPA
2. Choice of DPA is made by subject him- or herself
3. Subject's wishes have been discussed with DPA
4. Assigned DPA understands his or her responsibilities and is willing to execute discussions if or when subject becomes too impaired

choosing the relative risk of research involvement. For instance, a DPA designee might approve a treatment with potential benefit that would be unavailable without a research protocol. Or, the DPA might approve a patient's participation in research simply to help advance the frontiers of science, with no direct personal benefit.

Participating in research to learn more about the patient's illness might be rewarding enough if that type of participation had been the pattern and intention of the individual before the cognitive impairment limited the consent process. Then, the research is free to proceed under the supervision of the DPA designee.

When considering research consent by proxy or surrogate decision maker, attention must be paid to possible conflicts of interest. Although the individual's desires should dictate participation in research, other involved figures include the family, the researcher, and the institution itself. Each of these participants brings possible elements of bias that must be considered by the DPA designee before agreeing to research participation. For example, the family may be eager to encourage participation if it means 2–3 months of institutional care for their loved one and a break or respite from their duties as caregivers. Researchers and institutions have the built-in safeguards of IRBs to help ensure protection of patients, but they must be vigilant in monitoring the risk-benefit balance and avoiding the temptation to become overeager in enrolling subjects. The DPA designee is responsible for assessing the risks of each research protocol and ensuring that the patient's wishes are carried out, much as that individual would do if he or she were still competent.

Risk-Benefit Analysis

Two key elements in the decision to participate in research are the *level of risk* and *potential of benefit* associated with any protocol. In practice, risk levels have been divided into the categories of minimal risk and more than minimal risk. Similarly, there are two major characterizations of benefit: prospect of direct benefit and no prospect of direct benefit.

For research with children, special guidelines have been developed for the following risk-benefit combinations (Department of Health and Human Services 1991, 45 *CFR* 46.401–46.409):

1. *Category 1:* Research not involving greater than minimal risk
2. *Category 2:* Research involving greater than minimal risk but presenting the prospect of direct benefit to individual subjects
3. *Category 3:* Research involving greater than minimal risk and no prospect of direct benefit to individual subjects

a. Minor increase over minimal risk

b. More than minor increase over minimal risk

These risk categories are the focus of discussion by any IRB when deliberating about a research protocol for children. Although the legal and moral obligations of parents consenting for children may seem quite different from the substituted judgment of a surrogate or DPA designee for a once-competent adult, there are many similarities. Therefore, with relatively little adjustment, these risk categories could function for cognitively impaired subjects. Instead of parents or guardians, the patient representative would be the DPA designee, surrogate decision maker, or court-appointed guardian. With a DPA, the principal investigator and IRB would be able to consider both the best interest, or substituted judgment of the individual, and the explicit wishes and/or previous research decisions of the individual before he or she was cognitively incapacitated.

Indeed, it might be useful to institute an assent process for all cognitively impaired subjects modeled after the federal guidelines for children. Although such a procedure is not yet required by any federal or state law, it would further ensure the protection of cognitively impaired individuals in research settings. The control for research participation would rest in the hands of the DPA designee and the patient him- or herself (through assent), under the protection of the local IRB. How one would define assent in the absence of adequate verbal communications is not clear, but it might well revolve around the concept of doctor-patient cooperation in the research procedures. As in other research arenas, the principal investigator would be responsible for explaining the research procedures and any associated risks to the patient and the DPA designee, who would monitor the assent during the research program.

Researcher Guidelines

Investigators face many different situations when dealing with cognitively impaired subjects, and it is thus imperative to recognize the research options available. The first task is to assess the level of cognitive impairment and determine whether it is reversible, stable, or progressive. This assessment generally includes clinical observations, neuropsychological consultation, and specific cognitive testing. Although many cognitive batteries have been developed and hundreds of specific cognitive tests are available, clinicians and researchers often summarize their findings with a simple mild, moderate, or severe classification. (A more complete review of standards for determining competence can be found in Chapter 4.)

Next, it must be determined whether the subject will be signing his or her own consent independently or with a surrogate decision maker. If the investigator is considering obtaining research consent directly from a mildly cognitively impaired subject, the research opportunities are time limited. Although minimal risk or even more than minimal risk research might be possible at this point, it is likely that disease progression will affect direct informed consent options in the relatively near future. On the other hand, if a mildly impaired subject has chosen a DPA designee, the options for continuing research during progressive stages of cognitive impairment are much broader. The various options for initiating research plans at the NIH are summarized in Table 5–2.

Another approach to deciding about research participation of cognitively impaired subjects involves assessing the level of risk associated with the proposed study. In general, research with a greater degree of risk is less possible as

TABLE 5–2. Options for initiating research at the National Institutes of Health during various stages of cognitive impairment assuming no previous AD or DPA surrogate assigned

	Level of cognitive impairment			
Consent options	None	Mild	Moderate	Severe
1. Independent research discussions	Yes	Possible[a]	NA	NA
2. Enter longitudinal research without DPA	Yes	Possible[a]	NA	NA
3. Determine AD	Yes	Possible[a]	Limited possibility[b]	NA
4. Assign DPA independently	Yes	Possible[a]	Limited possibility[b]	NA
5. DPA with ethics consultation	NA	Yes	Possible[b,c]	NA
6. Court-appointed guardianship	NA	Yes	Yes[d]	Possible[d]

Note. AD, advance directive; DPA, durable power of attorney; NA, not appropriate.
[a]Possible option if cognitive impairment does not impede the informed consent process.
[b]Assuming cognitive impairment does not impede ability to choose surrogate decision maker (DPA or AD execution).
[c]Assuming that ethics consultation supports choice of surrogate and that the level of research risk is not more than slightly above minimal risk.
[d]Assuming level of risk is not more than slightly above minimal risk.

individuals' cognitive impairment increases. The introduction of ADs and DPAs, however, has altered this situation somewhat, as summarized in the risk outline in Table 5–3. This decision grid is based on current practices at the NIH Clinical Center, and it presumes the existence of a bioethicist in the hospital who can serve as an independent voice in complicated cases. Although not all researchers have the luxury of working with hospital-based or community bioethicists, alternative independent observers may be found in the medical community or recommended by the local IRB to aid in difficult situations. Alternatively, the court system is always available. Unfortunately, court-appointed guardianship is often an expensive and time-consuming process, and it has generally been restricted to use in clinical rather than research decisions in medical care.

Who Makes the Final Decisions?

Assuming for the moment that a cognitively impaired subject has already appointed a DPA for research and that the local IRB has approved a research procedure for cognitively impaired subjects, who makes the final decision about research participation? For the purposes of informed consent, the DPA designee gives the authorization for the IRB-approved research as explained by the principal investigator and witnessed by an observer of the informed consent process. In practice, however, the patient must still assent to the research at his or her level of cognitive capacity and then willingly participate in whatever procedures are involved. Without that assent, the preparation and surrogate decision making are jeopardized. When appropriate consent is ensured, the research can proceed unimpeded.

CONCLUSION

Obtaining informed consent is always a complicated process involving researchers, medical staff, and patients and their families. It becomes even more difficult when the patient is cognitively impaired. In this chapter, we have reviewed some of the major issues (summarized in Table 5–4) that must be addressed before research can proceed with cognitively impaired patients.

In particular, we have reviewed the use of surrogate decision making with a DPA for research, as practiced at the NIH Clinical Center. Although the DPA is currently unique to the Clinical Center, the principles could well be applied in other university- and hospital-based research facilities. Of course, following the objectives of the DPA or other ADs does not reduce the risk of proposed

TABLE 5–3.   Research options for subjects with and without previously assigned surrogates according to level of research risk

| | Classification of research by level of risk | | | |
| | Minimal risk research | More than minimal risk with prospect of direct benefit | More than minimal risk without prospect of direct benefit | |
Level of cognitive impairment			Slight increase	More than slight increase
1. No impairment	Yes	Yes	Yes	Yes
2. Mild impairment				
Without DPA	Yes	Yes[a]	Possible with EC[a]	Possible with EC
With DPA	Yes	Yes	Yes	Yes[b]
3. Moderate impairment				
Without DPA	Possible[a] + kin	Possible with EC	Possible with EC	NA
With DPA	Yes	Yes	Yes	NA
4. Severe impairment				
Without DPA	Possible with EC + kin	Possible with EC + guardianship	Possible with EC + guardianship	NA
With DPA	Yes	Yes	Yes[b]	Yes[b]

Note.   DPA, durable power of attorney; EC, ethics consultation; NA, not appropriate; kin, family consent from next of kin.
[a]If informed consent process is fully intact.
[b]If subject had advance directive for higher levels of risk or if previous research record demonstrates willingness to participate in this level of research risk (local IRBs and state law may have more explicit regulations).

TABLE 5–4.   Practical objectives for research evaluating cognitively impaired subjects

1. Characterize the specific cognitive impairment
2. Establish whether the cognitive impairment is transient, stable, or progressive
3. Estimate the severity of the cognitive impairment
4. Identify the potential surrogate/proxy candidates
5. Determine level of research risk potentially available for the subject
6. Ensure the subject's consent for any research procedure

research or eliminate the possibility of investigator bias; however, the guidelines ensure additional safeguards beyond the IRB and offer extra protections for patients, their families, and the investigators themselves.

REFERENCES

American Psychiatric Association: Diagnostic and Statistical Manual of Mental Disorders, 4th Edition. Washington, DC, American Psychiatric Association, 1994

Baergen R: Revising the substituted judgment standard. J Clin Ethics 6:30–38, 1995a

Baergen R: Surrogates and uncertainty. J Clin Ethics 6:372–377, 1995b

Biros MH, Lewis RJ, Olson CM, et al: Informed consent in emergency research: consensus statement from the Coalition Conference of Acute Resuscitation and Critical Care Researchers. JAMA 273:1283–1287, 1995

Cruzan v Director, Missouri Department of Health, 497 US 111 L Ed 2nd 224 100 S Ct 2841 (1990)

Department of Health and Human Services: Rules and Regulations for the Protection of Human Research Subjects, 45 Code of Federal Regulations 46 (1991)

DeRenzo E: Surrogate decision making for severely cognitively impaired research subjects: the continuing debate. Camb Q Healthc Ethics 3:539–548, 1994

Emanuel LL, Emanuel EJ: The medical directive. JAMA 261:3288–3293, 1989

Emanuel LL, Barry MJ, Stoeckle JD, et al: Advance directives for medical care: a case for greater use. N Engl J Med 324:889–895, 1991

Finucane TE, Beamer BA, Roca RP, et al: Establishing advance medical directives with demented patients: a pilot study. J Clin Ethics 4:51–54, 1993

Fletcher JC, Wichman A: A new consent policy for research with impaired human subjects. Psychopharmacol Bull 23:382–385, 1987

Grisso T, Appelbaum PS: Comparison of standards for assessing patients' capacities to make treatment decisions. Am J Psychiatry 152:1033–1037, 1995

Gutheil T, Appelbaum P: The substituted judgment approach: its difficulties and paradoxes in mental health settings. Law, Medicine, and Health Care 1:61–64, 1985

High DM: Research with Alzheimer's disease subjects: informed consent and proxy decision making. J Am Geriatr Soc 40:950–957, 1992

Keyserlingk EW: Proposed guideline for the participation of persons with dementia as research subjects. Perspect Biol Med 38:319–362, 1995

Maryland Health Care Decisions Act. Health—General Article: Annotated Code of Maryland. Chapters 591 and 540 of the Acts of 1984, §§20–107 (1984)

President's Commission for the Study of Ethical Problems in Medicine and Biomedical and Behavioral Research: Deciding to Forgo Life-Sustaining Treatment. Washington, DC, U.S. Government Printing Office, 1983

Seckler AB, Meier DE, Mulvihill M, et al: Substituted judgment: how accurate are proxy predictions? Ann Intern Med 115:92–98, 1991

Sehgal A, Galbraith A, Chesney M, et al: How strictly do dialysis patients want their advance directives followed? JAMA 267:59–63, 1992

Smith DG, Nunn S: Substituted judgment: in search of a foolproof method; a response to Baergen. J Clin Ethics 6:184–186, 1995

Wichman A, Sandler AL: Research involving subjects with dementia and other cognitive impairments: experience at the NIH, and some unresolved ethical considerations. Neurology 45:1777–1778, 1995

Clinical Center Policy on the Use of Advance Directives in Health Care

I. PURPOSE

This policy directs the efforts of the Clinical Center (CC) towards (1) educating adult patients and research subjects, families, staff, and the community regarding advance directives (ADs) in health care decision making, and (2) implementing ADs for those patients who request assistance in the process. This policy is consistent with the 1990 federal legislation, "Patient Self-Determination Act," which requires that health care institutions inform patients of their right to participate in and direct health care decisions by implementing advance directives. This policy is based on an ethical foundation of respect for individuals and recognizes the importance of patient participation in health care decisions.

II. GLOSSARY of DEFINITIONS

A. *Adult Patient*

For the purposes of this policy, an adult is a person who is (1) 18 years or older, or (2) an emancipated minor. An emancipated minor is a person under the age of 18 years who is married or has a child. The term "patient" in this policy refers to patients and research subjects (including healthy volunteers) admitted to the hospital or an outpatient unit.

B. *Advance Directives for Health Care Decisions*

Formal advance directives (ADs) are written documents specifying a person's preferences concerning medical treatment, including life-sustaining treatment, in advance of a medical condition or cognitive impairment that may render the person incapable of making such health care decisions at the appropriate time. Two legally recognized forms of ADs are the "Living Will" and the "Durable Power of Attorney for Health Care." These types of ADs are not mutually exclusive and, in some instances, may be best implemented together. ADs may be changed or canceled at any time and are valid indefinitely unless changed or canceled. They allow for decisions in health care only.

C. *Living Will*

A Living Will is an AD in which a person specifies which medical interventions/measures he/she would want instituted, continued, withheld, or withdrawn in the event that the individual is diagnosed as suffering from a terminal condition and is no longer capable of making health care decisions. The definition of "terminal condition" may vary from state to state; however, it is generally defined as a condition from which, within a reasonable degree of medical certainty, there can be no recovery and death is imminent.

D. *Durable Power of Attorney for Health Care (DPA)*

A Durable Power of Attorney for Health Care is an AD in which a person appoints a surrogate to make health care decisions for him/her in the event that he/she becomes incapable of doing so. The DPA becomes effective only if and when the designating person becomes unable to make health care decisions. Unlike the Living Will, operation of the DPA is not limited to cases where the person is diagnosed with a terminal condition.

E. *The Clinical Center (CC) Durable Power of Attorney Form*

The CC DPA form documents the appointment by an adult CC patient of a surrogate decision maker. The CC DPA form is a legal document at the Clinical Center only, although it may provide some guidance as to a person's wishes once he/she leaves the CC. Patients implementing a DPA will be educated about this limited usefulness and will be given information about how they can implement a legally binding AD in their home state. The CC form is to be completed with the assistance of designated personnel in each Institute. Proper completion includes the signature of a witness.

III. POLICY

A. All adult CC in- and out-patients will be provided with information concerning ADs. If requested, they will receive additional assistance in the implementation of ADs from designated and trained CC staff.

B. The CC will not condition the provision of care or research participation on the execution of an AD except as stipulated by an IRB consistent with CC policy, "Consent Process in Research Involving Impaired Human Subjects."

C. In most states, the Living Will is not applicable to health care decision-making until the person is diagnosed as being in a terminal condition. Given such limitations of the Living Will and because unique health care and research decisions face CC patients, the Medical Board endorses and prefers the use of the DPA. However, this policy is not intended to discourage the use of Living Wills. Patients will be provided with information on the strengths and weaknesses of each AD to help them decide which AD is best for them in light of their care at the CC.

D. If a patient admitted to the CC has a valid DPA or Living Will already in existence, it will be honored, documented in the progress notes of the medical record, and placed in the patient's medical record. An existing AD will be considered valid within the NIH if, to the knowledge of the patient, it was executed in keeping with the laws of the patient's home state. In addition, patients with valid ADs will be encouraged but not required to implement a CC DPA.

IV. IMPLEMENTATION

The Clinical Director of each Institute is responsible for designating appropriate individuals to provide information and assistance in the implementation of ADs to patients in his/her Institute. The decision about the appropriate personnel for this task should be made in light of the particular Institute's needs and in consultation with other health care disciplines, such as social work and nursing. Designated personnel may include physicians, nurses, social workers, physician assistants, or others.

V. EDUCATION

A. *Designated personnel*

The CC will provide formal training, educational materials, and on-going instruction and support for those individuals designated to provide education and assistance in the implementation of ADs.

B. *Other Clinical Center staff*

All clinical care personnel will receive this policy and other information on ADs.

C. *Community education*

At the direction of the Medical Board, the CC Ethics Committee, CC Communications Office, and other appropriate departments will co-ordinate community outreach educational activities on ADs.

VI. PROCEDURES

A. *Pre-admission*

During the pre-admission phone interview by the admissions clerk, patients will be asked if they have already implemented an AD. Patients with ADs will be asked to bring them to the CC when admitted.

B. *Initial admission*

1. Upon initial admission to the CC, every patient will be:
   a. provided with information in the admission packet about patients' rights to make health care decisions.
   b. asked whether he/she has an AD in existence. If he/she does not and requests more information or wants to implement an AD, the patient will be referred to the designated individual(s) in the admitting Institute for further information and assistance in implementing the CC DPA.
2. For patients with an AD in existence:
   a. designated personnel will discuss the AD with the patient in order to determine its validity (see III., D.) and content. If valid, it will be filed in the medical record under "Authorization." If it is not valid, individuals will be provided information about and assistance in implementing a CC DPA.

b. in addition, patients with a valid AD will be encouraged (but not required) to implement a CC DPA as well.

C. *Re-admission*

At the time of each re-admission, patients will be asked if they want their AD from the previous admission to stay in the medical record. Any answer other than "yes" will prompt referral to designated personnel. Patients without ADs will be referred to appropriate personnel.

D. *Documentation*

1. *Completion/distribution of ADs:*
   a. CC DPAs will be properly completed and the original will be filed in the medical record under "Authorization." Copies will be given to (1) the patient, (2) the individual designated as surrogate, and (3) the Institute Clinical Director.
   b. Valid non-Clinical Center ADs will also be filed in the medical record under "Authorization."

E. *Special Concerns*

Situations may arise in which a variety of ethical and legal issues relative to ADs need to be addressed. These may include questions about the interpretation and application of ADs already in existence or the cognitive ability of the patient to execute an AD. Questions and concerns relating to the consent process in research involving cognitively impaired human subjects should be made in concert with the Durable Power of Attorney (see Appendix 5–2). The Bioethics Program is available for consultation on issues related to ADs in the CC.

VII. SUPERVISION

Responsibility for this policy's implementation, effectiveness, and evaluation rests with the Medical Board, with the assistance of its various subcommittees, most notably the CC Ethics Committee.

National Institutes of Health Clinical Center Policy on the Consent Process in Research Involving Impaired Human Subjects

PURPOSE

I. Research Review of Studies Involving Impaired Human Subjects

A. General

The Institute Clinical Research Subpanel (ICRS) is authorized by Federal regulation to protect the rights and welfare of subjects of research who are temporarily or permanently impaired, by including "appropriate additional safeguards" (45 CFR 46.111 (b)). This policy specifies how the ICRS can approve "additional safeguards" for the consent process with impaired human subjects and their legally authorized representatives.

B. Procedures

1. Investigators who plan research with human subjects who are or will become cognitively impaired must include a written section in the protocol which:
   a. describes the risks of the proposed research;
   b. describes the prospect of direct benefit(s) of the research to the subject, or if direct benefit to the subject is not expected, describes the importance of the knowledge sought by the research;
   c. describes the anticipated degree of clinical impairment of subjects during their participation; and,
   d. requests ICRS approval to use a Durable Power of Attorney (DPA) for the consent process, when appropriate.
   (The DPA is a legal document by which a prospective research subject appoints a surrogate to make decisions for the subject about his or her participation in research at the NIH.)
2. In reviewing the research, the ICRS shall specify, in consultation with the principal investigator, the level of risk involved in the proposed research. The minutes of the ICRS shall record the assessment of risk level and approval of the planned use of the DPA.
3. Three levels of research risks, as described in Federal regulations and set forth below, are permitted in NIH intramural research involving impaired subjects, provided that the consent process described in Section II, following, is used.

LEVEL 1. Research having minimal risk, i.e., where the risks of harm anticipated are not greater, considering probability and magnitude, than those ordinarily encountered in

daily life, e.g., non-invasive procedures; psychometric tests; medical record reviews; venipuncture; medical tests or procedures carried out in the routine physical examination, diagnosis and treatment of patients; etc.

LEVEL 2. Research having greater than minimal risk but presenting the prospect of direct benefit to individual subjects, e.g., a drug trial with minimal side effects; tests involving minimal radiation but providing useful diagnostic information (CAT Scan), etc.

LEVEL 3. Research having greater than minimal risk with no prospect of direct benefit to subjects, but likely to yield general knowledge about the subject's disorder or condition, e.g., added lumbar punctures or ionizing radiation done for research, etc.

II. *Consent Process with Impaired Human Subjects*

A. General

Clinical Center (CC) policy is that consent of impaired subjects is necessary but is not sufficient to begin research. More must be done to provide the best substituted judgment that the subject would consent to the research if he or she were not impaired.

When the subject is not seriously impaired, he or she shall be asked to appoint the surrogate decision-maker. The patient may select the person of choice, not necessarily a relative. The DPA is the official record of the subject's choice. When the subject is so seriously impaired as to be incapable of understanding the intent or meaning of the DPA process, a next-of-kin surrogate may be chosen by the physician. However, a consultation is required from the CC Bioethics Program about the suitability and willingness of the prospective surrogate to serve in this role.

Further, the policy provides that if higher levels of research risk and impairment are involved, a higher degree of monitoring will be required. Three levels of monitoring are embodied in the policy: 1) notification of Institute and CC officials of the use of the DPA, 2) required bioethics consultations in five of eight types of cases, and 3) family-initiated court appointment of a guardian in two types of cases.

B. Procedures

1. Patients with a valid DPA prepared elsewhere or with a court-appointed guardian need not execute a new DPA. Also, the DPA is valid for all research and clinical care involving the patient during his or her entire NIH stay.
2. The physician caring for the research subject is responsible for all phases of the DPA procedure: (a) securing consultation if needed, (b) explaining the DPA to the subject and the surrogate, (c) completing the DPA and placing it in the chart, and (d) notifying designated officials by sending carbon copies as indicated.
3. DPA forms with instructions are available from all unit nursing stations and from the Bioethics Program.

4. Consultation on ethical problems in the consent process with impaired human subjects or answers to questions about the DPA policy can be obtained by calling the CC Bioethics Program.

SELECTED CASE EXAMPLES:

Case 1: The subject is capable of understanding the DPA, and the research risk is minimal. The DPA is executed, notification given, and research can proceed. Notification is done by sending copies of the signed and witnessed DPA forms to those designated on the carbons (Chair, ICRS; Institute Clinical Director; CC Bioethicist).

Case 2: The subject is incapable of understanding the DPA, and the research risk is minimal. The physician shall request an ethics consultation for the selection of a next-of-kin surrogate. After positive consultation report, the substituted proxy consent of the relative can be obtained, and research can proceed.

Case 3: The subject is capable of understanding the DPA, and the research risk is greater than minimal but with a prospect of direct benefit to the subject. The physician shall request an ethics consultation to assure that the person appointed by the subject is capable of understanding the risks and benefits of the study. After the DPA is executed, notification shall occur, and research can proceed.

Case 4: The subject is capable of understanding the DPA, and the research risk is greater than minimal but with no prospect of benefit to the subject. The physician shall request an ethics consultation to assure that the person appointed by the subject is capable of understanding the purpose and risks of the study. After the DPA is executed, notification shall occur, and research can proceed.

Case 5: The subject is incapable of understanding the DPA, and the research risk is greater than minimal with a prospect of direct benefit to the subject. No court-appointed guardian exists, but family members desire the patient's participation in the research. The physician shall request an ethics consultation for the family members to assure their understanding of the risks and benefits and also of the CC's policy requiring court appointment of a guardian. Research shall not proceed until family members initiate court proceedings and a court-appointed guardian can give consent for the research.

Case 6: The subject is incapable of understanding the DPA, and the research risk is greater than minimal with no prospect of benefit to the subject. No court-appointed guardian exists, but family members desire the subject's participation in the research. The physician shall request an ethics consultation for the family members to assure their understanding of the risks and lack of benefit in this case. Research shall not proceed until family members initiate court proceedings and a court-appointed guardian can give consent for the research.

Case 7: The subject is incapable of understanding the DPA, and the research risk is greater than minimal with a prospect of direct benefit to the subject. The subject does not have an intact family; i.e., either no relatives are alive or none are able to act as surrogate decision makers. Research can proceed if the situation is a medical emergency, when a physician may give therapy, including experimental therapy, if in the physician's judgment it is necessary to protect the life or health of the patient.

Case 8: The subject is incapable of understanding the DPA, and the research risk is greater than minimal with no benefit to the subject. The subject does not have an intact family or relatives. Research is prohibited in this case.

CHAPTER 6

Informing Subjects of Risks and Benefits

JOSEPH P. MCEVOY, M.D., AND RICHARD S. E. KEEFE, PH.D.

A n investigator seeking informed consent must convey to a prospective research participant the facts that a reasonable individual would need to
know about a study to make a decision about participation. In this chapter, we
use the Federal Policy for the Protection of Human Subjects: Notices and Rules
(reprinted in Appendix 6–1) as a basis for discussing the content areas (the
what and *why*) that must be covered during an informed consent presentation.
We discuss the pros and cons of different approaches for dealing with each
content area and provide and critique sample paragraphs. We stress the use of
clear and simple language in consent presentations because investigators often
speak and write to the reading level of their colleagues rather than to that of
their patients (Grundner 1980; Riecken and Ravich 1982). Appendix 6–2 contains two simple tests of the reading level of written presentations (Flesch 1948;
Fry 1968). Appendix 6–3 includes examples, written for high school–level read-
ers, of descriptions of research procedures that are commonly utilized in studies
in psychiatry and the behavioral sciences.

Even if an investigator has thoughtfully selected, organized, and transmitted
all of the information that must be conveyed to patients, patient reception of
information is not ensured (Robinson and Merav 1976). Therefore, we also
review the *who, where, when,* and *how* of informed consent, which may influence
patients' reception of information and suggest methods to help patients understand the consent information conveyed to them. When a study involves
more than minimal risk, or a patient's capacity to process new information is
not optimal, use of these methods is especially important (Bonnie 1997; Dresser
1996; Faden and Beauchamp 1986; Hirschfeld et al. 1997).

As Faden and Beauchamp (1986, p. 308) point out, "Disclosure should only
serve to *initiate* the communication process necessary for substantial understanding." The investigator cannot be sure that a patient has understood what

has been conveyed without some form of checking (Miller and Willner 1974), nor can the investigator identify all issues of material import to a patient without offering the patient an opportunity to bring up these issues (Lidz et al. 1984). Therefore, we urge investigators to invite questions from patients and engage in discussions with patients when seeking informed consent. In addition, we suggest methods and a manner of disclosure that may permit patients to best incorporate and use what is disclosed.

FACTORS INFLUENCING PATIENTS' UNDERSTANDING OF CONSENT INFORMATION

Who Presents the Consent Information?

The principal investigator and coinvestigators are ultimately responsible for providing information about the research to the patient, assessing the patient's understanding, and obtaining informed consent. If the research involves more than minimal risk, one of the investigators should be involved personally in the consent process. However, it may be helpful, both to patients and to the investigator, if other research staff provide initial information (e.g., review the consent form, show diagrams of the study procedures, and answer initial questions) (Tankanow et al. 1992). Other research staff are likely to have more time to spend with the patient, and the patient may know these staff members better and feel more comfortable with them. At regular intervals, the investigator should accompany these staff members and observe them providing consent information to ensure the consistency and completeness of presented information. The investigator should also encourage staff members to invite active participation by patients (Faden and Beauchamp 1986). By asking questions that elicit the concerns and interests of the patient, the staff member presenting information can ensure that the patient has all of the information he or she needs.

Informed Consent in Stressful Situations

When questioned about the informed consent process, patients complain that consent discussions often occur at inappropriate or stressful times (Advisory Committee on Human Radiation Experiments 1995). Many clinical studies are carried out during diagnostic evaluation or initiation of treatment (Ockene et al. 1991). The context in which the investigator seeks informed consent may be unfamiliar to the patient (Hewlett 1996). The patient usually also has other concerns (e.g., the costs of medical care, lost work, and separation from family and friends). Competing concerns and painful emotions can limit a patient's attention to consent information, thereby compromising understanding. Acute decisional stress may explain why the potential risks of a procedure or study tend to be less well remembered than any other category of information (Bergler et al. 1980; Robinson and Merav 1976).

> Who would want, on the eve of surgery, after having disrupted one's life, gath-
> ered one's courage, and entered the hospital, to change one's mind? And thus
> who would want to pay attention to information that challenges the wisdom of
> the decision? (Faden and Beauchamp 1986, p. 325)

Investigators doing research involving acute exacerbations of illness usually must seek informed consent during stressful times. When an investigator seeks consent in stressful situations, it is important to use the methods discussed in the following sections (e.g., repeated presentation of the information, multiple methods of presentation, involvement of family, and feedback testing) to enhance patients' capacities to incorporate and weigh the information.

Information Overload

When questioned about the informed consent process, patients also complain that consent forms contain too much technical information that is difficult to read and understand (Advisory Committee on Human Radiation Experiments 1995). Only a limited amount of information can be retained in short-term memory long enough to relate it to old information and weigh it relative to the consent decision (Mozley et al. 1996).

> [T]he practice of adding detail to consent forms as a way of further informing
> potential subjects who often have a difficult time understanding risks, benefits,
> and purposes of research, is unacceptable; by confusing subjects, it offers less
> rather than greater protection. (Advisory Committee on Human Radiation Ex-
> periments 1995, p. 762)

It is important for investigators to realize that they are not required (Lidz et al. 1984), nor in most cases is it helpful, to communicate everything medically known about an illness, procedure, or intervention (Epstein and Lasagna 1969). Investigators are required to disclose only the information about a proposed study that a reasonable person in the patient's situation would consider material to a decision about whether to participate.

Because patients with severe psychiatric disorders have impairments of verbal memory (Grisso and Appelbaum 1995; Jones 1995; Olin and Olin 1975), communicating less information during the informed consent process may be better than communicating too much. Studies using the California Verbal Learning Test, which requires subjects to immediately recall 16 common words, have found that patients with schizophrenia can recall, on average, 5 words, whereas control subjects without psychiatric disorders can recall, on average, 10 words (Saykin et al. 1991). Therefore, patients with severe psychiatric disorders may do best with an informed consent process that provides them with about half as much information as control subjects without psychiatric disorders would be expected to remember; of course, this information must be thoughtfully selected and include the critical facts about the study.

It may help patients to meaningfully group the consent information by using a preamble, as suggested by Faden and Beauchamp (1986, p. 323):

> I am going to tell you about the purpose of the research, what your involvement would be like, the risks of participation, and then the benefits. First, the purpose of the study . . .

Informed Consent Takes Place Over Time

The process of obtaining information and the process of assimilating and understanding information are not instantaneous; these processes often occur over days, weeks, or even months (Lidz et al. 1988). As optimally implemented,

> Informed consent is an ongoing process of communication between researchers and the subjects of their research. It is not simply a signed consent form and does not end at the moment a prospective subject agrees to participate in a research project. (Advisory Committee on Human Radiation Experiments 1995, p. 181)

Patients with severe psychiatric illnesses frequently have reduced cognitive processing capacities (Gold et al. 1997), so that they are able to focus on only small amounts of information at one time. It is important that patients proceed through the informed consent process at their pace, not the investigator's (Dresser 1996). To attend to and process relevant information, most patients require that consent issues be covered slowly, with plenty of pauses and repetition. To prevent shortcutting of attention to consent information, the patient must believe that sufficient time is available to make an adequate decision (Faden and Beauchamp 1986).

Of course, studies of acute conditions cannot wait weeks or months to begin

(Ockene et al. 1991). Therefore, after a patient has provided initial consent to participate, the baseline and subsequent assessment visits and the implementation of study procedures should be used as opportunities to again explain what is being done and why (Dresser 1996).

Repeated presentation of information will especially benefit patients with limited processing capacities whose verbal learning abilities are intact. Although these patients may not retain much information the first time they are exposed to it, they may recall far more with repeated exposures (Grisso and Appelbaum 1995; Taub and Baker 1984).

Providing Consent Information via Multiple Methods

Some individuals understand spoken information better than written information, whereas others gain the most from written information. It may be best to present information in an oral form first and then later in a written form. When information is presented orally, more feedback can occur (e.g., through questions and puzzled looks) to indicate what patients understand or do not understand (Lidz et al. 1984). When information is presented in writing, consistency and completeness can be ensured, and patients can refer to the material when they wish.

It is not wise to present spoken and written information simultaneously. Because of the reduced cognitive processing capacities of some patients with severe psychiatric disorders, simultaneous spoken and written presentations may be overwhelming (Serper et al. 1990).

One way to communicate novel and specialized (e.g., medical) information to patients is to draw analogies (or, even better, to help the patient to draw analogies) between the novel information and ordinary events with which the patient is likely to be familiar (Faden and Beauchamp 1986).

Certain information can be conveyed better through pictures than through words. Pictures of equipment involved in diagnostic or assessment procedures (e.g., magnetic resonance imaging [MRI] scanners) may be more informative than verbal descriptions (Faden and Beauchamp 1986; Taub and Baker 1984). Simple diagrams that display the sequential flow of study activities may be helpful to some patients (see Figure 6–1). In addition, brief videotapes, such as those used to review safety procedures on commercial airliners, can ensure consistent and complete coverage of consent information (Dresser 1996).

Involvement of Patients' Families

Patients who have had to make informed consent decisions in stressful situations report that they often relied on family members to help process the information

Baseline	2 Weeks	4 Weeks	6 Weeks
Questionnaires	Questionnaires	Questionnaires	Questionnaires
Blood and urine samples	Blood and urine samples	Blood and urine samples	Blood and urine samples
MRI brain scan			MRI brain scan

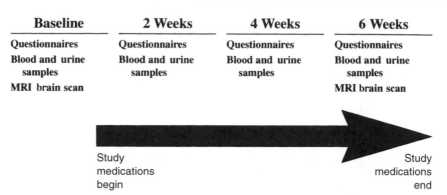

Study
medications
begin

Study
medications
end

FIGURE 6–1. Outline of study procedures. MRI = magnetic resonance imaging.

conveyed (Lidz et al. 1984). Family involvement provides a safeguard for patients who may be too overwhelmed to process new information adequately (Dresser 1996). A family member can review the pertinent features of the study with the patient at the patient's preferred pace, and the family member is also likely to know the medium through which the patient can best incorporate information (Gostin 1995). Paranoid patients may be better able to focus on the content of the information, with less distracting suspicion, when a family member is present.

Involving a family member (and documenting this involvement in the record) also safeguards the investigator from claims that the family was unaware that the patient was involved in the study or that the investigator took advantage of the patient when the patient could not adequately process the informed consent information.

Feedback Testing

> Professionals and subjects and patients cannot be assured that they have understood one another—especially in the case of persons already known to suffer problems of comprehension—without some form of checking. (Faden and Beauchamp 1986, p. 329)

Exchanges that test whether each party correctly understood what the other said must be used. The investigator can initiate the feedback discussion using a free-recall paradigm (asking patients to restate in their own words what they have just been told by the investigator) or a recognition paradigm (involving multiple-choice or true-false questions about the study) (Miller and Willner

1974; Robinson and Merav 1976). Gathering this information from the patient helps the investigator to see information areas that require repeating and more detailed explanation (Taub and Baker 1984). At repeated intervals during the provision of consent information, the investigator should offer the patient opportunities to question and clarify what the investigator has said.

CONTENT OF THE CONSENT INFORMATION

In 1981 the President's Commission for the Study of Ethical Problems in Medicine and Biomedical and Behavioral Research recommended specific rules for obtaining informed consent. Ten years later, these recommendations were mandated for federally funded research and research performed at institutions in which research is subject to a multiple project assurance (Federal Policy for the Protection of Human Subjects 1991; see Appendix 6–1). We review in this section the specific content areas mandated as basic elements of informed consent.

Statement That the Study Involves Research

Surveys of patients involved in clinical research reveal that these patients have only limited understanding of the systematic features of research design (e.g., random assignment to different treatments or to inactive placebo treatment) and how these design features may determine treatment decisions in their particular cases (Appelbaum et al. 1987). Patients may find it difficult to believe that clinical staff are not specifically guiding treatment toward individual patients' best interests in all circumstances (Lidz et al. 1984). Although when specifically asked, many patients involved in treatment research can distinguish procedures done for research purposes from clinical procedures, they report that they do not regularly make such distinctions between research and medical treatment (Advisory Committee on Human Radiation Experiments 1995).

To highlight that the investigator is inviting the patient to participate in research, an introductory statement such as

We are asking you to participate in a research study

may be helpful. It may also be helpful to begin paragraphs describing study procedures with statements similar to the following:

If you agree to participate in this research study, procedures A and B will take place.

Subtle shifts to statements about treatment or therapy should be avoided unless all patients will receive interventions of proven effectiveness—that is, no unproven interventions or placebo assignments are involved (Advisory Committee on Human Radiation Experiments 1995).

Consider the differences between the following introductory statements to an early phase II, placebo-controlled trial of a potential (efficacy not yet demonstrated) antidepressant. (The goals of early phase II trials include identifying conditions or symptoms that seem responsive to the drug and estimating the appropriate clinical dosage, dosage regimen, and duration of effect [Lasagna 1994].)

> We are asking you to help us in a study of new drug treatment for depression.

> We are asking you to participate in research to determine whether a new drug is helpful and safe for people with depression.

The latter statement more accurately reflects the actual situation and the purposes of the study.

On the other hand, investigators need not use language connoting a less well reasoned or more hazardous protocol than is actually the case. The obligation to ensure a patient's understanding that the study involves research permits communication of the care taken in crafting the project to protect participants and of the hoped-for gains in knowledge (Cassileth et al. 1982).

Explanation of the Purposes of the Research

Most clinical studies address a diagnostically restricted population. It may be reasonable to begin an explanation of the purposes of the research with a clear statement of the patient's diagnosis and some of the criteria used to reach it (Lidz et al. 1984):

> We are asking you to participate in this study because you have received a diagnosis of schizophrenia. Individuals with schizophrenia may hear voices when no one around them is talking, may be very suspicious, or may have difficulty organizing their thoughts.

The investigator may acknowledge that the research team will have to confirm the diagnosis and may wish to discuss the specific signs and symptoms suggesting the diagnosis in the particular patient's case.

Subsequently, the investigator lays out the specific purposes of the study in simple and parsimonious language, such as is found in both of the following statements:

> to find the highest dose of a new drug, X, that a person with a generalized anxiety disorder can take without uncomfortable side effects

> to find out whether a new drug, X, can decrease some of the symptoms of schizophrenia (voices, suspiciousness) and to discover what side effects the new drug has

If the investigator is doing the research as part of a larger study whose primary purpose is to gain knowledge for the sake of future patients (as in the example of the maximum tolerated dose study discussed earlier), with little, if any, likelihood of benefit to the present patient, these terms should be stated:

> *The results from this study will help to pick doses of the new drug, X, that seem to be helpful without uncomfortable side effects. Future studies will use these doses to find out whether X is really helpful for patients with generalized anxiety disorder.*

Statement About Expected Duration of Subject's Participation, Description of Procedures, and Identification of Experimental Procedures

The goal of this section of the consent process is to provide patients with a clear understanding of the time course and procedures involved in the study (i.e., "the realities of what it would be like to participate in the proposed research" [Advisory Committee on Human Radiation Experiments 1995, p. 701]). Key elements to cover in this section include the setting, duration, diagnostic and assessment procedures, and investigational and control interventions.

The major pitfalls to be avoided in this aspect of consent are excessive detail and highly technical language (Epstein and Lasagna 1969). Here, more than anywhere else in the consent process, simple visual aids such as pictures or flow diagrams can be helpful.

Setting

The investigator should make clear what portions of the study, if any, require inpatient status, as well as the frequency of visits to the outpatient clinic, research area, or other sites (e.g., imaging facility). Any planned visits by research staff to the patient's home are detailed here.

Duration

The investigator should state the overall duration of the study, including any baseline, lead-in period:

If you agree to participate, you will have to stay in the hospital for 10–13 days. During the first 3 of those days, we will do procedures A, B, and C to assess your illness. After that, you will start taking the study medication. The dose of study medication will increase from 1 pill/day to 4 pills/day over 6–7 days, if you do not experience any uncomfortable side effects. About 1 in 5 people report low blood pressure and feeling faint when starting the study medication. If that happens, it usually takes slightly longer (about 10 days) to reach the dose of 4 pills/day.

During the first month after you leave the hospital, we will ask you to return to the clinic once each week for a visit lasting approximately 1 hour. After that, we will ask you to return once each month for a 1-hour visit.

The total duration of the study, from when we begin until the final visit, will be 1 year.

In addition, the investigator should provide estimates of the duration of each assessment, intervention, or procedure required by the study:

The tests of your memory and attention span will take about 45 minutes.

Diagnostic and Assessment Procedures

Procedures to determine whether patients meet entry (inclusion/exclusion) criteria are clustered at the start of the study and may be done only once:

We must confirm your diagnosis of depression and be sure that you are not addicted to any drug of abuse (e.g., alcohol or cocaine). We will review your medical record and ask you a series of questions about psychiatric symptoms and addicting drugs. The interview will last about 45 minutes.

Other procedures may be done as repeated measures to determine whether change occurs over time:

We will draw a tube of blood from your arm on five occasions—once before you start the medication and again 7, 14, 21, and 28 days after you begin taking the medication—to check the level of the study medication in your blood.

If any diagnostic or assessment procedures are investigational, they should be described as such:

We will draw a tube of blood from your arm before you start medication and again 2 and 4 weeks after you start taking medication. We are investigating whether the level of a hormone (cortisol) in your blood changes during treatment.

If an assessment procedure uses complicated equipment that is difficult to describe (e.g., cerebral blood flow scanners), it may be more informative to show a picture of the equipment.

Interventions

The central thrust of many studies is a comparison between two or more treatments. The investigator often needs to discuss the presence of, and reason for, random assignment and blinding of the particular treatment the patient receives:

> *On four mornings in a row, you will wear a skin patch from 6:00 A.M. until 12:00 noon. There are four different skin patches. Each skin patch contains a dose of nicotine, 0 mg (placebo, no nicotine), 7 mg, 14 mg, or 21 mg. You will receive these four doses in random order (decided by chance, like rolling dice). Neither you nor the doctor rating your response to each patch will know what dose you receive on any given day so that you can report its effects without being biased.*

In other studies, the central question is the relative responsiveness of two different diagnostic groups of patients to a single, standardized intervention. Here the investigator can describe the intervention in a straightforward manner:

> *You will receive treatment with lithium. We will adjust the dose to produce lithium levels of 0.8–1.0 mEq/L in your blood. These levels produce the best treatment effect for most patients with a minimum of uncomfortable side effects.*

The investigator should clarify the experimental nature of any untested interventions:

> *We are studying the new medication, X, to find out whether it is helpful and safe for people with depression.*

Description of Any Reasonably Foreseeable Risks or Discomforts to the Subject

The investigator is obligated to tell patients, based on reasonable projections, chances that bad outcomes may ensue from research participation and what those possible bad outcomes are. In this section we discuss physical, psychological, and financial risks and review aspects of the presentation of these risks (i.e., detail in describing risks, presentation of probabilities, and framing of effects) that may influence how the risks are understood.

Physical Risks

It may help patients to understand and weigh risks if the risks are clustered under useful rubrics. Common side effects, even if minor (e.g., pain from venipuncture) should be listed, as well as uncommon side effects that are dangerous (e.g., agranulocytosis during clozapine treatment). Patients should also be told everything they can do to limit the risks:

> Most patients experience brief pain or pressure as the spinal needle goes in for the spinal tap. We will first inject a numbing medication into your skin to reduce the pain caused by the spinal needle. You may get a headache after the spinal tap (about 1 in 3 patients do), and the headache may be severe. Drinking lots of fluid and lying down in bed for an hour or more after the spinal tap can decrease the likelihood of a headache. Very rare (1 in 100 patients or fewer) but serious dangers include damage to a nerve by the spinal needle or infection in the spinal fluid.

It may be useful to tell patients how to identify unwanted side effects early and bring them to the staff's attention. They should also be informed of what procedures the staff will employ to identify side effects and intervene:

> The medication may cause your blood pressure to drop when you get up quickly. If you feel faint or your heart starts pounding when you get up from a sitting or lying position, please let the staff know right away. The staff will check your blood pressure lying down, and again standing, every day to catch this problem early if it occurs.

If patients are removed from their ongoing standard treatments, their condition may worsen, even if the ongoing treatments have only limited and unsatisfactory therapeutic efficacy (Appelbaum 1997). The investigator must warn patients of this possibility:

> Before we begin this study, we will gradually decrease and then stop your present medications. If the new medication does not help you or if you receive the placebo (inactive pill) your depression may worsen.

When the research involves new interventions that have been administered to only a limited number of normal volunteers or patients, the investigator may wish to include a statement that unexpected side effects may occur.

Psychological Risks

Common psychological reactions to diagnostic or interventive procedures include weariness from filling out long questionnaires and anxiety during stressful procedures (e.g., the enclosed space and noise of an MRI scanner). More distressing psychological reactions can occur in protocols designed to elicit and study such reactions:

> *You will see a movie with realistic war scenes. The action and sounds will be similar to what you experienced in combat. Some of the painful feelings and flashbacks that you have had since being in combat may resurface during the movie.*

The findings of a study may provoke psychological distress, especially if these findings confirm the presence of, or risk for, a serious illness:

> *The genetic test can tell whether you are at high, moderate, or low risk for developing Huntington's chorea as you grow older. If the test suggests that you have a moderate or high risk, you may become anxious or sad. Staff will be available to answer your questions and provide support. If you wish, we can also refer you for help with legal or financial planning or for treatment of anxiety or depression.*

Patients may have concerns about their performance on cognitive tests and should be reassured:

> *Some of these tests are very difficult. Most people do not get all of the answers right. Being tired, anxious, sad, or bored may make it harder to do the tests. If you have concerns about how you did, one of the research staff can discuss the tests with you after you have completed the study.*

Financial Risks

Any charges to the patient for participation in the study should be clearly detailed. Frequently, patients are charged for their routine care but not for research procedures:

> *There will be no charge to you for treatment, examinations, or tests done for research reasons. Treatments, examinations, or tests that are part of your routine medical care may be charged to you or your insurance company. We will tell you what is paid for by the study and what is not.*

Detail in Describing Risk

Detailing every remote risk will hinder, not help, informed consent: "such exhaustive treatment may serve only to overwhelm and numb patient-subjects" (Advisory Committee on Human Radiation Experiments 1995, p. 715).

The following example reflects excessive detail:

> *When used regularly at the doses required to treat high blood pressure, meca-mylamine may cause side effects of diarrhea, constipation, vomiting, nausea, loss of appetite, dizziness on standing, fainting, inflammation and fluid in the lungs, urinary retention, impotence, blurred vision, weakness, fatigue, sedation, tremor and numbness or prickling sensations, soreness of the tongue, and dry mouth. Rarely, intestinal blockage and convulsions may occur.*

This paragraph also demonstrates another problematic approach to informing patients about risks: "the risks are not summarized, and risks of particular relevance to the particular research project are not highlighted" (Advisory Committee on Human Radiation Experiments 1995, p. 715). The paragraph could be rewritten thus:

> *At the usual doses required to treat high blood pressure, mecamylamine may (in 1 in 10 patients) decrease your appetite, upset your stomach, or alter your bowel habits. More commonly (in 2 in 10 patients) you may feel faint if you stand up suddenly or feel tired. Less common side effects (in 1 in 100 patients) include impotence or fluid collecting in your lungs. Rare (in less than 1 in 1,000 patients) but serious side effects include convulsions or a blockage of your bowel.*

Presentation of Probabilities

Numeric expressions of probability that are a part of the language of the investigator may be meaningless to patients unfamiliar with such expressions. The investigator should strive for clear statements of incidence in simple terms. Faden and Beauchamp (1986, p. 322) contrast the following two examples in communicating risk:

> *The risk for (the problem) when having this surgery is between 0.2% and 0.3%.*

> *The risk for this problem is that out of every 1,000 patients who have this surgery, 2 to 3 will get (the problem) and 997 to 988 will not.*

The latter is more palpable, even for the numerically sophisticated.

Nonnumeric expressions of probability may also help in communicating risk. However, because different people have different definitions for *rare, uncommon, unlikely, infrequent,* and other such descriptors, these terms should not be used alone. Rather, they can be used in combination with a numeric description as in the second example given earlier.

Framing Effects

Patients' choices between risky alternatives can be strongly influenced by the way information is presented (Faden and Beauchamp 1986). The following two

examples present similar information. The first highlights the benefits of clozapine relative to the risks. The second highlights the risks of clozapine relative
to the benefits:

> *Out of 10 patients who take clozapine, 3 to 5 experience substantial relief from
> suspiciousness or painful voices that are not relieved by other drugs. In rare
> cases (1 in 100) clozapine may also cause a serious drop in the white cells
> in your blood. Very rarely (1 in 10,000) this condition has been fatal. We
> will monitor your white cell count weekly to detect this problem early if it
> occurs.*

> *Although clozapine may help your psychotic symptoms (voices or suspiciousness
> diminish in 3 to 5 of 10 patients who take clozapine), it also has a serious
> side effect. Approximately 1 in 100 patients who take clozapine experience
> a dangerous drop in the number of white cells in their blood. Although
> careful monitoring of white blood cell counts every week can detect most
> such cases early, some patients (approximately 1 in 10,000 who take clo-
> zapine) have died from this side effect.*

Faden and Beauchamp (1986, p. 321) recommend providing patients with
"*both sides* of the story—the half-full and half-empty presentations, the mortality and survival frames—in the hope of avoiding the gaps in understanding
that framing effects may produce."

> *Clozapine offers important benefits that other drugs for the treatment of schizo-
> phrenia cannot provide.*

> *However, clozapine has a serious side effect.*

A patient deciding whether to participate in treatment research with a potential
for substantial benefit as well as serious adverse outcomes will be in the best
position to make an informed decision if framing of effects is limited.

Description of Any Benefits That May Reasonably Be Expected From the Research

For most patients who participate in clinical research, the research procedures
are, in fact and in their minds, interwoven with routine clinical care. Psychiatric
patients, in particular, may show indifference to the particulars of which assessments or interventions represent clinical care and which are for research.
Investigators must be careful to avoid statements about benefits that cannot be
guaranteed from investigational interventions.

Many patients hold strong hopes that research interventions will offer
greater benefit than prior standard therapies (Daugherty et al. 1995; Penman et

al. 1984). Patients may agree to participate in research in the hope of gaining access to new agents available only in investigational trials (an especially important factor for patients who have failed treatment with conventional agents) or because they expect better staffing and closer attention in the research environment.

Actual Benefit

As a new pharmaceutical agent proceeds through development, more data become available on its potential benefits; these data can be cautiously summarized for the patient when discussing late phase II or phase III trials. (The goals of late phase II and phase III trials include demonstrating convincingly that therapeutic benefit can be derived from the compound and quantifying the comparative efficacy and side effect liability of the drug when comparing it with a placebo or standard treatment [Lasagna 1994].) However, in random assignment studies comparing the new agent with a standard treatment or placebo, access to the new agent cannot be guaranteed to the patient. Nevertheless, in some situations the investigator can guarantee access to the new agent in open label follow-up trials after the double-blind, random assignment phase is completed:

> About 550 patients have already participated in studies of the new medication, X. These studies suggest that X can decrease symptoms of schizophrenia (voices, suspiciousness) and that X causes less muscle stiffness, shaking, and restlessness than standard medications such as haloperidol.
>
> If you agree to participate in this study, you will receive one of three different doses of X, or haloperidol, or an inactive pill (placebo) for up to 4 weeks.

In essentially all phase I trials, and in many early phase II trials, efficacy is unproven, and it is disingenuous to speak in terms of treatment or therapy with these medications.

Altruism

A purpose of all research studies, and the only purpose of some, is to advance knowledge for the sake of future rather than present patients:

> Studies in animals suggest that the new medication, X, may diminish anxiety without causing sleepiness or dizziness. The purpose of this study is to identify the best dose range to test in people. The information from this study will help us to decide whether this new drug is helpful and safe for patients with anxiety. You may not be helped by participating in this study, but what is learned could help others.

When questioned, most patients report altruistic motives as one of the reasons they agree to participate in clinical studies (Cassileth et al. 1982). An investigator can honestly communicate his or her excitement about the importance of the study:

> This willingness of patients to be altruistic should be tapped explicitly when recruiting participants for research, since it might help to underscore for patients that the primary objective of research is to create generalizable scientific knowledge rather than to simply offer them a chance for some medical benefit. In the end it is only the benefit of furthering knowledge that can be honestly guaranteed to a potential research subject. (Advisory Committee on Human Radiation Experiments 1995, p. 749)

Inducements

In minimal risk studies, inducements (e.g., monetary reward) may be offered in the hope of increasing patient participation and effort. Faden and Beauchamp (1986) suggest two criteria for protecting informed consent when inducements are offered: 1) the inducement is welcomed and 2) it is of small enough value that it can be easily resisted.

> *We are comparing two questionnaires for rating how sad a person feels. Each questionnaire takes about 30 minutes to complete. If you agree to participate, we will pay you $5.00 to complete each of the questionnaires (total $10.00).*

Disclosure of Appropriate Alternative Procedures or Courses of Treatment

The disclosure of information, especially relating to alternative procedures that may be advantageous for the subject, can be a difficult area for investigators. Clinicians normally select the technically best treatment for a patient's condition (Lidz et al. 1984), and it is rare that two or more equally effective treatment alternatives are available for a given patient. Clinicians do not usually describe the alternatives they have already judged to be less preferable to patients, who have less training in how to select among alternatives.

Investigators must inform patients that they have the alternative of *not* participating in the study. This statement serves to remind both the investigator and the patient that informed consent is fundamentally an act of *authorization* by the patient for the investigator to include the patient in the study procedures (Faden and Beauchamp 1986).

The investigator should briefly review examples of the most commonly used standard treatments for the patient's condition, listing their relative benefits and risks:

> *You do not have to participate in this study. Other standard treatments are available to treat schizophrenia, including Haldol, Prolixin, Thorazine, and others. These standard medications have been proven to help patients with schizophrenia. However, they may cause stiffness, tremor, or restlessness.*

Statement Describing the Confidentiality of Records

The investigator must describe the specific procedures to be used to safeguard records and to avoid identifying personal details about patients when results are presented or published. This description should also include information about how confidential records will be maintained and note the possibility that the U.S. Food and Drug Administration (FDA) may inspect the records. It is important to clarify that certain individuals will have access to records (e.g., monitors from sponsoring organizations or the FDA) but that all of these individuals must sign confidentiality agreements:

> *We will store the information from this study in a locked file cabinet on a locked research wing. Staff from the pharmaceutical company that makes the new medication, X, and representatives of the U.S. Food and Drug Administration will have access to this information and to your medical record (including information containing your identity) to check the accuracy of the research files. All of these individuals have agreed to maintain patients' confidentiality. If we talk or write about the information from this study, we will not identify you in any way.*

Explanation About What Options Are Available If Injury Occurs

Individuals participating in research involving more than minimal risk should be informed about whether any compensation or medical treatments are available if they are injured in the course of the study. The investigator should describe the degree to which the research institution and the sponsoring organization will provide a safety net for patients who experience an untoward outcome related to participation in the study. Information should be provided about whom to contact in case of injury and available financial compensation for additional necessary care, lost wages, and so forth if a patient's condition deteriorates during the study (e.g., if the patient is assigned to placebo) or if a serious side effect occurs:

> *Dr. A, the investigator, and PPP, Inc., the sponsor of the study, will make every effort to prevent injury resulting from the study. There is no provision for free medical care or monetary compensation for any such injury from UUU University or HHH Hospital. If during the course of the study any injury should occur to you as a direct result of your taking the study drug, PPP, Inc., agrees to pay all medical expenses necessary to treat such injury. Reimbursement for things such as lost wages is not routinely available. You will not give up any legal right by signing this form.*

Attorneys for sponsoring organizations often participate in writing the paragraphs about compensation, which may result in language that is more complicated than would otherwise be used.

Explanation of Whom to Contact

Subjects should be given a listing of whom to contact in case of research-related injury or for answers to pertinent questions about the research and research subjects' rights. The investigators at the study site, as well as specific contact persons independent of the research program who are associated with the involved Human Subjects Committees, should be listed:

> *If you have questions about the study, please discuss them with your doctor. You may also contact the doctor in charge of the study, Dr. W, at 611-1111. If you are injured during the study, please call the UUU University Risk Management Office at 622-2222 or the HHH Hospital Research Office at 633-3333.*

Statement That Participation Is Voluntary

Potential subjects must be informed that participation is voluntary, that refusal to participate will involve no loss of benefits to which the subject is otherwise entitled, and that the subject may discontinue participation at any time without penalty or loss of benefits to which the subject is otherwise entitled. This final, repeated acknowledgment that the investigator seeks authorization from the patient is usually placed immediately above where the patient signs the consent form:

> *Participation in this study is voluntary. If you refuse to participate you will not lose any benefits to which you are entitled. If you agree to participate, you*

may stop participating at any time without losing any benefits to which you are entitled.

ADDITIONAL ELEMENTS OF INFORMED CONSENT

Federal policy also directs that, when appropriate, investigators should provide information about one or more of the following topics to potential participants.

Statement About Currently Unforeseeable Risks

Investigators should notify potential subjects that a particular treatment or procedure may involve risks to the subject (or to the embryo or fetus, if the subject is or may become pregnant) that are currently unforeseeable:

> *Because the new medication has been given to only about 500 people so far, there may be side effects that are not yet known.*

Description of Investigator-Initiated Termination of Subject Participation

A subject should be informed of any anticipated circumstances under which his or her participation may be terminated by the investigator without regard to the subject's consent:

> *You may be dropped from the study, without your consent, by your doctor or PPP, Inc., for failure to follow your doctor's instructions. If in your doctor's opinion you are not doing well, or your safety or well-being is in question, you will be dropped from the study. If this should happen, your doctor will ask that you have a final study evaluation consisting of all of the tests administered at the beginning of the study.*

Disclosure of Any Additional Costs to the Subject That May Result From Participation in the Research

> *You will have to come to the clinic twice each month over the next 6 months for research visits, which is more frequently than you would routinely come. You will have to pay the transportation costs.*

Statement About Consequences of and Procedures for Subject-Initiated Withdrawal From the Study

Situations in which information about consequences of early withdrawal is important include the use of treatments that, if discontinued abruptly, could be associated with withdrawal or rebound phenomena and situations in which the research staff have been the patient's primary caregivers:

> *You may withdraw from the study at any time. However, if one of the study medications (clonidine) is stopped suddenly, your blood pressure may rise rapidly. If you decide to withdraw, we will decrease your study medication gradually over 4–6 days before stopping it, and we will check your blood pressure carefully.*

Statement About Release of New Findings

Significant new findings developed during the course of the research that may relate to the subject's willingness to continue participation will be provided to the subject:

> *We will tell you and your doctor about any new findings that come from this research that might affect your willingness to participate in the study.*

Disclosure of Approximate Number of Subjects Involved in the Study

> *A total of 250 patients with depression will take part in this study.*

CONCLUSION

We have reviewed the specific content areas that must be covered during the informed consent process and suggested ways of communicating this information that will permit patients to successfully incorporate and use it.

In most cases, the investigator will better serve the intent of informed consent by selecting and highlighting a small number of important points particular to the study rather than scrupulously (but to little real purpose) going over every detail and possible eventuality. Both the investigator's time and the patient's time are valuable, and for simple studies of inconsequential risk the process of informed consent can be efficiently completed. As the demands and/ or risks of participation in a study increase, it becomes more important that approaches likely to enhance patients' understanding and capacity for reasoned choice be included in the consent process (e.g., offering adequate time and repeated presentations of information, involving family, feedback testing).

REFERENCES

Advisory Committee on Human Radiation Experiments: Final Report. Washington, DC, U.S. Government Printing Office, October 1995

Appelbaum PS: Rethinking the conduct of psychiatric research. Arch Gen Psychiatry 54:117–120, 1997

Appelbaum PS, Lidz CW, Meisel A: Informed Consent: Legal Theory and Clinical Practice. New York, Oxford University Press, 1987

Bergler JH, Pennington AC, Metcalfe M, et al: Informed consent: how much does the patient understand? Clin Pharmacol Ther 27:435–440, 1980

Bonnie RJ: Research with cognitively impaired subjects. Arch Gen Psychiatry 54:105–111, 1997

Cassileth BR, Lusk EJ, Miller DS, et al: Attitudes toward clinical trials among patients and the public. JAMA 248:968–970, 1982

Daugherty C, Ratain MJ, Grochowski E, et al: Perceptions of cancer patients and their physicians involved in phase I trials. J Clin Oncol 13:1062–1072, 1995

Delis DC, Kramer JH, Kaplan E, et al: California Verbal Learning Test, Research Edition. Cleveland, OH, Psychological Corp, 1983

Dresser R: Mentally disabled research subjects: the enduring policy issues. JAMA 276:67–72, 1996

Epstein LC, Lasagna L: Obtaining informed consent. Arch Intern Med 123:682–688, 1969

Faden RR, Beauchamp TL: A History and Theory of Informed Consent. New York, Oxford University Press, 1986

Federal Policy for the Protection of Human Subjects: Notices and Rules. Federal Register 56 (June 18, 1991):28002–28032

Flesch R: A new readability yardstick. J Appl Psychol 32:221–233, 1948

Fry E: A readability formula that saves time. Journal of Reading 11:513–516, 1968

Gold JM, Carpenter C, Randolph C, et al: Auditory working memory and Wisconsin Card Sorting Test performance in schizophrenia. Arch Gen Psychiatry 54:159–165, 1997

Gostin LO: Informed consent, cultural sensitivity, and respect for persons. JAMA 274:844–845, 1995

Grisso T, Appelbaum TS: The MacArthur Treatment Competence Study, III: abilities of patients to consent to psychiatric and medical treatments. Law and Human Behavior 19:149–174, 1995

Grundner TM: Two formulas for determining the readability of subject consent forms. Am Psychol 33:773–775, 1978

Grundner TM: On the readability of surgical consent forms. N Engl J Med 302:900–902, 1980

Hewlett S: Consent to clinical research: adequately voluntary or substantially influenced? J Med Ethics 22:232–237, 1996

Hirschfeld RMA, Winslade W, Krouse TL: Protecting subjects and fostering research. Arch Gen Psychiatry 54:121–123, 1997

Jones GH: Informed consent in chronic schizophrenia? Br J Psychiatry 167:565–568, 1995

Lasagna L: Decision processes in establishing the efficacy and safety of psychotropic agents, in Clinical Evaluation of Psychotropic Drugs: Principles and Guidelines. Edited by Prein RF, Robinson DS. New York, Raven, 1994, pp 13–28

Lidz CW, Meisel A, Zerubavel E, et al: Informed Consent: A Study of Decision Making in Psychiatry. New York, Guilford, 1984

Lidz CW, Appelbaum PS, Meisel A: Two models of implementing informed consent. Arch Intern Med 148:1385–1389, 1988

Miller R, Willner HS: The two-part consent form. N Engl J Med 290:964–966, 1974

Mozley LH, Gur RL, Gur RE, et al: Relationships between verbal memory performance and the cerebral distribution of fluorodeoxyglucose in patients with schizophrenia. Biol Psychiatry 40:443–451, 1996

Ockene IS, Miner J, Shannon TA, et al: The consent process in the Thrombolysis in Myocardial Infarction (TIMI–phase I) Trial. Clin Res 39:13–17, 1991

Olin GB, Olin HS: Informed consent in voluntary mental hospital admissions. Am J Psychiatry 132:938–941, 1975

Penman DT, Holland JC, Bahna GF, et al: Informed consent for investigational chemotherapy: patients' and physicians' perceptions. J Clin Oncol 2:849–855, 1984

President's Commission for the Study of Ethical Problems in Medicine and Biomedical and Behavioral Research: Protecting Human Subjects: The Adequacy and Uniformity of Federal Rules and Their Implementation. Washington, DC, U.S. Government Printing Office, 1981

Riecken HW, Ravich R: Informed consent to biomedical research in Veterans Administration hospitals. JAMA 248:344–348, 1982

Robinson G, Merav A: Informed consent: recall by patients tested post-operatively. Ann Thorac Surg 22:209–212, 1976

Saykin AJ, Gur RC, Gur RE, et al: Neuropsychological function in schizophrenia: selective impairment in memory and learning. Arch Gen Psychiatry 48:618–624, 1991

Serper MR, Bergman RI, Harvey PD: Medication may be required for the development of automatic information processing in schizophrenia. Psychiatry Res 32:281–288, 1990

Tankanow RM, Sweet BV, Weiskopt JA: Patients' perceived understanding of informed consent in investigational drug studies. Am J Hosp Pharm 49:633–635, 1992

Taub HA, Baker MT: A re-evaluation of informed consent in the elderly: a method for improving comprehension through direct testing. Clin Res 17–21, 1984

Federal Policy for the Protection of Human Subjects: Notices and Rules, 56 Federal Register 28002–28032; June 18 1991

50.25 Elements of informed consent.

   (a) **Basic elements of informed consent.** In seeking informed consent, the following information shall be provided to each subject:

      (1) A statement that the study involves research, an explanation of the purposes of the research and the expected duration of the subject's participation, a description of the procedures to be followed, and identification of any procedures which are experimental.

      (2) A description of any reasonably foreseeable risks or discomforts to the subject.

      (3) A description of any benefits to the subject or to others which may reasonably be expected from the research.

      (4) A disclosure of appropriate alternative procedures or courses of treatment, if any, that might be advantageous to the subject.

      (5) A statement describing the extent, if any, to which confidentiality of records identifying the subject will be maintained and that notes the possibility that the Food and Drug Administration may inspect the records.

      (6) For research involving more than minimal risk, an explanation as to whether any compensation and an explanation as to whether any medical treatments are available if injury occurs and, if so, what they consist of, or where further information may be obtained.

      (7) An explanation of whom to contact for answers to pertinent questions about the research and research subjects' rights, and whom to contact in the event of a research-related injury to the subject.

      (8) A statement that participation is voluntary, that refusal to participate will involve no penalty or loss of benefits to which the subject is otherwise entitled, and that the subject may discontinue participation at any time without penalty or loss of benefits to which the subject is otherwise entitled.

   (b) **Additional elements of informed consent.** When appropriate, one or more of the following elements of information shall also be provided to each subject:

      (1) A statement that the particular treatment or procedure may involve risks to the subject (or to the embryo or fetus if the subject is or may become pregnant) which are currently unforeseeable.

      (2) Anticipated circumstances under which the subject's participation may be terminated by the investigator without regard to the subject's consent.

      (3) Any additional costs to the subject that may result from participation in the research.

(4) The consequences of a subject's decision to withdraw from the research and procedures for orderly termination of participation by the subject.

(5) A statement that significant new findings developed during the course of the research which may relate to the subject's willingness to continue participation will be provided to the subject.

(6) The approximate number of subjects involved in the study.

(c) **The informed consent requirements in these regulations are not intended to preempt any applicable Federal, State, or local laws which require additional information to be disclosed for informed consent to be legally effective.**

(d) **Nothing in these regulations is intended to limit the authority of a physician to provide emergency medical care to the extent the physician is permitted to do so under applicable Federal, State, or local law.**

Tests for Determining the Reading Level of Consent Forms (Grundner 1978)

THE FLESCH READABILITY FORMULA (FLESCH 1948):

1. Collect three 100-word samples from important sections of the consent form (e.g., the purpose of study, procedures, and risk and benefit sections). If possible, start each sample at the beginning of a paragraph. Count contractions and hyphenated words as one word. Count numbers or letters separated by spaces as words.
2. Count the total syllables in each of the 100-word samples. Count the number of syllables in symbols and figures the way they are read aloud (e.g., 144 has seven syllables). Calculate the average number of syllables per 100 words, i.e., word length (WL).
3. Find the sentence that ends nearest the 100-word mark in each sample (this could be the 95th word or the 107th word). Count the number of sentences up to that point. Divide the number of words in those sentences by the number of sentences, and average this across the three samples to get the average sentence length (SL).
4. Insert the word length (WL) and sentence length (SL) terms into the following formula

$$RE \text{ (Reading ease)} = 206.835 - .846 \text{ WL} - 1.015 \text{ SL}$$

The result will be a number between 0 and 100. Lower figures represent more difficult reading, i.e., longer words and longer sentences. For example, scores of 0–30 represent very difficult reading as may be found in specialty scientific journals. Scores of 60–70 suggest that average adult reading abilities are required. Scores from 70 to 100 represent easier reading, with 90–100 at comic book level.

FRY READABILITY SCALE (FRY 1968):

1. Collect three 100-word samples as described above for the Flesch formula.
2. Count the total number of sentences in each 100-word sample, estimating to the nearest tenth of a sentence, and average these across the three samples.
3. Count the total number of syllables in each 100-word sample, and average these across the three samples.
4. On the graph shown below (Figure 6–2), plot the average number of syllables per 100 words along the X axis and the average number of sentences per 100 words along the Y axis. The approximate grade level equivalence can then be read off the curved line.

The point of the two tests can be summarized briefly: **shorter words and shorter sentences are usually associated with easier reading.**

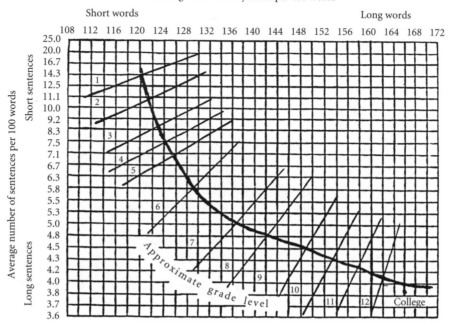

FIGURE 6–2. Graph for estimating readability (by Edward Fry, Rutgers University Reading Center). *Note.* The Readability Graph is not copyrighted. Anyone may reproduce it in any quantity, but the author and the editors would be pleased if this source were cited. *Source.* Fry E: "A Readability Formula That Saves Time." *Journal of Reading* 11:513–516, 1968.

Descriptions of Common Procedures

Venipuncture: We will draw _____ cc (_____ teaspoonsful) of blood by needle stick from a vein in your arm. This is momentarily painful. There is a small (1 in 10) chance of bruising (bleeding under the skin) or fainting. There is a very small chance of an infection (less than 1 in 100).

Intravenous Catheter: A small plastic tube (the catheter) will be inserted into a vein on your arm. There will be some pain as the needle containing the catheter goes through your skin and into the vein. The catheter will remain in your vein for _____ minutes/ hours. There is a small chance (1 in 10) of bruising (bleeding under the skin) where the catheter is inserted. There is a very small chance of an infection (less than 1 in 100).

Lumbar Puncture: See p. xx, this chapter.

Tryptophan Depletion: We are studying how serotonin, a naturally occurring chemical (amino acid), acts in the brain. If you agree to participate in this study, you will take two capsules and a chilled, chocolate-flavored drink. The capsules and drink contain many naturally occurring amino acids, but not the amino acid that becomes serotonin in your body. Taking the capsules and the drink lowers the amount of serotonin in your blood and brain for several hours.

Magnetic Resonance Imaging (MRI) Scan: The MRI scanning machine takes pictures of your brain without using x-rays. The scanner is shaped like a large box with a hole in one side. You lie on a bed that slides into that hole. You will have to lie still for 30–40 minutes for the scanning machine to take clear pictures. The scanning machine makes loud banging sounds as it is taking the pictures.

Positron Emission Tomography (PET) Scan: The PET scanning machine takes pictures of your brain that show how active each part of your brain is at the time. You will lie on a bed with your head inside a machine that looks like a large box. A doctor will inject a small amount of radioactive water into a vein in your arm. The machine will measure how much of this water travels in your blood to each part of your brain.

Pregnancy Exclusion Guidelines: FOR WOMEN WHO MAY BECOME PREGNANT: The medications (or other procedures, e.g., x-rays) used in this study may possibly be harmful to an unborn child. If you are pregnant or might become pregnant during the study, it is better that you not participate. We will draw a blood sample (two teaspoonsful from a vein in your arm) to check for pregnancy. To your knowledge, you are not pregnant at this time.

CHAPTER 7

Special Issues in Mental Health/Illness Research With Children and Adolescents

PETER S. JENSEN, M.D., CELIA B. FISHER, PH.D., AND
KIMBERLY HOAGWOOD, PH.D.

A s noted in the Institute of Medicine's *Research on Children and Adolescents With Mental, Behavioral, and Developmental Disorders* (1989), mental health research with children and adolescents has lagged behind research with adults. In part, this difference reflects difficulties in developing appropriate research methods and tools to study young populations. In addition, however, the research methods and tools for clinical investigation may pose unique ethical and safety concerns with children and adolescents, given their special circumstances. These factors have combined to limit research in this population, and as a result children have been described as "therapeutic orphans"—that is, less likely to reap the benefits of new knowledge on the safety and efficacy of various treatment alternatives. Recently, innovative research approaches and promising new tools that limit children's exposure to risk in the course of research have been developed, but progress is slow at best.

In this chapter we review special regulatory protections that apply to research on the mental disorders of children and adolescents, identify ethical challenges in the conduct of this research, and propose a way to address some of these challenges through reconceptualization of the relationships between investigators and families.

Research designed to describe, explain, and evaluate treatments for mental disorders in children and adolescents presents the possibility of both benefits and risks for participants. Ethical justification for the conduct of research therefore rests on demonstrating a favorable balance of risks to benefits for participating children, just as for adults. However, in research with children and adolescents, no risk is acceptable if the research does not have the potential to directly benefit the participant or enhance knowledge of the child's or adolescent's disorder or condition.

SPECIAL PROTECTIONS FOR CHILDREN INVOLVED IN RESEARCH

The federal guidelines for allowable research with pediatric populations, published in final form in 1983 by the Department of Health and Human Services (DHHS), were based principally on the work of the National Commission for the Protection of Human Subjects of Biomedical and Behavioral Research (1977). Recognizing the special vulnerability of child participants in human subjects research, these guidelines are designed to ensure that children's rights and welfare are protected, particularly when the research entails more than minimal risk. These guidelines, as described in the DHHS regulations 45 *Code of Federal Regulations [CFR]* 46, subpart D, are outlined in the following sections.

Minimal Risk Research

Research is considered minimal risk when "the probability and magnitude of harm or discomfort anticipated in the research are not greater in and of themselves than those ordinarily encountered in daily life or during the performance of routine physical or psychological examinations or tests" (Department of Health and Human Services 1991, 46.102[i]). Studies involving venipunctures and most psychological assessments routinely fit under this category. Often, one can further minimize risk by selecting the minimum levels of experimental manipulation necessary and, whenever possible, combining with procedures already being performed on subjects for diagnostic or treatment purposes.

Research Involving More Than Minimal Risk but Presenting the Prospect of Direct Benefit to an Individual Subject

When research involves more than minimal risk, investigators must justify the possible risks and associated discomforts in terms of the expected benefits to the child or to society as a whole. For example, in research involving an experimental drug with potential side effects, 45 *CFR* 46.405 requires the investigator to demonstrate that risks are justified by anticipated direct benefits to the participants, that the balance of these benefits and risks is at least as favorable to participants as that presented by available alternative approaches, and that adequate provisions are made for obtaining both the guardian's and the child's assent.

Research Involving More Than Minimal Risk With No Prospect of Direct Benefit to Individual Subjects but Likely to Yield Generalizable Knowledge About the Subject's Disorder or Condition

When research involving more than minimal risk holds no prospect of direct benefit to the child participants, an acceptable balance of risk and benefits must include the likelihood that the research will yield generalizable knowledge that is of vital importance for the understanding or amelioration of the subject's disorder or condition. In addition, the increased risk must represent only a *minor* increment over minimal risk, *and* the research risk must be reasonably commensurate with the risks inherent in situations the child would be expected to experience (such as biomedical tests consistent with the child's disorder or condition). Finally, adequate provisions must be made for obtaining both guardian consent and child assent (45 *CFR* 46.406).

Research Not Otherwise Approvable

Under exceptional circumstances, when research may provide understanding, prevention, or alleviation of a serious problem affecting the health or welfare of children, the secretary of DHHS may approve research not otherwise considered acceptable under the previously outlined regulations.

ETHICAL CHALLENGES IN PEDIATRIC RESEARCH

Minimal Risk

As noted by Kopelman (1989), the definition of minimal risk is "pivotal." Arnold et al. (1996) have suggested that some institutional review boards (IRBs) seem to interpret minimal risk as *no* risk. If *minimal risk* means that the risks of harm anticipated in the proposed research are no greater than those ordinarily encountered in daily life or during routine physical or psychological examinations or tests, then this definition implies that the everyday risks that parents and society routinely approve for children, such as bike riding or riding in a car, and even seasonally limited but otherwise daily activities such as swimming or skiing, must be taken into consideration. But opinions can be divided about this issue. Kopelman (1989, p. 92) points out that the phrase "ordinarily encountered in daily life" can be variously interpreted as "all the risks ordinary people encounter, or the risks all people ordinarily encounter, or the minimal risks all ordinary people ordinarily encounter." Because risk can be interpreted in divergent ways and no single viewpoint is acceptable in all cases, IRBs should be careful not to be too restrictive. Such restrictiveness can create unnecessary obstacles to children's participation in research. An approach to refining the concept of minimal risk has been offered by Arnold et al. (1996), who suggest differentiating between risk and aversiveness. A procedure can have associated risks without being aversive or uncomfortable; conversely, a procedure can be aversive without entailing any meaningful risks. For example, Kruesi et al. (1988) have found spinal taps to be no more aversive to children than attending school. Several authors (e.g., Castellanos et al 1994; Jay et al 1982) have noted that the psychological risk of aversiveness can be minimized by preliminary rehearsal and role-playing, such that in a well-run research protocol psychological risk and aversiveness tend to be minimal. Judgments concerning the appropriate balance of risks and benefits when using invasive biomedical procedures in pediatric research are frequently difficult. These judgments become even more problematic when biomedical procedures are employed in studies of normal pediatric populations; in such instances, controversy about the definitions of minimal risk is common, and opinions often vary across IRBs.

Confidentiality

Research on children and adolescents with mental disorders often elicits sensitive information that an individual may not have previously revealed to others or that could produce risk or harm if known beyond the research setting. Once a participant or his or her guardian has agreed to share personal information with a research team, investigators are obligated to ensure that the information is not divulged to others in a manner inconsistent with the participant's understanding of the original agreement. Routine procedures for maintaining confidentiality may not be sufficient for researchers investigating especially sensitive or potentially stigmatizing information such as drug or alcohol abuse, HIV infection, or illegal behaviors. Although special provisions are available to protect the confidentiality of patients divulging sensitive information, research situations may arise in which maintenance of confidentiality cannot be guaranteed. In general, such limitations on confidentiality should be noted in the consent form.

The Certificate of Confidentiality

When individual identifiers are required during the conduct of sensitive research (i.e., therapeutic or longitudinal research), routine procedures for assuring confidentiality may be insufficient to protect the participant from harmful disclosures. For example, data collected on violent behavior, substance abuse, or even parenting behaviors of individuals with mental disorders may be subject to subpoena stemming from criminal investigations or custody disputes. In these circumstances an investigator conducting biomedical, behavioral, clinical, or other research can apply for a certificate of confidentiality under section 301[d] of the Public Health Service Act. The certificate provides the investigator immunity from any governmental or civil order to disclose identifying information contained in research records. The certificate is granted when data to be obtained in a study involve sensitive information that if released could result in stigmatization, discrimination, or legal action or could damage an individual's financial standing, employability, or reputation (Hoagwood 1994).

The certificate does not, however, override state reporting laws on child abuse. Therefore, investigators should always consult appropriate state laws (see discussion about disclosure in the following section). The certificate can protect the confidentiality of information about past abuse divulged by research subjects, but it does not mitigate the researcher's requirement to disclose minor children's data to their parents; such protection can be ensured only through permission by the parent or guardian at the time of informed consent (Hoagwood 1994). When an investigator is granted a certificate, both the protections and the limitations of protection should be explained to child and adolescent participants and their parents.

Disclosures

Investigators studying mental disorders of childhood and youth may, during the course of research, become privy to information suggesting child abuse or threats of harm or violence to the participant or identified others. Following the 1976 Child Abuse Prevention and Treatment Act, all 50 states enacted statutes mandating the reporting of suspected child abuse or neglect. In all states, this law pertains to mental health professionals and in at least 13 states it pertains to researchers, as well as members of the general citizenry (Liss 1994).

Other states vary as to whether researchers are included in mandated reporting statutes. Thus, investigators need to review their own state laws to determine whether they or members of their research team are obligated to report child abuse and neglect (Fisher 1991, 1993; Liss 1994). At present, it is not clear whether researchers are legally required to release to authorities research records pertinent to the abuse after it is reported, and there are case examples of investigators withholding and releasing such records. However, once reporting obligations are determined, the principal investigator must ensure that research personnel are trained to recognize indicators of abuse and to follow appropriate procedures. Such obligations should be fully communicated to both parents and minor participants at the time of obtaining informed consent (Fisher 1993). Investigators may also choose not to ask specific questions about child abuse in situations in which the obligation to report such information might place the participant in greater social or physical risk.

Protecting Participants From Self-Harm

In the course of research, investigators interviewing or administering standardized tests to high-risk children and youth or those with disorders may come upon information suggesting that a minor is contemplating suicide. Investigators need to prepare for such circumstances by establishing specific criteria and procedures to be followed if research personnel suspect the possibility of self-harm. Participants and their guardians should be informed about these procedures before giving permission to participate, and investigators must be prepared to veto a child or adolescent's request that information not be released.

Protecting Third Parties From Harm

An issue particularly relevant to scientists who study family violence or delinquency is whether researchers share with practitioners the responsibility to protect third parties from dangers posed by patients (Fisher 1993). Investigators should examine whether their role in research meets requirements for a duty to protect as outlined by *Tarasoff v. Regents of the University of California* (1976): 1) a "special relationship" with a participant, 2) the ability to predict that violence will occur, and 3) the ability to identify the potential victim (Appelbaum and Rosenbaum 1989). The presenting problems of some research participants (e.g., pedophiles) require advanced planning to protect both the rights of the participants and the welfare of the community (Monahan et al. 1993). In recent years the obligation to protect identifiable third parties from potential harm caused by the unsafe sex practices of an HIV-positive research participant has been debated. Investigators should approach such a situation with extreme caution, taking into account the fact that some state laws prohibit certain licensed professionals from revealing a client's HIV status.

Parental/Guardian Consent

Consent procedures for children and adolescents require special consideration for several reasons. Children do not have the legal capacity to consent and, depending on the age of the child and the complexity of the research, may lack the cognitive capacity to comprehend the purpose, scope, or nature of the study (Fisher 1993; Melton et al. 1983; Thompson 1992). Children may also feel themselves incapable of refusing participation (Fisher and Rosendahl 1990; Koocher and Keith-Spiegel 1990; Levine 1986). Thus, to ensure that the rights of minors are protected, federal regulations require that adequate provisions be made for soliciting the consent of parents, legal guardians, or those who act *in loco parentis.* According to federal regulation 46.408[b], the permission of one parent is sufficient for minimal risk research or research involving more than minimal risk but presenting the prospect of direct benefit to the individual subject. Permission of both parents, where feasible, must be sought for research involving greater than minimal risk with no prospect of direct benefit and for research not otherwise approvable. Investigators working with children who are in the custody of state agencies may encounter practical difficulties in determining guardianship.

Child Assent

In addition to parental/guardian consent, the rights of minors are further protected through the requirement that adequate provisions be made for soliciting the assent of the child, when he or she is capable (45 *CFR* 46.408[a]). *Assent* assumes that a child has the requisite cognitive capacity and emotional maturity to understand the nature of the research and its risks and benefits and agrees to participate. Responsibility for determination of whether a child is capable of giving assent rests with the local IRB. Research with a very young child deemed not capable of providing assent may proceed with parental consent alone. However, the objection of a child of any age is binding, unless the research holds out the prospect of direct benefit that is important to the child and achievable only through the experimental procedures. In designing assent procedures, investigators need to take into account the child's maturity, cognitive abilities, and unique strengths and vulnerabilities, as well as the context (i.e., parent/ caretaker and child relationship) in which decision making will take place.

The informed consent procedures currently required by federal regulations and professional ethical codes are designed to protect participant autonomy by ensuring that the decision to participate is informed, rational, and voluntary. The investigator is obligated to fully disclose information about all procedures that might influence an individual's willingness to participate in a study. According to 45 *CFR* 46.116, such information must include the following: 1) an explanation of the purpose and duration of the research and a description of the procedures; 2) a description of any foreseeable risks or discomforts; 3) a description of potential benefits to the participant or others; 4) disclosure of alternative procedures or treatments that may be advantageous to the subject; 5) a description of the extent and limits of confidentiality; 6) for research involving more than minimal risk, information on compensation and the availability and nature of treatment if injury occurs; and 7) a statement describing the voluntary nature of the research and the right to refuse participation or withdraw from the study at any time without penalty. A further requirement of informed consent is that the information be presented in a manner that is appropriate to the language usage and comprehension level of the potential participant and/or his or her guardian (Office for Protection From Research Risks 1993).

In most cases federal guidelines require that informed consent be documented. However, under certain circumstances, such as when data are gathered from administrative records and no identifying information is transmitted, this requirement may be waived (45 *CFR* 46.117[c][1]). In cases in which the information to be gathered is sensitive, and reporting the information to authorities is legally mandated, subjects should be so informed before agreeing to participate in the study (Office for Protection From Research Risks 1993). The Office for Protection From Research Risks considers research in sensitive areas to include child abuse, illegal activities, and reportable communicable diseases.

Child Assent in the Absence of Parental Consent

Significant numbers of children and adolescents with mental disorders or at high risk for disorders have undetermined custody, nonrelative guardians, or state guardianship (Gibbs 1990; Hendren 1991). In addition, the adverse physical or social environments in which some children live may make obtaining parental consent difficult or dangerous for the child. Federal regulations provide guidelines to help investigators and IRBs determine the conditions under which requiring parental consent does not reasonably protect the welfare of minor research participants (45 *CFR* 46.408[c]). Children from neglecting or abusing families may be included in this category. In other types of research (e.g., studies on adolescent sexual activity or substance abuse), the solicitation of parental consent may violate a teenager's privacy or even jeopardize his or her welfare. Current state laws granting adolescents the autonomy to make decisions concerning treatment for venereal disease, drug abuse, or emotional disorders have been used as a model to determine the conditions under which guardian consent may be waived (Fisher 1993; Holder 1981).

In other situations, parental consent may be waived when the research cannot be practically carried out without a waiver. However, despite the availability of a waiver, respect for the importance of family involvement in children's lives dictates that (in addition to child assent procedures) parental notification be offered as both a courtesy and a mechanism for providing additional information (45 *CFR* 46.115[d]; Nolan 1992).

The Voluntary Nature of Consent

Families contacted while seeking services at a hospital, mental health center, or social service agency may be concerned that failure to consent will result in a loss of services for themselves or their children (Fisher 1991, 1993; Fisher and Rosendahl 1990) or that they may lose custody of their children altogether (Friesen and Koroloff 1990; Osher and Telesford 1996). Therefore, investigators studying children with mental disorders must be particularly sensitive to the potentially coercive nature of informed consent procedures. Investigators also need to guard against potential conflicts of interest that may restrict the perceived voluntary nature of participation. For example, in the United States, few services are available to treat children and adolescents (or adults) with mental disorders. As a rule, resources are sparse, and insurance companies and third-party payers have restricted access to the full range of mental health services thought necessary for adequate treatment for many conditions. In this context, parents may feel a great sense of urgency about obtaining care for their children. A university-based research program may appear to be a godsend, alleviating families' anxiety and concern about helping their children. They may be subject to the therapeutic misconception, the perception that their children's participation in the research will increase access to active and effective treatments. Yet given our current lack of knowledge concerning clinical treatments of many child and adolescent mental disorders, placebo treatments or other alternatives are critical in most if not all circumstances. Thus, families may be severely disappointed if active treatment is not included as a part of their children's participation in a research program.

Informed consent should be conceptualized as an ongoing educational process between the investigator and prospective participant. Consent should be monitored and discussed throughout the course of the study. This guideline is particularly relevant for longitudinal studies when the child's cognitive understanding and personal autonomy are increasing, when the nature of the assessment instruments may be modified to fit the changing developmental status of participants, and when issues of confidentiality may shift as a child participant reaches adolescence.

Passive Consent

Difficulties in acquiring guardian consent are not sufficient to waive the requirement for obtaining it simply as a means of overcoming low rates of parental response. In general, passive consent (when guardians are sent forms asking them to respond only if they do *not* wish their child to participate) should not be regarded as an ethical substitute for guardian consent, because this tactic does not meet the standards set by the principles of beneficence, respect for persons, and justice (Fisher 1993). The use of passive consent procedures with vulnerable, poor, and disenfranchised populations poses special ethical problems because it can create an unjust situation in which vulnerable children are deprived of the protections afforded by guardian consent more often than their less vulnerable peers.

Participant Advocates

When parental consent is waived or when children or adolescents are wards of the state, federal regulations (45 *CFR* 46) require that an advocate for the minor be present to 1) verify the minor's understanding of assent procedures, 2) support his or her preferences, 3) ensure that participation is voluntary, 4) check periodically to determine whether the youth wants to terminate participation, 5) assess reactions to planned procedures, and 6) ensure that debriefing addresses all participant questions and concerns (Office for Protection From Research Risks 1993). The participant advocate should have no investment in the research project or role in subject recruitment (Fisher 1993).

Incentives for Participation

Offering incentives for participation is often used as a means of recruiting subjects. The decision to offer inducements creates an ethical tension between fair compensation for the time and inconvenience of research participation and undue coercion to participate in procedures to which subjects might not otherwise consent. Investigators must be particularly cautious when deciding on appropriate inducements for impoverished persons, who may be willing to assume, or have their children assume, extraordinary burdens to receive payment (Levine 1986). Subject payments should reflect the degree of risk, inconvenience, or discomfort associated with participation (Office for Protection From Research Risks 1993). However, there is little consensus on what constitutes due and undue incentives for research participation (Macklin 1981).

Ensuring Fair Representation and Access to Research Benefits

Investigators working with diverse or disadvantaged populations have the responsibility to ensure that 1) minority and lower-socioeconomic populations have equal access to research benefits and 2) they are not exposed to unfair distribution of research risks because of their vulnerability. These responsibilities present special challenges to investigators assessing mental health services for children and adolescents, because there may be serious questions about the validity of existing measures to identify psychopathology in different populations. In such situations, investigators run the risk of under- or overdiagnosing children from minority and poor communities. As a result of diagnostic errors, minority and poor children may be unfairly excluded from potentially advantageous treatment studies or unfairly overrepresented in research, such as drug studies, which present more than minimal risk. Recruitment strategies for diverse populations can be enhanced through the establishment of advisory committees made up of minority representatives from the community and the mental health professions. The appropriateness of research inclusion and exclusion criteria and assessment approaches can be additionally enhanced by ensuring that such methods meet the highest standards for ecological and cultural validity.

ADDITIONAL CONSIDERATIONS IN PEDIATRIC RESEARCH

Technically, most of the requirements described previously apply only to research supported by DHHS, but the requirement that any proposed study be reviewed by an IRB to receive federal funding, as well as IRB review of all research at most institutions, essentially brings all research under the purview of these regulations. Above and beyond the formal requirements established for federally supported research, two other significant factors should be considered by all parties participating in mental health research with children and adolescents. The first of these issues is the effect of stigma on IRB members' assumptions and behavior, and the second is the need to reconceptualize the relationship between investigators and research participants as one guided not by procedures but by an ethical compact.

The Effect of Stigma on Child and Adolescent Mental Health Research

In our view, investigators and IRB members frequently hold subtle yet stigmatizing opinions and attitudes toward research participants who may be at risk for, or are afflicted by, a mental disorder. Too often, the presumption of incompetence seems to shape the views of investigators and IRB members. Thus, investigators and IRB members may feel the need to go to greater than usual lengths to protect the child with a mental disorder or disablement. This presumption of incompetence stems from the unsupported belief that emotional, behavioral, and developmental disorders impair persons' ability to comprehend information and meaningfully evaluate the risk-benefit ratio. However, no empirical evidence suggests that children with behavioral and emotional disorders (apart from those that frequently affect cognition, such as pervasive developmental disorders and autism) are less able than their age-matched counterparts to evaluate and participate in the assent process in research.

The presumption of incompetence also extends to the parents of children with such disorders, who are considered unable to evaluate research participation with regard to the best interests of their children, such that their children require greater than usual protection (e.g., a consent auditor or parent monitor) during the course of the research. The stigmatization of parents of children with mental disorders is based in part on unsupported biases concerning the ability of at-risk or distressed persons to give fully informed consent and in part on the historical assumption that parents cause their children's mental disorder. That parents of children with mental disorders are incompetent to provide rational and fully informed consent has not been demonstrated.

Stigma also affects investigators' and IRB members' assumptions about the kinds of questions and procedures to which children may be safely exposed in the course of research. For example, no evidence has demonstrated that asking children about suicidal feelings increases the likelihood of such feelings or gives a child passive permission to act out suicidal impulses; indeed, clinical experience suggests just the opposite, yet many IRBs assume that such questions may be dangerous or lead to untoward consequences. In fact, asking children and families such personal, highly confidential questions is acceptable for the vast majority of participating subjects and families (Lahey et al. 1996). In our experience, ongoing education and consultation are needed for IRB members to render knowledgeable and sophisticated judgments concerning the balance of risks and benefits of research for pediatric participants.

The Ethical Compact Between Investigators and Research Participants

In the deepest sense, a full and consensual understanding of the nature of the research and its potential risks and benefits must be shared between investigators and research participants. This shared understanding should form the basis of an *ethical compact* between the investigator and the participant, and the information sharing process should be one of candor, respect, and mutual trust. An ethical compact requires that the clinical investigator be aware of and fully communicate to prospective participants and their guardians his or her potential for conflicts of interest in the dual roles of a scientist embarked on a quest for knowledge and a clinician bound to work solely on behalf of the patient. The clinical investigator must be aware of this conflict of interest, which is inherent in therapeutic research, and recognize that his or her actions are shaped by two competing value systems. Full awareness of this conflict of interest is essential for trust between investigators and research participants. Honest communication at the initial stages of a research partnership can serve as a basis for a mutually respectful relationship, which can in turn enhance the ethical compact by overriding what in many instances may appear to be unequal power relationships.

Mutuality, candor, and shared participation in the research process are critical for maintaining the public's trust and goodwill toward the goal of advancing science for the benefit of all. Clearly, this ethical compact requires more than a single consent form signed under limited or less than optimal conditions. A research partnership bound by an ethical compact begins with the initial consent procedures, continues through the duration of the research, and ends with a thoughtful debriefing and a shared, final examination of the entire process. The process should be mutually and gladly undertaken by the investigator and the research participants. Thus, in the conduct of research, investigators should not just aim for IRB approval but try to reach a higher standard through a plan to address human subjects issues that considers all possible ramifications of the research enterprise, embedded in ethical principles and built on systematic efforts to increase trust in the investigator-participant relationship. Although IRBs cannot fully anticipate every eventuality that may arise during the course of research, if the investigator grasps the essential nature of the ethical compact, he or she can make appropriate adjustments at critical points of the study, ensuring that families' confidence in the research and the researcher increase during their mutual collaboration. Although systematic approaches to addressing these issues (e.g., data safety and monitoring boards and ongoing reviews of side effects and treatment outcomes during the course of clinical trials) have been developed, such formal mechanisms cannot replace the investigator's own concern for research participants' well-being and the active communication of this concern in interactions with families.

FUTURE RECOMMENDATIONS

We believe that increased efforts are needed to strengthen the links between investigators, IRBs, families, and communities. In the final analysis, the highest ethical standard cannot be obtained simply by an elegant, well-written, and explicit consent form. Although such consent statements are to be emulated whenever possible, they fall well short of an ethical standard that seeks to involve members of the larger community of citizens as research participants and collaborators in the goals of science and research. Although science should ultimately benefit the larger community, all too often investigators note that their research findings are not incorporated into current understandings and do not change the standards of practice. Upon reflection, this situation is not entirely surprising: the terms used to delineate the research questions and aims of research are often very different from the policy objectives of program planners or the more personal concerns of parents and families who are dealing with the immediate effects of a family member who has a disabling disorder.

To address these difficulties in research dissemination, members of the communities whom the research is intended to benefit must increasingly be a part of the early identification of research questions, determination of research procedures, selection of domains for assessment and specific terminologies, and dissemination of research findings. This action perspective more closely joins the interests of scientists, research participants, and the larger community and seems to us ethical in the deepest sense. Such an approach offers a comprehensive means of strengthening collaborations between scientists and research participants, engendering trust, developing relevant research that is well received by communities, and enhancing effective research dissemination. Such partnerships between scientists and the citizenry could yield a number of important benefits, including the development of consensus on levels of acceptable risk, the cultivation of a common will to address critical research gaps (particularly in the area of children and adolescents), and the reaffirmation of the importance of science in improving the lives of all citizens.

Given concerns about younger children's understanding of research procedures, investigators must pay great attention to engaging participants in the research enterprise. Such engagement entails creative and sustained attention to the process of obtaining and continuing informed consent, to developmental issues, and to therapeutic comprehensiveness. For example, investigators may want to use systematic staged consent, particularly if consent procedures are long or complex or the research procedures take place over a long period. In the area of therapeutic research, investigators need to consider using developmentally sensitive, yet scientifically sensible, designs. Given the nature of children's development and their needs over time and across multiple settings and contexts, children with an emotional or behavior disorder may require more comprehensive treatment approaches than simple placebo-controlled, double-masked designs can offer. Studies that involve comprehensive treatment strategies are likely to be more acceptable to families, offer a better basis for trust and shared commitment to the research process, and provide more sensible and generalizable findings to inform public policy and health practices.

Research with children poses special challenges in the areas of balancing risks and benefits, maintaining appropriate confidentiality, and ensuring developmentally sensitive child assent and parental consent. In part because of these challenges, children run the risk of becoming "therapeutic orphans," deprived of the benefits of medical research as a class of citizens. To illustrate, 80% of all medications approved for marketing in the United States have not been tested for safety and efficacy in children (Jensen et al. 1994). In many instances, novel strategies and special arrangements can be made to enable appropriate research with pediatric age groups (e.g., see Hoagwood et al. 1996). In our view, however, substantial progress will be possible only by increasing dialogue and building more effective coalitions among families, investigators, IRBs, policy makers, and the general public. Research cannot and should not be the province of science and scientists alone. Science, in the public trust and on behalf of the public health, is the province of us all.

REFERENCES

Appelbaum PD, Rosenbaum A: Tarasoff and the researcher: does the duty to protect apply in the research setting? Am Psychol 44:885–894, 1989

Arnold LEA, Stoff D, Cook E, et al: Biologic procedures: ethical issues in research with children and adolescents, in Ethical Issues in Mental Health Research With Children and Adolescents. Edited by Hoagwood K, Jensen PS, Fisher C. Hillsdale, NJ, Erlbaum, 1996, pp 89–111

Castellanos FX, Elia J, Kruesi MJP, et al: Cerebrospinal fluid monoamine metabolites in ADHD boys. Psychiatry Res 52:305–316, 1994

Department of Health and Human Services: Protection of human subjects: research involving children. Federal Register 48 (March 8, 1983):9814–9820

Department of Health and Human Services: OPRR reports: protection of human subjects. Federal Register 46 (June 18, 1991):1–17

Fisher CB: Ethical considerations for research on psychosocial interventions for high-risk infants and children, in Psychological Practice: Marketing, Legal, Ethical, and Current Professional Issues. Washington, DC, National Register, 1991, pp 92–94

Fisher CB: Integrating science and ethics in research with high-risk children and youth. Society for Research and Development Social Policy Report 7:1–27, 1993

Fisher CB, Rosendahl SA: Emerging ethical issues in an emerging field, in Annual Advances in Applied Developmental Psychology, Vol 4. Edited by Fisher CB, Tryon WW. Norwood, NJ, Ablex, 1990, pp 43–60

Friesen BJ, Koroloff NM: Family-centered services: implications for mental health administration and research. Journal of Mental Health Administration 17:13–25, 1990

Gibbs JT: Mental health issues of black adolescents: implications for policy and practice, in Ethnic Issues in Adolescent Mental Health. Edited by Stiffman AR, Davis LE. Newbury Park, CA, Sage, 1990, pp 21–52

Hendren RL: Determining the need for inpatient treatment, in Psychiatric Inpatient Care of Children and Adolescents: A Multi-Cultural Approach. Edited by Hendren RL, Berlin IN. New York, Wiley, 1991, pp 37–64

Hoagwood K: The certificate of confidentiality at NIMH: applications and implications for service research with children. Ethics and Behavior 4:123–131, 1994

Hoagwood K, Jensen P, Fisher C (eds): Ethical Issues in Mental Health Research With Children and Adolescents: A Casebook and Guide. Hillsdale, NJ, Erlbaum, 1996

Holder AR: Can teenagers participate in research without parental consent? IRB: Review of Human Subjects Research 3:5–7, 1981

Institute of Medicine: Research on children and adolescents with mental, behavioral, and developmental disorders (Publ No IOM-89-07). Washington, DC, National Academy Press, 1989

Jay SM, Elliot CH, Ozolins M, et al: Behavioral management of children's distress during painful medical procedures. Behav Res Ther 23:513–520, 1982

Jensen PS, Vitiello B, Leonard H, et al: Child and adolescent psychopharmacology: expanding the research base. Psychopharmacol Bull 30:3–8, 1994

Koocher GP, Keith-Spiegel PC: Children, Ethics, and the Law: Professional Issues and Cases. Lincoln, NE, University of Nebraska Press, 1990

Kopelman LM: When is the risk minimal enough for children to be research subjects? in Children and Health Care: Moral and Social Issues. Edited by Kopelman LM, Moskop JC. Boston, MA, Kluwer, 1989, pp 89–99

Kruesi MJP, Swedo SE, Coffey ML, et al: Objective and subjective side effects of research lumbar punctures in children and adolescents. Psychiatry Res 25:59–63, 1988

Lahey B, Flagg E, Bird H, et al: The NIMH Methods for the Epidemiology of Child and Adolescent Mental Disorders (MECA) study: background and methodology. J Am Acad Child Adolesc Psychiatry 35:855–864, 1996

Levine R: Ethics and Regulation of Clinical Research, 2nd Edition. Munich, Urban & Schwarzenberg, 1986

Liss M: State and federal laws governing reporting for researchers. Ethics and Behavior 4:133–146, 1994

Macklin R: "Due" and "undue" inducements: on paying money to research subjects. IRB: Review of Human Subjects Research 3:1–6, 1981

Melton GB, Koocher GP, Saks MJ: Children's Competence to Consent. New York, Plenum, 1983

Monahan J, Appelbaum PS, Mulvey EP, et al: Ethical and legal duties in conducting research on violence: lessons from the MacArthur Risk Assessment Study. Violence Vict 8:387–396, 1993

National Commission for the Protection of Human Subjects of Biomedical and Behavioral Research Involving Children: Report and recommendations (DHEW Publ No OS-77-0005). Washington, DC, U.S. Government Printing Office, 1977

Nolan K: Assent, consent, and behavioral research with adolescents. AACAP Child and Adolescent Research Notes, Summer 1992, pp 7–10

Office for Protection From Research Risks, Department of Health and Human Services, National Institutes of Health: Protecting Human Research Subjects: Institutional Review Board Guidebook. Washington, DC, U.S. Government Printing Office, 1993

Osher TW, Telesford M: Involving families to improve research, in Ethical Issues in Mental Health Research With Children and Adolescents. Edited by Hoagwood K, Jensen PS, Fisher CB. Hillsdale, NJ, Erlbaum, 1996, pp 29–39

Thompson RA: Developmental changes in risk and benefit: a changing calculus of concerns, in Social Research on Children and Adolescents: Ethical Issues. Edited by Stanley BL, Sieber JE. Newbury Park, CA, Sage, 1992, pp 31–64

CHAPTER 8

Clinical Research in Substance Abuse: Human Subjects Issues

David A. Gorelick, M.D., Ph.D., Roy W. Pickens, Ph.D., and Frederick O. Bonkovsky, Ph.D.

I n this chapter we review human subjects issues in clinical research on substance abuse—that is, research involving subjects who use (or have used) psychoactive substances and research investigating the actions of substances with abuse liability. Our aim is to increase awareness and stimulate discussion of relevant ethical issues, their impact on research protocols, and ethical principles that can be implemented. We start with the assumption that good science is ethical science. Our presentation of issues, descriptions of research practice, and suggestions about the conduct of research are intended to be informative rather than authoritative, prescriptive, or proscriptive. Few empirical studies on the clinical research process in substance abuse or systematic surveys of investigators and institutional review boards (IRBs) have been undertaken (with the exception of a recent mail survey of 91 clinical researchers funded by the clinical research divisions of the National Institute on Alcohol Abuse and Alcoholism [NIAAA] and the National Institute on Drug Abuse [NIDA]; [McCrady and Bux, in press]). Thus, it is impossible to be authoritative on the question of how human subjects issues are being handled currently or to prescribe definitive answers to ethical issues. An investigator's colleagues and local IRB are often the best source of information and advice.

Human subjects issues in substance abuse research are similar to those in other areas of psychiatric and medical research (Kleber 1989; Mendelson 1991), with ethical imperatives resting on the three fundamental principles of respect

We thank the anonymous and named reviewers who provided helpful comments. The views expressed in this chapter are solely those of the authors, and do not necessarily represent any official policies or guidelines of the National Institutes of Health or the National Institute on Drug Abuse.

for person (autonomy), beneficence, and equity enunciated in the Nuremberg Code (Beals et al. 1996 [see Appendix E]), the Declaration of Helsinki (World Medical Association 1997 [see Appendix A]), and the Belmont Report (National Commission 1978 [see Appendix B]). The legal and regulatory principles are also the same as those codified for U.S. researchers in the *Code of Federal Regulations (CFR)* (45 *CFR* 46, subpart A, first adopted in 1974 and revised in 1991 [see Appendix C]). As in any other clinical research study, a protocol in the area of substance abuse must have a favorable risk-benefit ratio—that is, "risks to subjects are reasonable in relation to anticipated benefits, if any, to subjects, and the importance of the knowledge that may reasonably be expected to result" (45 *CFR* 46.111[a][2]).

Clinical research in substance abuse encompasses a broad spectrum of scientific methods and types of subjects, ranging from epidemiologic surveys of substance use by college students to experimental studies of the effects of drug administration on physiological function. There is ample scope for both individual and societal benefits to flow from this research. Few broadly effective treatments are available for many abused substances (Gorelick 1993), and untreated substance abuse is associated with high rates of morbidity and mortality (Gronbladh et al. 1990) and with substantial societal and economic costs (Rice et al. 1990). Significant gaps remain in our knowledge of the etiology, development, and consequences of substance abuse, and much of this needed knowledge can be obtained only through clinical research (Gorelick 1992a). Extrapolation from in vitro or animal models to the human situation can rarely be done with absolute confidence, and some psychological and behavioral phenomena can be adequately studied only with human subjects. Validation of the safety and efficacy of new treatments always requires clinical research as the final step. Thus, both therapeutic research (i.e., with potential direct benefit to participating subjects) that evaluates the efficacy of new diagnostic and treatment methods and nontherapeutic research (i.e., without any direct benefit to participating subjects) that expands our basic knowledge of the pathophysiology of substance abuse and leads to future improvements in prevention, diagnosis, and treatment are needed.

The preceding notwithstanding, investigators must recognize and address the particular issues raised by clinical research in substance abuse. One issue is the substantial social and legal stigma still attached to substance use and abuse, especially use and abuse of illegal substances. This stigma is reflected in several ways that may hinder clinical research. For example, legal and regulatory oversight of substances with abuse liability, even when used for therapeutic purposes, can be stricter and more rigid than for other pharmaceuticals used in clinical research. Further, stigma may hinder the identification and recruitment of users of abusable substances, resulting in sample or selection bias.

A second issue is confidentiality, which takes on special importance when research entails the disclosure of past or present use of illegal substances. This issue is addressed in federal and state laws and regulations regarding the confidentiality and handling of clinical substance abuse–related information.

A third issue is the concept of addiction as a loss of control over behavior. Because voluntariness is one of the cornerstones of valid informed consent, this loss of control raises questions about the ability of addicted individuals to give informed consent to research participation. This question is particularly acute when the research involves the administration of substances with abuse liability (see section titled "Study Design: Administration of Abusable Drugs").

RECRUITMENT

Recruitment of research subjects involves the ethical principles of autonomy and equity. Autonomy requires that prospective subjects not be vulnerable to coercion or undue influence or unduly motivated to accept the risks of research participation. Federal regulations do not include individuals who abuse substances or are addicted to drugs among the classes of subjects considered especially vulnerable and therefore requiring special protection. The regulations mention "mentally disabled persons, or economically or educationally disadvantaged persons" as "likely to be vulnerable" and therefore likely to need additional safeguards (45 *CFR* 46.111[b]); however, the regulations do not specify what those additional safeguards might be (45 *CFR* 46.111[b]). Some individuals recruited for substance abuse research have other psychiatric conditions or are of low socioeconomic status or poorly educated and so would fall into these categories. Respect for autonomy suggests that recruitment efforts not preferentially target such individuals (Novick 1989).

Another issue related to subject autonomy in substance abuse research is whether addiction itself, or associated personality traits (e.g., risk taking), might render subjects unduly vulnerable to research recruitment. As noted earlier, addiction has been conceptualized by some as loss of control over drug-seeking and drug-taking behavior, reflected in consumption of more substance than initially intended, unsuccessful efforts to cut down or control substance use, or continued substance use despite knowledge of adverse consequences from such use (American Psychiatric Association 1994). Thus, an addicted individual might be considered unduly vulnerable to recruitment to studies involving administration of substances with abuse liability (Nahas 1990).

The ethical principle of social equity mandates that all population groups share fairly in both the benefits and the burdens of clinical research. This principle is now reflected in U.S. law (NIH Revitalization Act of 1993 [42 USC 289a–2]) and National Institutes of Health (NIH) guidelines (National Institutes of Health 1994a), which require all NIH-funded research to adequately represent women and minorities as subjects. Encouraging women and minority partici-pation is also good science. Substance abuse affects both males and females and all ethnic groups. Women and minorities must be included in samples to be able to validly generalize research findings to the broader population of sub-stance abusers. Gender and ethnicity are also known to influence many depen-dent variables in substance abuse research (e.g., treatment response [Gorelick 1992b]). Thus, ignoring issues of sociodemographic representation weakens a study. Interestingly, a recent review of published studies on phar-macological treatment of cocaine addiction found both under- and overrepre-sentation of various population subgroups as research subjects, suggesting the need for more attention to this issue (Gorelick et al. 1998).

Regulatory interpretation of "adequate representation" is not clear, how-ever, except in the case of a phase III clinical trial (Hohmann and Parron 1996; National Institutes of Health 1994b, 1994c). One interpretation is that the sub-ject sample should be representative of the national population with the con-dition being studied. This approach may be impractical for an investigator constrained to working in a particular geographic area but might be an appro-priate target for a large collaborative study with multiple sites. One factor in choosing study sites could be ensuring adequate subject representation in the sites taken as a whole, even when no single site itself has broad subject repre-sentation.

An appropriate recruitment target for the individual investigator might be subject representation comparable to the gender and ethnicity distribution in the population meeting the study's substance use eligibility criteria and living within the recruiting catchment area. The size of the recruiting catchment area may vary with the type of study and subject involved. A residential or inpa-tient study may recruit from a larger geographic area than an outpatient study, because the former may require only a single trip to the study site (for admis-sion), whereas the latter may require frequent trips for collection of data. Similarly, studies that involve subjects with ready access to automobiles or convenient public transportation may recruit from a wider area than those that do not.

The recruiting process should take into account both the practical issue of providing a sufficient number of subjects to allow meaningful statistical analysis and the ethical issue of avoiding undue recruitment of vulnerable subjects. Use of a variety of recruitment sources can help investigators achieve adequate rep-resentation of women and minorities as well as a sufficient flow of eligible subjects so that the project can be completed in a timely manner. Recruitment methods can include both direct solicitation in the community, such as by newspaper and radio advertisements and flyers, and outreach to community-based organizations (e.g., churches and social organizations) and to government and private health care facilities and social services agencies. Such outreach beyond the investigator's home institution may be especially important in recruiting underrepresented populations. Investigators who target recruitment only at previously used or obviously accessible sources run the risk of perpetuating past patterns of over- and underrepresentation.

One issue of ethical relevance to substance abuse research is whether the prospective research subject is interested in substance abuse treatment. Therapeutic research studies (i.e., those with potential direct benefit to subjects) may appropriately recruit individuals interested in substance abuse treatment, as long as the alternative available nonresearch treatments are fully disclosed. Nontherapeutic studies (i.e., those without any direct benefit to subjects) that recruit subjects interested in treatment should address the issue of whether research participation might delay or prevent subjects' entry into treatment. No direct empirical evidence suggests that research participation actually alters future treatment participation. One approach is to couple research participation with treatment that follows immediately, so that subjects volunteering for research are also committing to treatment. Another approach is to assess individuals' treatment interest at the time of recruitment and refer those expressing treatment interest to therapeutic studies or treatment programs, excluding them from nontherapeutic studies. Regardless of approach, the consent process for nontherapeutic studies should make clear the nontherapeutic nature of the study (to avoid the common therapeutic misconception by subjects that any medical study will be clinically beneficial to them [Appelbaum et al. 1987]) and disclose the treatment options available as alternatives to research participation.

An applicant's eligibility for participation in a substance abuse research protocol may depend on the validity of screening data collected by self-report, such as personal or family history of substance use. Two approaches have been used to help ensure the accuracy of such data. One is to use redundancy of data collection (i.e., information collected by different staff members using different instruments at different times), with the research team investigating any omissions or inconsistencies. Another option is to obtain objective verification of self-report data whenever possible, such as through drug testing to verify recent drug use.

INFORMED CONSENT

Consent to research participation is valid when three criteria are satisfied: 1) the individual must have the capacity (competence) to give consent (see Chapter 4),

2) the individual must be informed of and understand all of the relevant information (see Chapter 6), and 3) the individual must give consent voluntarily.

The issue of competence to give informed consent is similar for those who abuse substances and other types of research subjects. Some obvious substance-related conditions, such as acute intoxication and withdrawal and alcohol amnestic disorder (American Psychiatric Association 1994), may temporarily or permanently impair competence. These conditions must be considered when enrolling subjects. However, the mere existence of a psychiatric disorder does not of itself preclude the ability to give informed consent (Dresser 1996). Long-term studies involving subjects whose cognitive abilities (and thus competence to consent to research participation) might deteriorate over the course of a study (e.g., individuals with HIV infection or a progressive dementing disorder) might consider use of an advance directive or durable power of attorney (see Chapter 5). Such a document, executed at study entry when the subject is competent, makes possible continued research participation by taking into account potential changes in the subject's future cognitive status.

Several procedures can be used to help ensure that recruited subjects are competent to comprehend the relevant information and consent (McCrady and Bux, in press). Competence can be evaluated by clinical interview, mental status tests, or standardized cognitive tests. A minimum score (e.g., IQ level) may be set to qualify for research participation. The consent form should be written in nontechnical language at a reading level commensurate with that expected among potential subjects, so that subjects can easily comprehend the material (Davis et al. 1993; Philipson et al. 1995). Degree of comprehension can be evaluated by administering a short quiz as part of the consent process to assess subjects' understanding of and memory for the information just conveyed, with a minimum passing score required for research participation. Because some individuals are unaware of or reluctant to admit their difficulty with reading comprehension or memory, it may be appropriate to use such procedures with all subjects, regardless of their performance on initial interview. Reading the consent form aloud to a prospective subject can also lessen the problem of limited reading skills.

Informed consent is best considered a continual process over time rather than a one-time event occurring at the signing of the written consent form. Thus, investigators should be prepared to provide information, solicit and answer questions, and monitor understanding throughout subject screening and recruitment, as well as during the study itself. Researchers should pay attention to the possible influence of the consent process (including the consent form) on an applicant's likelihood of volunteering (selection bias) and on the data collected, especially self-report data on sensitive topics such as illegal drug use (Bok 1992; Trice 1987).

CONFIDENTIALITY

Substance abuse researchers should pay special attention to confidentiality issues. Their work is likely to involve the collection and recording of information about illegal activities including possession and use of illegal drugs and the criminal behavior engaged in by some who abuse substances. Because of these sensitive issues and the social stigma attached to substance abuse, federal regulations (42 *CFR* part 2) and many state laws and regulations accord special confidentiality protection to patient records related to alcohol and drug abuse; these regulations prohibit release of information by those to whom information has been transferred and provide criminal sanctions for breaches of confidentiality. Common steps taken to protect the confidentiality of research data include the use of code numbers rather than subjects' names on data collection forms and in databases, separate storage of research data and identifying information, storage of identifiable data in locked areas, and training of all research staff (including those not having contact with subjects) in the importance of confidentiality (McCrady and Bux, in press).

Investigators may avail themselves of additional protection through federal certificates of confidentiality issued under 42 *CFR* 1A, part 2a (see Appendix D). An investigator may obtain a confidentiality certificate for a specific research protocol by applying to the NIH institute funding the research (or within whose research mission the protocol would fall). The application must include a copy of the protocol, the IRB-approved consent form, and a list of all personnel having major responsibilities in the research project. Issuance of a certificate gives the investigator the authority to refuse to disclose the name or other identifying characteristics of a research subject in any federal, state, or local civil, criminal, administrative, legislative, or other proceeding. For example, the investigator can decline to respond to a civil or criminal court subpoena or request from a law enforcement agency. There are two explicit exceptions to the protection afforded by a confidentiality certificate. Information must be released to the U.S. Food and Drug Administration (FDA) when it has jurisdiction over a study and to auditors and program evaluators from the government agency funding a study. Investigators must disclose to subjects the existence of a certificate of confidentiality in the consent form. Care should be taken not to imply an absolute guarantee of confidentiality, because research data might still be leaked to an outside party and subjects should be informed of any limits to confidentiality (e.g., if data will be shared with an outside sponsor of the research or with noninvestigators participating in their medical care).

The periods before active research participation (i.e., during recruiting and screening) and after it (i.e., during follow-up) may be especially sensitive in terms of confidentiality. Care should be taken to avoid inadvertent breaches of confidentiality when contacting potential or former subjects. For example, the name of the study or research group may itself imply to others that a research subject has problems with substance abuse, thus compromising confidentiality. Such a situation can be avoided by making all contacts through a neutrally named individual or organization. If follow-up of research subjects is anticipated, it should be included in the approved study design and clearly described in the consent form (Robins 1977).

Substance abuse research may uncover information about other conditions and situations that are subject to mandatory reporting by licensed professionals under state law, such as certain communicable diseases (syphilis, HIV or AIDS, and tuberculosis), child abuse or neglect, elder abuse, and domestic violence. Reporting in compliance with such state laws may put the investigator in conflict with federal confidentiality law and jeopardize the trust and cooperation of the subject. Both statutory and case law may impose additional reporting requirements; for example, the targets of threats of violence made by patients in psychotherapy must be notified (Tarasoff doctrine) (Appelbaum and Rosenbaum 1989), and maternal drug use must be reported (on the grounds of child endangerment) (Harrison 1991). Although federal confidentiality law now allows reporting of suspected child abuse, there is no clear legal resolution to many of these dilemmas (see Fisher 1994; Siegal et al. 1993). During the consent process, investigators should fully disclose to subjects the boundaries of, and possible exceptions to, confidentiality protection, such as the reporting of infectious disease, suspected child abuse or neglect, or threat of imminent, serious harm to self or others.

COMPENSATION

Ethical principles allow compensation to research subjects but preclude excessive compensation that might become coercive. Subjects are compensated for their time, inconvenience, and discomfort, not for the risks they undertake. No a priori formula exists for calculating adequate, but not excessive, compensation. From one perspective, fair compensation might vary with the economic status of the potential subjects, and from another perspective fairness might call for all subjects in a particular study to receive comparable compensation. One way to estimate the influence of compensation is to divide the total compensation that could accrue by the total hours of subject participation to obtain an hourly compensation rate and then compare this rate with the typical hourly earnings of the subject or pool of potential subjects (Stricker 1991). Many re-

search institutions adopt a uniform compensation schedule for all clinical research, based on the time and procedures involved, thus ensuring consistency
across all research fields. When several research groups in the same geographic
area are competing for similar subjects, it may be advisable to exchange compensation information or cooperate in setting compensation rates so as to avoid
a bidding war for subjects in which subjects shop around for the best compensation when deciding whether to participate in studies.

An ethical issue in compensating substance abusers, especially those who
might be addicted, is whether they will use the compensation to buy an abused
substance. Although addicted individuals can often find a way to obtain their
drug of choice without having cash income, the availability of funds, regardless
of the source, can significantly influence the degree of drug use among both
casual or recreational users and heavy users (see Shaner et al. 1995). Several
payment procedures have been used to minimize the possibility of such influence. One approach is to limit the amount of compensation paid at any one
time, spreading out the payment of the full compensation due to the subject.
Another approach is to avoid cash payments altogether by paying in kind, perhaps by using vouchers or making payments to third parties on behalf of the
subject. Both of these approaches, however, have been criticized as paternalistic
and denying those with substance abuse problems the same access to their
compensation as is afforded other types of research subjects.

A related issue is when and under what circumstances to remit the compensation so as to minimize the chance of its misuse. One approach is to withhold payment if the subject appears acutely intoxicated or in withdrawal. The
subject can also be required to provide a substance-free urine sample or breath
test to receive payment. This regulation has the practical effect of making the
payment system a form of behavioral treatment (contingency management) for
substance use. The timing of payments in relation to the study itself is another
issue. Some investigators delay payment until the subject has ended his or her
study participation on the grounds that receipt of compensation during a study
may itself influence study results. This issue may be especially important in
outpatient treatment studies, in which subjects' income level could influence
treatment outcome.

Ideally, the compensation procedures used should strike a balance between
minimizing the potential for subjects' misuse of compensation in ways that
might be harmful to themselves or society and according those who abuse substances the same rights and respect for autonomy given other research subjects.
Regardless of the procedures adopted, their possible influence on study outcomes should be considered. Researchers should fully disclose to subjects in the
consent form the amount of compensation (including the likely maximum if
they complete the study) and the procedures and conditions under which it will

be paid. Consideration must be given to the potential influence of compensation procedures (as disclosed in the consent form) on recruitment and sample bias.

STUDY DESIGN

Although issues of study design are of a general nature (see Chapter 2), some have nuances specific to substance abuse research. Such issues include using placebo or no-treatment groups, testing for HIV status, handling follow-up and termination of research participation, and administering abusable drugs.

Use of Placebo or No-Treatment Groups

Ethical questions have recently been raised about the use of placebo or no-treatment groups in clinical research, especially when effective treatments for the disease under study are known (Lieberman 1996). In some areas of substance abuse research, use of placebo groups may not be an issue because there are no known broadly effective treatments (e.g., pharmacotherapy for cocaine abuse) (Gorelick 1993). In other areas, such as in studies of severe acute opiate or alcohol withdrawal, use of a placebo group would probably be considered unethical. Whenever possible, provision of some beneficial intervention (e.g., counseling) to all subjects is desirable.

HIV Testing

Because injection drug users and many other substance users are at risk for HIV infection, one benefit for such subjects is offering HIV antibody testing with appropriate pre- and posttest counseling (Centers for Disease Control and Prevention 1994; National Institute on Drug Abuse 1993). The NIDA strongly encourages such testing and counseling for any study it funds that involves as subjects injection drug users, smoked cocaine users, or sexually active drug users and their sexual partners (National Institutes of Health 1995). Public Health Service policy requires that all subjects tested for HIV infection in funded research be notified of the results, but the policy does not specify the timing of testing or notification (Des Jarlais and Friedman 1987). Various states' laws and regulations also affect the handling of HIV testing and its results. Further, the timing of notification may need to take into account possible disruption of the study, such as from the stressful effects on subjects of being told they are infected. Such possible disruption may be avoided by consistently testing and notifying all subjects at either the beginning or the end of study participation.

Termination and Follow-Up of Research Participation

Termination of research participation, especially in therapeutic studies, can raise ethical questions. If the subject or investigator believes that the subject is benefiting from the research treatment, it might be considered unethical to abruptly terminate the subject's access to the beneficial treatment, especially if no alternative effective treatments are known or the subject's access to other treatment providers is limited. Some protocols handle this situation by providing for a humanitarian extension of the protocol for such subjects. If the research treatment is potentially available elsewhere (as with a medication already marketed for another indication), the subject could be referred to a clinician who could provide the treatment as part of nonresearch clinical care.

Some pharmacological treatments (e.g., agonist maintenance medications such as methadone on which the subject has become physically dependent) cannot be abruptly terminated without potential harm to the subject. In such cases, a weaning period may be necessary until the subject can be referred to another source for treatment.

Administration of Abusable Drugs

Some scientific issues can be adequately addressed only by studies incorporating experimental drug administration. For example, this type of study design may be necessary for valid attribution of putative drug effects or observed abnormalities in those who use drugs to the pharmacological actions of the drug rather than to the numerous other confounding factors present when drugs are taken in the natural environment outside of an experimental setting (Gorelick 1992a). Possible confounding elements range from pharmacological factors such as route and rate of drug administration and drug dose and purity to subject factors such as medical and psychological condition at the time of intake and environmental factors such as time of day and setting. By allowing direct evaluation and manipulation of drug effects in a controlled research setting, drug administration studies help elucidate the mechanisms of drug action and further the development of new diagnostic tests or new treatments to counteract drug effects (Miller and Rosenstein 1997).

The potential risks associated with experimental administration of abusable drugs are in principle no different from those involved in any other pharmacological study. However, some illegal drugs do not have an extensive body of

medical safety data such as is generated to support approval for the legal marketing of a drug. Decisions about medical safety may thus have to be made in
the absence of systematic human safety data, and sometimes the relevant safety
data can be generated only by performing the controlled clinical study under
consideration. Such studies may require design features found in phase I studies
of pharmaceutical agents, such as dose escalation regimens (lower doses are
always administered before higher doses) or a preliminary dose challenge to
establish that the subject can safely tolerate the drug being used. It is always
prudent to use the lowest doses and safest routes of administration consistent
with the scientific aims of the study (Deitrich and Harris 1996; Miller and
Rosenstein 1997). Subjects should be thoroughly screened for any preexisting
conditions or physiological abnormalities known to be associated with adverse
reactions to the drug being administered, including any history of adverse reactions to the drug.

Administration of abusable drugs, because they are psychoactive, may be
associated with psychiatric risk (Miller and Rosenstein 1997). The effects of
abusable drugs may mimic or induce a variety of psychological symptoms,
especially in individuals with preexisting psychiatric problems. Care should be
taken during subject screening to identify such individuals. Further, researchers
should disclose the possibility of psychiatric risk during the consent process.
Provision should also be made for psychiatric monitoring during the course of
the study (and afterward, if persisting or delayed adverse effects are possible)
and for appropriate psychiatric treatment (or referral for treatment) should that
become necessary. The importance of these precautions varies depending on
the likelihood of drug administration producing noticeable psychological
effects.

Outpatient studies that administer a psychoactive drug may pose a behavioral or legal risk to subjects if they leave the research setting before returning
to their normal mental status (i.e., while still "under the influence") or before
body fluid concentrations of the administered substance are below legal limits
(which may be zero for illegal drugs). For example, subjects may be exposed to
the risk of driving under the influence or otherwise behaving in a dangerous or
inappropriate manner outside of the research setting. Subjects may face legal
or employment consequences if they test positive for illegal substances after
leaving the research setting. To minimize these risks, outpatient studies that
administer psychoactive substances may require all subjects to remain in the
research setting for a specified period after the substance is administered or
until specified behavioral, physiological, or pharmacokinetic variables are within
normal limits. The appropriate period or variable parameters depend on the
expected intensity and duration of drug effects. Investigators may take additional precautions such as maintaining custody of car keys, providing alternative

transportation (e.g., taxi or bus fare), or asking that subjects have someone else accompany them home from the research site. These issues should be clearly discussed during the informed consent process.

Another concern often raised about the administration of abusable drugs in clinical research is the addictive risk—that is, the risk that research participation will increase the subject's use of the abused drug or even create or worsen addiction (Nahas 1990). There are two different mechanisms for causing such addictive risk. First, administration of an abusable drug in the context of a research study, backed by the legitimacy of science and sanctioned by a research organization (often a prestigious university or government agency), might communicate or imply to the subject that taking the drug outside of the research context is also acceptable or safe (Nahas 1990; Stricker 1991). Second, exposure to the drug, especially if it produces positive psychological effects, might induce drug-seeking and drug-taking behavior outside of the research setting.

No scientific data exist on whether implied endorsement of drug taking actually plays a role in clinical studies administering abusable drugs. Investigators could collect such data by examining the attitudes of subjects (and potential subjects) before and after their recruitment for and participation in related clinical studies. One approach to minimizing this mechanism of producing addictive risk is to explicitly raise the issue during the consent process by emphasizing the scientific goals that justify drug taking within the research context. The offer of referral to drug abuse treatment during or at the end of research participation may also forestall this mechanism by emphasizing the researchers' endorsement of a drug-free lifestyle.

Some scientific data address the addictive risk from research exposure to abusable drugs. More than half a dozen published studies have followed several hundred alcoholic individuals for up to 2 years after their participation in clinical studies (both therapeutic and nontherapeutic) involving administration of alcohol (reviewed in Modell et al. 1993). All of the studies found that research participation produced no significant change in subjects' drinking behavior or any significant difference in alcoholism treatment participation. One unpublished study (Bigelow et al. 1995) has reported similar data based on 1-month follow-up of 25 individuals with histories of illegal drug abuse who participated in drug administration studies. No significant change was seen in their drug use or treatment participation when compared with their preresearch behavior. These findings suggest that with appropriate safeguards, administration of abusable drugs in clinical research does not significantly alter the course of substance use disorders, either for better or worse. That the substance use disorders remain unaffected by subject participation may be due to the relatively short duration (usually days or weeks) of research participation compared with subjects' prior histories of substance use (usually years) and to the relatively low doses and infrequent administration of drug as compared with what subjects use outside of the research setting.

There are no published studies on the addictive risk of administering an abusable drug to research subjects who have not used or rarely use drugs or to individuals who were dependent on drugs but are now in remission. However, several types of safeguards have been proposed to reduce the addictive risk from exposure to abusable drugs during clinical research. One approach is to recruit subjects who are already experienced users of the drug to be administered and whose recent pattern of drug use (dose, frequency, and route of administration) matches or exceeds in intensity that to which they will be exposed during the research. This approach is often taken by researchers who administer illegal drugs such as cocaine, heroin, and marijuana. The rationale is that the less intense drug exposure during research participation is unlikely to significantly influence the course of subjects' more intense drug use outside of the research context or to serve as undue inducement to subjects to consent to research participation to receive drug administration. This factor may explain why the studies cited earlier found no effect of research participation on subjects' subsequent substance use.

Another approach is to recruit subjects with no history of substance misuse or illegal drug use on the grounds that such subjects are at less risk for increased substance use or addiction in general and therefore at less risk from research exposure to abusable substances. Researchers who administer legal substances (e.g., alcohol and other sedative-hypnotics or stimulants such as methylphenidate) as part of pharmacological challenge studies often take this approach. The rationale has some circumstantial supporting evidence. Individuals with a history of heavy substance use are considered at risk for addiction (as reflected in FDA labeling of some classes of psychoactive medications), are likely to abuse opiate analgesics prescribed for pain control (Perry and Heidrich 1982), and are likely to report positive psychoactive effects from experimental administration of abusable drugs (Ciraulo et al. 1996; Evans et al. 1996). Individuals without such a history are unlikely to become addicted even with chronic exposure to abusable drugs such as opiates and sedatives as part of medical treatment (Boethius and Westerholm 1977; Brown et al. 1996; Medina and Diamond 1977; Porter and Jick 1980).

Several organizations have developed guidelines to help investigators conducting studies that involve administration of abusable substances. The National Advisory Council of the NIAAA issued such guidelines for alcohol administration in 1989 (see Appendix 8–1). NIDA's National Advisory Council has recently developed analogous guidelines for the administration of drugs (see Appendix 8–2). The College on Problems of Drug Dependence (1995), a leading research organization in the field, has published a position paper on human subject issues in drug abuse research. The American College of Neuropsychopharmacology has issued "A Statement of Principles of Ethical Conduct for Neuropsychopharmacologic Research in Human Subjects" (see Appendix F).

REFERENCES

American Psychiatric Association: Diagnostic and Statistical Manual of Mental Disorders, 4th Edition. Washington, DC, American Psychiatric Association, 1994

Appelbaum PS, Rosenbaum A: Tarasoff and the researcher: does the duty to protect apply in the research setting? Am Psychol 44:885–894, 1989

Appelbaum PS, Roth LH, Lidz C, et al: False hopes and best data: consent to research and the therapeutic misconception. Hastings Cent Rep 17:20–24, 1987

Beals WB, Sebring HL, Crawford JT: The Nuremberg Code. JAMA 276:1691, 1996

Bigelow GE, Brooner RK, Walsh SL, et al: Community outcomes following research exposure to cocaine or opioids (abstract). NIDA Res Monogr 153:354, 1995

Boethius G, Westerholm B: Purchases of hypnotics, sedatives, and minor tranquillizers among 2,566 individuals in the county of Jamtland, Sweden. Acta Psychiatr Scand 56:147–159, 1977

Bok S: Informed consent in tests of patient reliability. JAMA 267:1118–1119, 1992

Brown RL, Fleming MF, Patterson JJ: Chronic opioid analgesic therapy for chronic low back pain. J Am Board Fam Pract 9:191–204, 1996

Centers for Disease Control and Prevention: HIV Counseling, Testing, and Referral Standards and Guidelines. Atlanta, GA, Centers for Disease Control and Prevention, May 1994

Ciraulo DA, Sarid-Segal O, Knapp C, et al: Liability to alprazolam abuse in daughters of alcoholics. Am J Psychiatry 153:956–958, 1996

College on Problems of Drug Dependence: Human subject issues in drug abuse research. Drug Alcohol Depend 37:167–175, 1995

Davis TC, Jackson RH, George RB, et al: Reading ability in patients in substance misuse treatment centers. International Journal of Addictions 28:571–582, 1993

Deitrich RA, Harris RA: How much alcohol should I use in my experiments? Alcohol Clin Exp Res 20:1–2, 1996

Department of Health and Human Services: Confidentiality of Alcohol and Drug Abuse Patient Records, 42 Code of Federal Regulations, part 2 (1987)

Department of Health and Human Services: Rules and Regulations for the Protection of Human Research Subjects, 45 Code of Federal Regulations, part 46[a] (1991)

Des Jarlais DC, Friedman SR: AIDS prevention among IV drug abusers: potential conflicts between research design and ethics. IRB: Review of Human Subjects Research 9:6–8, 1987

Dresser R: Mentally disabled research subjects: the enduring policy issues. JAMA 276:67–72, 1996

Evans SM, Griffiths RR, de Witt H: Preference for diazepam, but not buspirone, in moderate drinkers. Psychopharmacology 123:154–163, 1996

Fisher CB: Reporting and referring research participants: ethical challenges for investigators studying children and youth. Ethics and Behavior 4:87–95, 1994

Gorelick DA: Pathophysiological effects of cocaine in humans: review of scientific issues. J Addict Dis 11:97–110, 1992a

Gorelick DA: Sociodemographic factors in drug abuse treatment. J Health Care Poor Underserved 3:49–58, 1992b

Gorelick DA: Overview of pharmacologic treatment approaches for alcohol and other drug addiction: intoxication, withdrawal, and relapse prevention. Psychiatr Clin North Am 16:141–156, 1993

Gorelick DA, Montoya ID, Johnson EO: Sociodemographic representation in published studies of cocaine abuse pharmacotherapy. Drug Alcohol Depend 49:89–93, 1998

Gronbladh L, Ohlund LS, Gunne LM: Mortality in heroin addiction: impact of methadone treatment. Acta Psychiatr Scand 82:223–227, 1990

Harrison M: Drug addiction in pregnancy: the interface of science, emotion, and social policy. J Subst Abuse Treat 8:261–268, 1991

Hohmann AA, Parron DL: How the new NIH guidelines on inclusion of women and minorities apply: efficacy trials, effectiveness trials, and validity. J Consult Clin Psychol 64:851–855, 1996

Kleber HD: Drug abuse liability testing: human subjects issues. NIDA Res Monogr 92:341–356, 1989

Lieberman JA: Ethical dilemmas in clinical research with human subjects: an investigator's perspective. Psychopharmacol Bull 32:19–25, 1996

McCrady BS, Bux DA Jr: Ethical issues in informed consent with substance abusers. J Consult Clin Psychol (in press)

Medina JL, Diamond S: Drug dependency in patients with chronic headaches. Headache 17:12–14, 1977

Mendelson JH: Protection of participants and experimental design in clinical abuse liability testing. British Journal of Addiction 86:1543–1548, 1991

Miller FG, Rosenstein DL: Psychiatric symptom-provoking studies: an ethical appraisal. Biol Psychiatry 42:403–409, 1997

Modell JG, Glaser FB, Mountz JM: The ethics and safety of alcohol administration in the experimental setting to individuals who have chronic, severe alcohol problems. Alcohol Alcohol 28:189–197, 1993

Nahas GG: The experimental use of cocaine in human subjects. Bull Narc 42:57–62, 1990

National Commission for the Protection of Human Subjects of Biomedical and Behavioral Research: The Belmont Report: ethical principles and guidelines for the protection of human subjects of research (DHEW Publ No OS-78-0012). Washington, DC, U.S. Government Printing Office, 1978

National Institute on Drug Abuse, Division of Clinical and Services Research: The NIDA HIV Counseling and Education Intervention Model: Intervention Manual. Rockville, MD, National Institute on Drug Abuse, 1993

National Institutes of Health Revitalization Act of 1993, Public Law 103-43, part I, subtitle B

National Institutes of Health: Guidelines on the inclusion of women and minorities as subjects in clinical research. NIH Guide for Grants and Contracts. 59 Federal Register, No 59 (March 28, 1994a):14508–14513

National Institutes of Health: Outreach Notebook for the NIH Guidelines on Inclusion of Women and Minorities as Subjects in Clinical Research. Bethesda, MD, National Institutes of Health, August 1994b

National Institutes of Health: Questions and Answers Concerning the 1994 NIH Guidelines on the Inclusion of Women and Minorities as Subjects in Clinical Research. Bethesda, MD, National Institutes of Health, September 7, 1994c

National Institutes of Health: HIV/AIDS Counseling and Testing Policy for the National Institute on Drug Abuse. NIH Guide Grants Contracts 24(21), June 9, 1995

Novick A: Clinical trials with vulnerable or disrespected subjects. AIDS Public Policy Journal 4:125–130, 1989

Perry S, Heidrich G: Management of pain during debridement: a survey of U.S. burn units. Pain 13:267–280, 1982

Philipson SJ, Doyle MA, Gabram SGA, et al: Informed consent for research: a study to evaluate readability and processability to effect change. J Investig Med 43:459–467, 1995

Porter J, Jick H: Addiction rare in patients treated with narcotics (letter). N Engl J Med 302:123, 1980

Rice DP, Kelman S, Miller LS, et al: The economic costs of alcohol, drug abuse, and mental illness, 1985 (DHHS Publ No ADM-90-1694). Washington, DC, U.S. Government Printing Office, 1990

Robins LN: Problems in follow-up studies. Am J Psychiatry 134:904–907, 1977

Shaner A, Eckman TA, Roberts LJ, et al: Disability income, cocaine use, and repeated hospitalization among schizophrenic cocaine abusers: a government-sponsored revolving door? N Engl J Med 333:777–783, 1995

Siegal HA, Carlson RG, Falck R, et al: Conducting HIV outreach and research among incarcerated drug abusers: a case study of ethical concerns and dilemmas. J Subst Abuse Treat 10:71–75, 1993

Stricker G: Ethical concerns in alcohol research. J Consult Clin Psychol 59:256–257, 1991

Trice AD: Informed consent, VIII: biasing of sensitive self-report data by both consent and information. Journal of Social Behavior and Personality 2:369–373, 1987

World Medical Association: Declaration of Helsinki: recommendations guiding physicians in biomedical research involving human subjects. JAMA 277:925–926, 1997

APPENDIX *8–1*

National Institute on Alcohol Abuse and Alcoholism Recommended Council Guidelines on Ethyl Alcohol Administration in Human Experimentation

Available on the NIAAA Web site: http://silk.nih.gov/silk/niaaa/

Prepared by the National Advisory Council on Alcohol Abuse and Alcoholism

Revised June 1989

U.S. DEPARTMENT OF HEALTH AND HUMAN SERVICES
Public Health Service
Alcohol, Drug Abuse, and Mental Health Administration

NOTE: The National Advisory Council on Alcohol Abuse and Alcoholism advises the National Institute on Alcohol Abuse and Alcoholism (NIAAA) and the Secretary of the Department of Health and Human Services (DHHS) on program and policy matters in the field of alcohol abuse and alcoholism. The recommended Council Guidelines represent National Advisory Council recommendations for consideration by research grant applicants, Institutional Review Boards, Initial Review Groups, and others in the alcohol research field. The recommended Council Guidelines are not official Federal NIAAA or DHHS regulation or policy.

RECOMMENDED COUNCIL GUIDELINES ON ETHYL ALCOHOL ADMINISTRATION IN HUMAN EXPERIMENTATION

Table of Contents

Medical and Psychological Screening
Pregnancy Screening
Medical Services
Alcohol-Naive Individuals
Alcohol Dose Levels
Use of Deception and Incomplete Disclosure
Subject Accommodation and Retention
Need for Follow-up
Subject Payment
Method of Payment

Part V.   CONCLUSION

APPENDIX   Membership of the National Advisory Council on Alcohol Abuse and
Alcoholism and the Ad Hoc Council Subcommittee on Ethyl Alcohol
Administration in Human Experimentation

The Belmont Report, April 18 1979 [see Appendix B]

I. PREAMBLE

It is recognized that much of our knowledge of biological and behavioral actions of alcohol
(all references to alcohol in the context of this document are limited to ethyl alcohol),
including knowledge relevant to treatment and prevention of alcoholism and alcohol
problems, has been attained through research involving alcohol ingestion by human
subjects (see Endnote 1). The National Advisory Council on Alcohol Abuse and Alcoholism (see Endnote 2) fully recognizes the need for research with human subjects including, as appropriate, research which involves consumption of alcohol by humans. The
Council views such research as essential for an understanding of alcohol's actions,
including reinforcement, tolerance, and dependence. Such research is critical to development of more effective prevention and treatment programs for alcohol abuse and
alcoholism. This research must be developed with full attention paid to the fundamental
ethical principles which govern all research with human subjects.

Fundamental ethical principles for research involving human subjects include the
concepts of respect for persons, beneficence, and justice. These principles have been well
summarized in a report issued by the National Commission for the Protection of Human
Subjects of Biomedical and Behavior Research, titled "Ethical Principles and Guidelines
for the Protection of Human Subjects of Research" (The Belmont Report), (OPRR Reports, NIH, PHS, DHHS, April 1979, FR Doc. 79-12065). The general principles of ethics
in human investigation are also addressed in such documents as the Nuremberg Code
of 1946, The Helsinki Declaration of 1964 (revised in 1975 and again in 1983), in guidelines from professional organizations, such as the American Psychological Association,
and in a number of relevant books including Ethics and Regulation of Clinical Research,

authored by Robert J. Levine (Urban and Schwarzenberg, Baltimore-Munich, Second Edition 1986). As a comprehensive presentation of the fundamental ethical principles of research is beyond the scope of the Council guidelines, The Belmont Report is provided. It can be located at the following Web site: http://helix.nih.gov:8001/ohsr/mpa /belmont.phtml.

From these ethical principles, important aspects of research practice are derived. From "respect for the person" is derived requirements for attainment of meaningful informed and voluntary consent. From "beneficence" is derived the principles of not doing harm and, wherever possible, promoting the well-being of the research subjects and other individuals with a similar disease, or society as a whole. From "justice" is derived principles related to the selection of research subjects: to not place specific subjects at risk merely because of convenient access to a population, a compromised position of the subjects, or the potential of the individuals to be manipulated; to not unduly involve persons in research protocols (when there is more than minimal risk) who are unlikely to be among the beneficiaries of subsequent applications of the research.

The Council notes that responsibility for development and implementation of ethical research protocols falls upon more than one individual or group. It rests first with the principal investigator and next with the Institutional Review Board (IRB), as required by the Code of Federal Regulations (CFR), 45 CFR Part 46, "Protection of Human Subjects." The IRB reviews all HHS conducted or funded research protocols involving human subjects, and IRB approval is required for research involving human subjects. The subsequent levels of review (for projects supported by the Institutes of the Public Health Service) are, in turn, the Initial Review Groups (IRGs) and the National Advisory Council. Though these bodies are not provided the same extensive detail on human subject protocols as provided to IRBs, they are required to call attention to any issues for which there may be ethical concerns. Human subject concerns raised by either the IRG or Council are conveyed to the principal investigator as well as to the applicant's institution. The program staff of the Institute, in consultation with the Office for Protection from Research Risks (OPRR), of the National Institutes of Health, have the responsibility for resolving Council human subject concerns, before any study involving human subjects can be undertaken.

II. PURPOSE OF THE GUIDELINES

The Council guidelines focus on issues related to experimentation involving alcohol administration to human subjects in the context of the ethical principles noted above. The Council guidelines are intended to identify potential problematic issues, and to serve as a guide to help ensure that appropriate consideration is given to relevant issues in the development and review of research protocols involving alcohol administration.

The guidelines are not intended to supplant the functions of the IRB, or of OPRR. The guidelines are advisory to applicants, IRBs, IRGs, and others; they are not codified and do not constitute Federal regulation. Rather, the guidelines are intended to reflect a sensitive, ethical approach which is also consistent with current research practices and experience in the field of alcohol research.

It has been observed that not all IRBs have addressed issues surrounding adminis-tration of alcohol uniformly. IRBs, as well as applicant sensitivity to the issues, are often related to prior experience with similar issues in alcohol or related research. The Council suggests that IRBs should consider obtaining outside expertise when they do not have sufficient familiarity with alcohol research issues.

The recommendations contained within the guidelines are in no way meant to interfere with the recovery for any individual for any disease, including alcoholism. Ac-cordingly, it is recognized at this time that the accepted and appropriate goal of alco-holism treatment is abstinence.

III. GENERAL ISSUES

The Council recommends consideration of a number of general issues applicable to all alcohol research involving human subjects, regardless of the specific population. These issues are presented here:

Risk/Benefit: A careful appraisal of the risk/benefit ratio is a critical aspect in the assessment of the appropriateness of a research protocol. This need derives from the ethical principle of beneficence (see above). In most contexts, the risk pertains to the research subject though, in some circumstances, it could be broader and encompass the group or society. Benefit must be considered first in the context of the research subject. Benefit may also encompass the broader context of other individuals with a similar disease (where applicable) or of humankind. There must be a reasonable balance of risk against potential benefit; without such a reasonable balance, a research protocol cannot be jus-tified ethically. For example, even a minimally invasive study involving merely the draw-ing of one milliliter of blood may be considered to have an unfavorable risk/benefit ratio in a poorly conceived study. Alternatively, more highly invasive procedures could be judged to have an acceptable risk/benefit ratio in a well-developed and important study.

The qualifications and experience of the research team must be considered in weigh-ing risk/benefit. Depending on the level of expertise of the research team, a project may not be judged to have an acceptable risk/benefit ratio even if the project has a sound scientific hypothesis and a good research design.

Similarly, the site for conduct of the research may influence the risk/benefit decision.

Within this context, the Council recommends consideration of the appropriateness of the qualifications of those who assess the risk/benefit ratio. Such individuals should be experienced and/or knowledgeable in clinical research issues. A particular degree (M.D., Ph.D., etc.) neither qualifies nor disqualifies an individual from participation in this assessment process.

The Council also notes that it is appropriate that the principal responsibility for approval of a research project involving human subjects rests with the IRB. Though both the IRG and Council have a responsibility to consider human subject issues, it is the local institution, and its IRB, which are most aware of the many subtle factors involving the research team's qualifications in similar studies, the suitability of the research site, and local policies and norms affecting the acceptability of proposed procedures.

Informed Consent: The Council reiterates the basic principle that the investigator has the responsibility of assuring that the informed consent process gives the research subjects all the information they need to make a voluntary and informed decision. IRBs, as well, should assure that the informed consent documents convey all relevant information in language readily understandable by the research subject or guardian. The Council also believes it appropriate that every informed consent form should indicate that the drug, alcohol, is a toxin and a reinforcing agent which may cause changes in behavior, including repetitive or excessive consumption. Such a statement would appropriately acknowledge that alcohol is not an innocuous substance, and that everyone who drinks alcohol is at some risk.

Also, the Council recommends that due consideration should be given to the cognitive, physiologic, and motivational states of the individuals in terms of their ability to fully understand the context of the informed consent. Individuals who are severely intoxicated or in a confusional withdrawal state are unable to give true informed consent. Alternatively, a blood alcohol concentration (BAC) of zero for the potential subject may not be a required prerequisite, depending upon cognitive capabilities of the individual at that time. If there is a question of a potential subject's ability to give meaningful informed consent, an independent clinician, ethical consultant, or uninvolved third party with appropriate qualifications may be asked to evaluate this ability.

Subject Selection: The Council emphasizes the need for care in subject selection so that appropriate subjects are utilized to address the research question and so that adequate safeguards are followed to prevent unnecessary risk to subjects. Included under this issue is the need to avoid using subjects merely because of their easy availability, low social or economic status, or limited capacity to understand the nature of the research. Also included under this category is the need to consider the subject's age, sex, familial or genetic background, prior alcohol use, other drug use, and general medical and psychological condition, including, if appropriate, alcoholism recovery status. The issues relating to subject selection are addressed in more detail in the following section on specific issues.

Confidentiality: Investigators should be aware that once alcohol histories are placed in charts, such charts have to be handled with the same confidentiality afforded other alcohol records for which requirements sometimes go beyond those for many other medical or research records.

Special Federal requirements that apply to certain alcohol records used in research are addressed in the Code of Federal Regulations (CFR) under 42 CFR Part 2, "Confidentiality of Alcohol and Drug Abuse Patient Records."

IV. SPECIFIC ISSUES

The Council believes that many of the issues are best expressed in the context of questions to be considered by applicants and IRBs. These are issues which the applicant should be addressing in the context of the risk/benefit analysis. Discussion of these issues is provided immediately following each question.

Question: Is the investigator assessing whether the potential subjects have a current or prior drinking problem, and whether or not the subjects are or have been in treatment?

Council Comment: These types of factors must be taken into consideration when subjects are recruited. Appropriate care should be taken to not unduly place any individual at risk.

Question: Will the protocol involve alcoholics (alcohol-dependent individuals)?

Council Comment: Experimentation which requires individuals who are alcohol-dependent or alcoholics to be exposed to alcohol clearly warrants special attention. There are a number of extremely important principles which need to be addressed by anyone considering or evaluating requests to undertake such research. It is noted that these issues differ to a degree, depending on where in the disease/rehabilitative/recovery process the potential subjects are. Further, it is useful to distinguish between these stages in addressing some of the key issues. For example, the likelihood that a subject would otherwise be encountering the agent (alcohol) would clearly differ, depending upon their disease or recovery status. The risk of the investigator inflicting harm is clearly greater when the probability that the subject would be otherwise exposed to alcohol is lower.

When potential subjects include alcoholics who are current, active drinkers, the screening procedures must clearly include a medical examination to assure the absence of any medical or mental condition for which further alcohol exposure at the dose contemplated would be contraindicated. Further, the Council stresses that it is incumbent on the investigator, or his/her agent, to make a serious and concerted effort to link such individuals with treatment. This linkage should be active in bringing together the subject with alcoholism treatment personnel, and not passive as in only providing names of treatment programs and phone numbers to the research subject. Whether or not the subject chooses to remain in the treatment program, it is incumbent on the investigator to actively facilitate entry of the research subject into the program.

The use of subjects who have completed the initial phase of treatment and progressed into rehabilitation or recovery would require an extremely strong scientific justification and risk/benefit assessment. Different factors will need to be considered, including at what stage they are in the rehabilitation program and the alcohol dose employed. Both the research staff and the treatment personnel must consider the potential for untoward effects on the treatment/recovery process. There should be a continuation of treatment after conclusion of research participation for a sufficient period to ensure continued recovery.

At the present time (1989), it is considered inappropriate to administer alcohol to any recovering alcoholic who is abstinent and living a sober life in the community. In taking this position, the Council believes that the issue of risk for relapse outweighs any consideration which may be afforded to the willingness of the subjects to participate in the project through informed and voluntary consent, or the unique requirements within a study to include recovered alcoholics to address the hypothesis posed. This position is derived from an assessment of risk, since the risk of the exposure eliciting relapse (or other health problems) is considered too great to warrant the recovering alcoholic's participation.

Question: Is the applicant obtaining a family history in order to determine (and, as appropriate, exclude) individuals who may carry a heightened familial or genetic risk to develop alcohol dependency?

Council Comment: It is recognized that, as a group, individuals with a familial or genetic history of alcoholism are at higher risk for the development of alcoholism. Thus, special consideration needs to be given to the risk/benefit assessment before exposing such individuals to alcohol, and even more so when either dosage levels exceed the normal drinking practice of the subject, or when the alcohol-naive individual is proposed as the subject (see below). It is appropriate to relate both in the assessment of the risk/benefit and in the informed consent process that, in the context of alcoholism, familial or genetic risks do not mean predestiny or predetermination. Rather, the risk translates into vulnerability which should appropriately suggest extra caution on the part of any individual with a family history of alcoholism in the context of any drinking situation, including, but not limited to, the research study.

Question: Has the age of the subjects been considered?

Council Comment: Alcohol is unique as a beverage because its availability and/or consumption is licit for a substantial segment of the population (in most States, those age 21 or older), but illicit below this age. It is the Council's opinion that persons who are under the State's legally set drinking age should normally not be given alcohol in research protocols. If the hypothesis under test clearly requires the involvement of individuals from that age group, and the risk/benefit assessment is strongly favorable, investigators must be sure to (1) obtain any underage subject's assent to participate in the research; (2) obtain permission from the parent(s) or guardian for the underage subject to participate in the research; and (3) comply with applicable laws of the jurisdiction in which the research is being conducted. As with all research, investigators and IRBs must adhere to the additional requirements for protection of children involved as subjects for research, as contained in HHS Regulations for Protection of Human Subjects, 45 CFR Part 46, Subpart D.

The principles for all research with children dictate that the research first begin with animals or adults before involving children. In addition, the investigative team should include individuals or the access to individuals who are sensitive to the needs of children, such as, as appropriate, social service professionals, pediatricians, or psychologists.

Question: Has the need been considered for medical and psychological evaluation of subjects prior to participation in a study?

Council Comment: Medical and psychological screening may be appropriate for given studies, depending on the nature of the study, the maximal doses of alcohol used, the subject population, and whether or not they are alcohol-dependent or using other drugs.

Question: Has the possibility of pregnancy been assessed for potential female subjects of childbearing age?

Council Comment: The possibility of pregnancy should always be assessed and a standard hormonal pregnancy test included. While menstrual and contraceptive history may be useful, the assessment of a pregnancy status should not be made solely by self-reported information. At the present time (1989), risk/benefit considerations almost always preclude administration of alcohol to pregnant women as this may endanger the fetus.

Question: Has the need for access to medical backup services been considered? Has there been discussion of the potential medical consequences and services necessary?

Council Comment: Depending on dose and subject population, the nature of the medical backup service will vary. In minimal circumstances, a nurse or physician available "on call" may be appropriate. This may be amplified to require the presence of a nurse with a physician available "on call," to the requirement of the presence of a physician if higher doses of alcohol are used or if there are other issues pertaining to the study population.

Question: Will alcohol-naive individuals be used?

Council Comment: The inclusion of alcohol-naive individuals in a protocol would need to be very strongly justified within the context of both the requirement that such individuals be included to answer the research question posed and a strongly favorable risk/benefit assessment including consideration of benefits for other individuals with the disease or society as a whole.

There are critically important issues which must be borne in mind when considering a protocol involving the exposure of the nondrinking individual to alcohol. It is recognized that the addictive liability of alcohol varies among individuals and is quite likely a function of genetic, psychological, and environmental factors. While those from a genetic or family background with alcoholism are more likely to be at risk, at present the science to identify those individuals with a high addictive liability does not exist. A risk/benefit assessment must include consideration of the likelihood that the individual would otherwise be encountering the agent (alcohol). This likelihood is not necessarily zero; it may depend on a number of factors relevant to the individual, including the environment in which the individual lives and personal decisions of the individual. In any event, the risk/benefit assessment should be strong and compelling before alcohol-naive individuals are used in research, and the potential subject should clearly understand the risks (as discussed above in the context of informed consent) before his/her consent is obtained.

Question: With reference to potential subjects who are either occasional or regular consumers of alcoholic beverages, will the subject ingest or be administered larger amounts of alcohol than they would normally consume in their own drinking contexts?

Council Comment: Such an activity should be justified within the context of both the requirements for the scientific questions posed and the risk/benefit assessment.

There is a class of studies that the Council believes should be commented upon under this heading so as to avoid confusion or misinterpretation; these are investigations where the dependent variable under study is the level of alcohol consumption itself. Distinct from protocols where the subject ingests a fixed amount of alcohol, in these studies the impact of various environmental or other factors on the extent of drinking is assessed. The Council notes that the context of the question stated here is not intended to convey that such research is inappropriate.

Question: If the study protocol requires an element of deception or incomplete disclosure, has the consent form indicated the amount of alcohol that would be consumed if the subject receives alcohol rather than a placebo? Is there a thorough debriefing of the subject following the study, explaining why the incomplete disclosure of information was necessary and the usefulness of it?

Council Comment: It is recognized that an element of deception or incomplete disclosure of information about the research methods or goals is sometimes required in alcohol as well as other research; for example, in the elucidation of expectancy and placebo effects. Research subjects are, however, entitled to a full debriefing when it was necessary to deceive them. The consent form should clearly indicate that they may receive alcohol and the amount of alcohol they may receive. Information about risks should never be withheld for the purpose of eliciting the cooperation of subjects, and truthful answers should always be given to direct questions about the research (see also the Informed Consent section of The Belmont Report).

Question: Are appropriate provisions made to accommodate the subjects receiving alcohol at the research sites until the alcohol dose has been effectively eliminated?

Council Comment: One concern which emerges is the possibility that individuals who have consumed alcohol in a study will, upon leaving the laboratory, drive or operate dangerous equipment. Providing transportation or escorting a subject back to a place of residence (or employment) does not assure that the individual will not engage in hazardous activities.

In addition to having observable behavior return to normal, it is frequently considered appropriate for the BAC to fall below 0.02 gram percent. In environments where the risk of engaging in hazardous activities is minimal, a level of 0.04 may be considered acceptable, again, conditioned upon other observable behavior having attained sufficient normalcy to preclude such immediate concerns as those stated above as well as upon other factors.

It may also be prudent to require the subject with other than zero BAC and no apparent impairment to state in writing that he/she will not drive a car or operate other machinery for several hours after each experimental session.

The consent form should address the estimated period of time that the subject will likely have to stay at the research facility. When dismissed from the laboratory (even with a BAC of 0.02), subjects should be informed of the estimated time that it will take to reach a zero BAC and counseled on the potential performance impairments to be expected during this period.

Given the large variability in pharmacokinetic clearance rates between individuals, the BAC should be determined with a certified or properly calibrated breathalyser, and not solely on the basis of pharmacokinetic-derived formulas, graphs, or tables. (BAC measurements may not be necessary when subjects are retained overnight.)

It is recognized that participants in a study, even if encouraged to remain at the testing facility, are free to leave the research setting at any time. Should subjects leave prematurely, they should be escorted back to their residence. Further, the consent form should address this contingency in a statement similar to the following: "If you choose to leave in the middle of the session, you will be sent home with care, by a conveyance provided by us." In some circumstances, consideration may also be given to the use of so-called Ulysses contracts in which subjects agree before the experiment begins to be temporarily restrained (in terms of leaving the facilities) even though they might protest the restraint later, when their BAC is above the safe limits.

Question: Does any aspect of the study dictate the need for follow-up of subjects? If so, is this done?

Council Comment: Depending on the nature of the study and the subject, it may be appropriate to determine if there will be any delayed reaction from participation in the study. This would be appropriate in some circumstances when (and as otherwise appropriately justified, see above) subjects are alcohol-dependent or the offspring (adult or otherwise) of an alcoholic. It is recognized that such follow-up may be difficult and/ or unattainable with some subject types. When this is true, however, the applicant should explain why the particular study population must be used.

Question: In the context of the proposed subject population, is the proposed payment to participants likely to be a coercive element in recruitment?

Council Comment: Payment to research subjects for their time and inconvenience is an acceptable practice in alcohol as well as other biomedical research. Nonetheless, the payment should not be coercive in the sense of tempting individuals to participate.

Question: Is the method of payment appropriate for the subject population?

Council Comment: In those unusual studies where alcohol-dependent individuals are used as subjects (see above), immediate cash payments are easily convertible for the purchase of alcoholic beverages and, thereby, may not be appropriate. Therefore, care should be given to the manner of payment: Who will get the payment? Where and in what form will payment be made? Can payment be made in a form other than money to avoid purchases of alcoholic beverages?

V. CONCLUSION

These guidelines represent a brief summary of basic principles and issues relating to the administration of alcohol to human subjects. Further information on human subject research may be obtained from the Office of Protection from Research Risks and from staff of the National Institute on Alcohol Abuse and Alcoholism at the following locations.

National Institutes of Health
Office for Protection from Research Risks
Cliff Scharke, D.D.S., M.P.H.
6100 Executive Boulevard, Room 3B01
Bethesda, MD 20892
301/402-5218

National Institute on Alcohol Abuse and Alcoholism
Office of Scientific Affairs
Willco Building, Suite 409
6000 Executive Boulevard
Bethesda, Maryland 20892-7003
301/443-3860

Endnotes:

1) As used in the context of this document, administration of alcohol to human subjects is intended to include studies which involve administration of alcohol by an inves-

tigator to a research subject by the oral or any other route, or voluntary oral consumption by a subject in a research setting.
2) The National Advisory Council on Alcohol Abuse and Alcoholism advises the National Institute on Alcohol Abuse and Alcoholism (NIAAA) and the Secretary of the Department of Health and Human Services on programs on policy matters in the field of alcohol abuse and alcoholism.

APPENDIX

June 1989

National Advisory Council on Alcohol Abuse and Alcoholism
National Institute on Alcohol Abuse and Alcoholism
Alcohol, Drug Abuse and Mental Health Administration

Chairperson
Enoch Gordis, M.D.
Director
National Institute on Alcohol Abuse and Alcoholism

Executive Secretary
James F. Vaughan
Deputy Director, Office of Scientific Affairs
National Institute on Alcohol Abuse and Alcoholism

Members

Martha Alexander
Executive Director
Charlotte Council on Alcoholism and Chemical Dependency
100 Billingsley Road
Charlotte, North Carolina 28211

Susan B. Blacksher
Deputy Director
Alcohol Program
California Department of Alcohol and Drug Programs
111 Capitol Mall, Room 223
Sacramento, California 95814

Bernell N. Boswell
Executive Director
The Cottage Program International, Inc.
736 South 500 East
Salt Lake City, Utah 84102

Carlton K. Erickson, Ph.D.
Professor of Pharmacology and Toxicology
College of Pharmacy
University of Texas
Austin, Texas 78712

Donald M. Gallant, M.D.
Professor of Psychiatry
Department of Psychiatry and Neurology
Tulane University School of Medicine
1430 Tulane Avenue
New Orleans, Louisiana 70112

Charles S. Lieber, M.D.
Professor of Medicine and Pathology
Mount Sinai School of Medicine (CUNY)
Director, Alcohol Research and Treatment Center
Liver Diseases and Nutrition Section
GI-Liver Training Program
Veterans Administration Medical Center
130 W. Kingsbridge Road
Bronx, New York 10468

George D. Lundberg, M.D.
Editor
Journal of the American Medical Association
535 Dearborn Street
Chicago, Illinois 60610

John P. McGovern, M.D.
Clinical Professor of Pediatrics and Microbiology
Baylor College of Medicine
Clinical Professor of Medicine
University of Texas School of Medicine at Houston
President, The John P. McGovern Foundation
6969 Brompton Street
Houston, Texas 77025

Roger E. Meyer, M.D.
Chairman
Department of Psychiatry
University of Connecticut Medical School
Farmington, Connecticut 06032

Sheldon I. Miller, M.D.
Professor and Chairman
Department of Psychiatry
UMDNJ/New Jersey Medical School
185 South Orange Avenue, E-561
Newark, New Jersey 07103-2757

Rudolf H. Moss, Ph.D.
Research Career Scientist and Director, Health Services Field Program
Veterans Administration Medical Center
Palo Alto, California
Professor
Department of Psychiatry and Behavioral Sciences
Stanford University School of Medicine
Stanford, California 94305

Roger D. Walker, M.D.
Professor
Department of Psychiatry and Behavioral Science
University of Washington School of Medicine and
Chief, Substance Abuse Treatment Programs
Veterans Administration Medical Center, 116ADTP
1600 South Columbian Way
Seattle, Washington 98108

Ex-officio Members

Peter Brock
Senior Policy Analyst and Special Consultant
on Alcohol and Drug Abuse
Room 3D-200, Pentagon
Office of the Assistant Secretary of Defense (Health Affairs)
Washington, DC 20301

Richard T. Suchinsky, M.D.
Associate Director for Mental Health and Behavioral Sciences
(Alcohol and Substance Abuse)
Department of Veterans Affairs
Central Office (116A1), Room 911
810 Vermont Avenue, N.W.
Washington, DC 20420

National Advisory Council on Alcohol Abuse and Alcoholism Ad Hoc Council Subcommittee on Development of Guidelines for Administration of Alcohol to Human Subjects

Chairperson
Sheldon I. Miller, M.D.
Professor and Chairman
Department of Psychiatry
UMDNJ/New Jersey Medical School
185 South Orange Avenue, E-561
Newark, New Jersey 07103-2757

Members

Mary Jeanne Kreek, M.D.
Associate Professor and Physician
The Rockefeller University
1230 York Avenue
New York, New York 10021

Charles S. Lieber, M.D.
Chief, Alcohol Research and Treatment Center
Liver Diseases and Nutrition Section
GI-Liver Training Program
Veterans Administration Medical Center
130 W. Kingsbridge Road
Bronx, New York 10468

Lawrence Lumeng, M.D.
Director
Division of Gastroenterology
Department of Medicine
Indiana University Medical School
Emerson Hall 421
545 Barnhill Drive
Indianapolis, Indiana 46223

George D. Lundberg, M.D.
Editor
Journal of the American Medical Association
535 Dearborn Street
Chicago, Illinois 60610

Alan Marlatt, Ph.D.
Professor of Psychology
Addictive Behaviors Research Center
Department of Psychology
University of Washington
Seattle, Washington 98195

Technical Advisors

Alison Wichman, M.D.
Bioethics Program Chief
Clinical Center, NIH
Room 2C-202, Building 10
9000 Rockville Pike
Bethesda, Maryland 20892

Zelig Dolinsky, Ph.D.
Assistant Professor of Psychiatry
University of Connecticut Medical School
Farmington, Connecticut 06032

National Advisory Council on Drug Abuse Recommended Guidelines for the Administration of Drugs to Human Subjects

PREAMBLE

The National Advisory Council on Drug Abuse recognizes the importance of research involving the administration of drugs to human subjects. This research produces the scientific knowledge that is essential to understanding and addressing problems of drug abuse and addiction, and is particularly important in the development of effective, scientifically-based treatment and prevention strategies.

Research involving the administration of drugs to research participants must be designed, reviewed, and conducted within the fundamental ethical principles governing all biomedical and behavioral research with human subjects. These principles have been articulated in the Belmont Report, which provides a broad framework for establishing and evaluating specific aspects of ethics in research with human subjects. While a complete reading of the Belmont Report is required for a full understanding of these principles and their application in complex ethical issues involved in research on human subjects, the principles can be summarized as follows:

Respect for Persons—Individuals must be given the opportunity to choose what shall or shall not happen to them and their decisions must be informed and protected. Persons with diminished autonomy or capacity are entitled to protection.

Beneficence—Researchers must go beyond the obligation to avoid inflicting harm and maximize the potential benefits of the research to individuals and society.

Justice—Fairness and equality must guide the distribution of the benefits and burdens of research involving human subjects.

The general principles of ethics in human investigation are also addressed in such documents as the Nuremberg Code of 1947, The Helsinki Declaration of 1964 (most recently revised in 1989), in guidelines from professional organizations, such as the American Psychological Association, and in a number of relevant books including Ethics and Regulation of Clinical Research, authored by Robert J. Levine (Urban and Schwarzenberg, Baltimore-Munich, Second Edition 1986).

The Council notes that responsibility for development and implementation of ethical research protocols falls upon more than one individual or group. It rests first with the principal investigator and next with the Institutional Review Board (IRB), as required by the Code of Federal Regulations (CFR), 45 CFR Part 46, "Protection of Human Subjects." IRBs review all HHS conducted or funded research protocols involving human subjects, and IRB approval is required for research involving human subjects. The subsequent levels of review (for projects supported by the Institutes of the National Institutes of Health) are, in turn, the Initial Review Groups (IRGs) and the National Advisory Councils. Although these bodies are not provided the same extensive detail on human subject protocols as is provided to IRBs, they are required to call attention to any issues for which there may be ethical concerns. Human subject concerns raised by either the IRG or Council are conveyed to the principal investigator as well as to the applicant's institution. The program staff of the Institute, in consultation with the Office for Protection from Research Risks (OPRR), of the National Institutes of Health, have the responsibility for resolving human subject concerns before any study involving human subjects can be undertaken. Program staff are responsible for requesting and OPRR is responsible for negotiating assurances of compliance with institutions that will be engaged in the research and for which no assurances covering the research are in place at the institutions.

PURPOSE OF THESE GUIDELINES

These Council guidelines focus on the issues that arise in research involving drug administration to human subjects in the context of the ethical principles noted above. The principles are intended to identify issues to be considered in the development and review of research protocols involving drug administration.

The guidelines are not intended to supplant the functions of either the IRB or OPRR. The guidelines are *advisory* to applicants, IRBs, IRGs, and others. They are not codified and do not constitute Federal regulation. Rather, the guidelines are intended to encourage a sensitive, ethical approach which is also consistent with the best current practices and experience in the field of drug abuse research.

Not all IRBs have uniformly addressed issues surrounding administration of drugs. IRB, as well as researcher, sensitivity to the issues are often related to prior experience with similar issues in drug abuse or related research. The Council suggests that IRBs, consistent with 45 CFR 46.107(f), consider obtaining outside advice when they do not have sufficient familiarity with drug abuse research issues.

GENERAL ISSUES

The Council recommends consideration of a number of general issues applicable to drug administration research involving human subjects, regardless of the specific population. These issues are:

Risk/Benefit

Research with volunteer participants begins with a careful appraisal of the risks and benefits. Considerations include importance and validity of the scientific information to be gained, degree of risk to research participants, and availability of alternative research approaches and information sources. There must be a favorable balance of risk against potential benefit; without a favorable balance, a research protocol cannot be justified ethically.

In assessing the risks and benefits, the IRB should also take into account the qualifications and experience of the research team, the appropriateness and adequacy of the research design, and the suitability of any site where the administration of drugs and other interventions occur. Depending on the level of expertise of the research team, a project may not be judged to have an acceptable risk/benefit ratio even if the project has a sound scientific hypothesis and research design. Similarly, the site of the research may influence risk/benefit decisions.

The Council also notes that the principal responsibility for approval of a research project involving human subjects rests with the IRB. Though both the IRG and Council have a responsibility to consider human subject issues, it is the local institution and its IRB which are most aware of the many complex factors involving the research team's qualifications and experience in conducting similar studies, the suitability of the research site, and local policies affecting the acceptability of proposed procedures.

Informed Consent

The Council reiterates the basic principle that the investigator has the responsibility for assuring that the informed consent process gives potential participants all the information they need to make a voluntary and informed decision. IRBs, as well, should assure that the informed consent documents convey all relevant information in language readily understandable by the research participants and/or guardians. Also, the Council recommends that the investigator give adequate consideration to the mental and physical conditions and motives of the individuals in terms of their ability to fully understand the context of the informed consent. If there is a question about a potential subject's ability to give meaningful and informed consent, an independent clinician, ethical consultant, or uninvolved third party with appropriate qualifications should be asked to evaluate this ability if the subject is to be entered or continued in the study.

Subject Selection

The Council emphasizes the need for care in subject selection so that appropriate participants are recruited to address the research question and to ensure that adequate safeguards are followed to prevent unnecessary risk. The issues relating to subject selection are addressed in more detail in the following section on specific issues.

Confidentiality

Investigators should be aware that once drug abuse histories are placed in patient records, such records must be handled with the same confidentiality afforded other drug abuse records. These confidentiality requirements sometimes go beyond those for many other medical or research records. Further, investigators and IRBs should be aware that special Federal requirements may apply to certain drug abuse records used in research. Information about this may be found in the Code of Federal Regulations (CFR) under 42 CFR Part 2, "Confidentiality of Alcohol and Drug Abuse Patient Records."

Investigators should also be aware that the Secretary may authorize persons engaged to biomedical, behavioral, clinical, or other research to protect the privacy of individuals who are the subject of such research by withholding from all persons not connected with the conduct of such research the names or other identifying characteristics of such individuals. Persons so authorized to protect the privacy of such individuals may not be compelled in any Federal, State, or local civil, criminal, administrative, legislative, or other proceedings to identify such individuals (42 CFR Part 2a). Investigators, research participants, and IRBs should be aware that there are no absolute guarantees of confidentiality.

SPECIFIC ISSUES

The Council recommends that these important issues be considered in the development and review of research involving the administration of drugs to human subjects:

Informed consent

Investigators should thoroughly assess the research participants' ability to participate in the informed consent process, i.e., to understand the risks and benefits of participating in the study. Investigators should include only participants who are competent and authorized to give informed consent or for whom there are properly appointed guardians who can legally act in that capacity.

Medical and psychological screening and services

Medical and psychological screening procedures must be carried out to ensure that participants chosen for the study will not be harmed by drug administration. To further assure this, appropriate monitoring and medical support services must be available during the study. The amount of medical support necessary will depend on the study protocol (e.g., drug(s) under study, route and rate of drug administration). At a minimum, a nurse or physician available "on call" may be appropriate. This may be amplified to require a nurse to be present with a physician available, or to require a physician to be present, if the demands of the study require it.

Administration of drugs to individuals who have never used drugs

It is expected that research involving the administration of drugs to individuals who have never used drugs prior to study participation would occur only in the rarest of circumstances and with the strongest justification. Such research must be very strongly justified within the requirement that (1) the question under study cannot be reasonably or validly answered without their participation and (2) there exists a strongly favorable risk/benefit assessment. It should be remembered that a wide range of potentially abusable drugs may be the focus of drug administration research—from caffeine and nicotine to cocaine and opiates. Depending on the drug, limited and investigator-controlled exposure to these drugs have very different levels of risk for potential participants.

Involvement of individuals currently addicted to drugs

Research which requires individuals who are addicted to drugs to be administered drugs warrants special attention. As stated above, investigators should thoroughly assess the participant's ability to provide informed consent and take into consideration current, recent, and past drug use. There are a number of extremely important principles which need to be addressed by anyone considering or evaluating requests to undertake such research. These include a thorough assessment of the risks entailed if participants are to be exposed to higher dose, rate of administration, and/or new route of administration than they would normally encounter by their own choice in their usual circumstance; inclusion of medical examination and screening to assure the absence of any medical or mental condition for which further drug exposure would be contraindicated; and a serious and concerted effort be made to link these individuals to drug abuse treatment.

Drug doses and routes of administration

To minimize the risk, participants should be exposed to the least amount of drug necessary to achieve the purpose of the study. Sometimes it may be necessary for participants to be administered new drugs, doses of drugs greater than that they would normally consume by their own choice in their usual circumstance, or to be exposed to a new route of administration. Under those circumstances, the rationale for exposure to new drugs, to higher doses, or to new routes of administration should be clear and compelling.

Prior and current drug treatment status

Whereas, in general, in-treatment or treatment-seeking individuals should not be given drugs of abuse, there can be compelling circumstances in which such research is appropriate. In-treatment or treatment-seeking individuals who have an addiction history may be uniquely appropriate for some types of research. Investigators have a special burden to establish a compelling rationale for the inclusion of these participants. Investigators also have an additional burden for ensuring proper participation in the informed consent process. Among current and past drug users, special issues arise regarding their interest in, and level of commitment to, abstinence. Priority must always be given to what is in the best interest of the research participant. Participants should not be recruited simply for the convenience of the investigator.

Pregnancy

Women of childbearing potential should not be routinely excluded from participation in clinical research. The NIH policy is that women must be included in all NIH-supported biomedical and behavioral research projects involving human subjects, unless a clear and compelling reason shows that inclusion is inappropriate. Risk/benefit considerations would normally preclude administration of drugs to pregnant women as this may endanger the fetus. Therefore, it is the responsibility of the investigator to take adequate precautions, throughout the study, to prevent inappropriate administration of drugs to women who are pregnant. Pregnancy must always be assessed using an acceptable pregnancy test. While menstrual and contraceptive history may be useful, the assessment of pregnancy status should not be made solely by information which is self-reported. As with all research, investigators and IRBs must adhere to the additional requirements pertaining to research involving fetuses, pregnant women, and human in vitro fertilization as contained in HHS Regulations for the Protection of Human Subjects, 45 CFR Part 46, Subpart B.

Age of research participants

If the hypothesis being tested requires the involvement of individuals under age 18 and the risk/benefit assessment is favorable, the investigator must: (1) obtain the individual's consent and/or assent to participate in the study; (2) obtain permission from the parent(s) or guardian for the individual to participate in the study, as appropriate; and (3) comply with any applicable local laws governing such research. As with all research, investigators and IRBs must adhere to the additional requirements for the protection of children involved as subjects in research, as contained in HHS Regulations for Protection of Human Subjects, 45 CFR Part 46, Subpart D.

Study personnel training and experience

Care should be taken to ensure that those study personnel who are administering the drug(s) have had the proper training and experience in administering drugs to humans. Investigators should specify the level of training and experience study personnel must have prior to their direct involvement in drug administration.

HIV risk reduction counseling and testing

Drug abuse and behaviors that transmit HIV are linked, and HIV risk reduction interventions have been demonstrated to effectively reduce these behaviors. Therefore, NIDA has established a policy (NIH Guide for Grants and Contracts, June 9 1995) that strongly encourages NIDA-funded researchers to make HIV risk reduction counseling and HIV testing available to research subjects at high risk for acquiring or transmitting HIV.

Safety of research participants outside of the research site

A concern is the possibility that individuals who have been administered drugs in a study will, upon leaving the laboratory, if still affected by the drug, drive or engage in behavior that may be harmful to themselves or others. The consent form and research protocol should address the estimated period of time that the research participant will likely have to stay at the research facility. Participants must be kept under observation for that period and when dismissed from the laboratory, participants should be informed of the potential performance impairments to be expected during this period. Investigators should also determine, depending on the nature of the study and the subject, the likelihood of any delayed reaction from participation in the study.

Discharge personnel should have the necessary training and experience to determine whether the subject is impaired. If it is determined that the subject is impaired, provisions should be made to provide the appropriate treatment.

Referral to treatment

Investigators should be knowledgeable about available drug abuse treatment options and, where medically indicated, offer research participants referral to treatment before, during, and at the conclusion of study participation. Investigators who identify comorbid or coincident diseases in study participants should provide or refer them to appropriate medical care.

Incomplete disclosure

On relatively rare occasions, an element of deception or incomplete disclosure of information about the research methods or goals may be justified in drug abuse as well as other research; for example, when researching expectancy and placebo effects. Any such withholding which results in the exclusion or alteration of some or all of the elements of informed consent in 45 CFR Section 46.116(a) must be approved by the IRB in accordance with the waiver requirements of 45 CFR Section 46.116(c) or (d). Research participants should have a full debriefing when incomplete disclosure is necessary. The consent form should clearly indicate that they may receive drugs, what types of drugs, and information on the amount they may receive. Information about risks must never be withheld for the purpose of eliciting the cooperation of volunteer participants. Truthful answers must always be given to direct questions about research. (See also Appendix B, "The Belmont Report.")

Payment for participation in research

Payment to research participants for their time and inconvenience is an acceptable practice in drug abuse as well as other biomedical research. The payment should not be exploitive or coercive in the sense of unduly tempting individuals to participate. In this regard, alternatives to cash payments should be considered. For example, can the payment be made in installments? Where and in what form will payment be made? Can payment be made in a form other than money (e.g., vouchers for food, movies, clothing, etc.)?

CONCLUSION

These principles represent a brief summary of basic issues relating to research involving the administration of drugs to human subjects. It should be recognized that there are benefits in addition to risks to individuals who participate in research. Such benefits may include medical and psychological evaluation, HIV counseling and testing, and referral to drug abuse treatment.

Further information on human subject research may be obtained from the Office for Protection from Research Risks and from the National Institute on Drug Abuse at the following locations.

National Institutes of Health
Office for Protection from Research Risks
6100 Executive Boulevard, Suite 3B01
Rockville, MD 20892-7507
(301) 496-7005

National Institutes of Health
Office of Human Subjects Research
Office of Intramural Research
9000 Rockville Pike
Building 10, Room 1C116 (MSC 1154)
Bethesda, MD 20892-1154
(301) 402-3444

National Institute on Drug Abuse
Office of Science Policy and Communications
Parklawn Building, Room 10A-55
5600 Fishers Lane
Rockville, MD 20857
(301) 443-6036

*National Advisory Council on Drug Abuse Ad Hoc Subcommittee to Develop
Guidelines for the Administration of Drugs to Human Subjects*

William L. Dewey, Ph.D.
Vice President for Research and Graduate Affairs
Virginia Commonwealth University
Box 568
Richmond, Virginia 23298

June Osborn, M.D.
President
Josiah Macy, Jr. Foundation
44 East 64th Street
New York, New York 10021

Marian Fischman, Ph.D.
Professor of Behavioral Biology
Department of Psychiatry
College of Physicians and Surgeons of Columbia University
722 West 168th Street
New York, New York 10032

Reese T. Jones, M.D.
Professor of Psychiatry
School of Medicine
University of California, San Francisco
401 Parnassus Avenue, Room A-322
San Francisco, California 94143

G. Alan Marlatt, Ph.D.
Professor of Psychology and Director
Addictive Behaviors Research Center
Department of Psychology
College of Arts and Sciences
University of Washington
Seattle, Washington 98195

A. Thomas McLellan, Ph.D.
Professor of Psychology in Psychiatry
Center for Studies of Addiction
School of Medicine
University of Pennsylvania
Bldg. 7, PVAMC
University and Woodland Avenues
Philadelphia, Pennsylvania 19104

For additional information about NIDA send e-mail to Information@lists.nida.nih.gov

CHAPTER 9

Consumer and Family Concerns About Research Involving Human Subjects

Laura Lee Hall, Ph.D., and Laurie Flynn

W hy do individuals with serious brain illnesses, such as schizophrenia and bipolar disorder, participate in research? How well do these patients and caregiving family members understand the research protocols in which they are participating and the risks and benefits involved? Are individuals with serious brain disorders satisfied with their experience as research subjects? Are their caregiving family members satisfied?

Little empirical evidence is available to answer these questions directly. We can only surmise, based on anecdotes, an appreciation of the clinical realities that people with serious brain disorders face and evaluation of the experiences of human subjects in other areas of research, the results of organizational oversight of research, and the voice of advocates who represent people with these illnesses and their families.

The information from these sources provides a complex picture of consumers' and families' concerns. In this chapter we describe the patient and family view of research involving human subjects and detail the history of the work in this area by the National Alliance for the Mentally Ill (NAMI). We build a case for enhanced attention to research participants and their caregiving families and for real partnerships between researchers and the patients and families with whom they work.

NAMI'S INTEREST IN RESEARCH ETHICS

The 185,000 consumers with severe mental illnesses, including schizophrenia, bipolar illness, major recurrent depressive illness, obsessive-compulsive disorder, and panic disorder, and their family members who are members of NAMI strongly support research. Like most people who face serious illness, the members of NAMI know that research is essential to advance our understanding and treatment of these illnesses. Indeed, biomedical research has yielded remarkable breakthroughs in the understanding and treatment of severe mental illnesses. Because of these advances, it is important to maintain a climate conducive to biomedical research on severe mental illnesses and to acknowledge the need for studies that involve human subjects. NAMI members not only accept the critical necessity for research using human subjects but honor the important contribution of individuals who volunteer to participate in research. Without their contribution, research progress would be greatly curtailed.

Strong and unequivocal support for research must be balanced by unequivocal support for the protection of the individuals who participate as human subjects in this research and for their families. A patient's dignity, let alone health, can never be the cost of a research project. Because individuals with serious brain disorders may have significant mental impairments and disabilities and are often vulnerable, their rights and well-being are matters of critical importance. Voluntary and uncoerced participation of individuals with serious brain disorders in research, full and comprehensible disclosure of risks and benefits to them and—as appropriate—their family members, and quality clinical care in conjunction with the research protocol are all important principles. NAMI recognized these principles in its first policy statement on the protection of individuals with serious brain disorders who participate as human subjects in research, which was approved by the NAMI board in February of 1995:

> NAMI accepts the critical necessity for research using human subjects, acknowledges the important contribution of persons who become human subjects, and affirms that all such research should be conducted in accordance with the highest medical, ethical, and scientific standards. (National Alliance for the Mentally Ill 1997, p. 22)

Although widespread problems in research involving patients with serious brain disorders are not assumed, and indeed no pervasive or widespread problem has been documented, these issues are too important to ignore. Several incidents in the past few years have suggested that problems can arise (Berg 1996). Federal policy on the protection of human subjects in research is incomplete in addressing people with serious brain disorders whose impairments diminish consent capacity (Berg 1996; Bonnie 1997; Dresser 1996; Shamoo and Irving 1993). Federal regulations were developed to protect all of the vulnerable subject populations identified by national and president's commissions except individuals with serious brain disorders. Research projects that involve discontinuing lifesaving medication for seriously ill patients require intensive and on-going dialogue and evaluation.

The NAMI policy—10 points on the protection of persons with serious brain disorders who are research subjects—addresses the issue of regulation and strives to achieve a balance between the requirements of research and pro-tection of the rights of individuals who participate in research and their families (National Alliance for the Mentally Ill 1997).

The policy sets forth standards for many aspects of the research process including informed consent procedures, patients' and families' roles on insti-tutional review boards (IRBs), substitute consent procedures when individuals are incompetent to provide informed consent, researchers' responsibility to link individuals who terminate participation in research protocols with necessary and appropriate care, and mechanisms for ensuring that individuals who par-ticipate in protocols involving assessment of new medications have continuing access to those medications.

In the remainder of this chapter we describe the key issues identified by NAMI in its policy on research involving human subjects with serious brain disorders and examine some issues unresolved by NAMI's policy. First, however, we discuss the reason that patients and their families might participate in re-search—an important perspective to keep in mind as we consider research involving human subjects with serious brain disorders.

Research May Be the Only Road to Treatment

People participate in research for altruistic reasons—they want to see improved care, if not for themselves, then for others in their situation. But people also participate in research for their own personal benefit or the benefit of a loved one (Cassileth et al. 1982; Daugherty et al. 1995; Newburg et al. 1992; Penman et al. 1984).

The clinical and treatment system realities that many people with serious brain disorders encounter make it clear why people would seek therapeutic benefit from research. Despite extraordinary medical advances, individuals with serious brain disorders too often experience terrible clinical conditions. The incompleteness of the current brain illness pharmacopoeia is one issue: as many as a third of individuals with schizophrenia do not significantly respond to available medication (Hall and Mark 1995). Some patients are hamstrung by such debilitating side effects that medication cannot be continued. Even for those who respond to existing medications, the side effects and incomplete relief offered by these medications make them imperfect palliative agents and certainly not curative ones. Further, some of the most promising medications may be available only through research trials. Finally, many service systems fail to provide the minimum level of effective treatments and supports for consumers with severe mental illnesses (Lehman et al. 1998).

Research has documented the current clinical situation of people with brain disorders as a rationale for participating in clinical studies. In one study, it was observed that the choice of a research unit was usually made under acute family stress related to the patient's need for hospitalization or failure to respond to hospital treatment (Sturges and Sternberg 1985).

It is not simply our science but also nationally erected barriers that limit access to effective treatment of serious brain disorders. At least one study has noted that one of the most common reasons for choosing a research setting is financial (Sturges and Sternberg 1985). Patients and families whose insurance coverage and financial resources have been depleted are relieved to find a psychiatric unit affiliated with a prestigious university that has no fee and no time limit for a hospitalization that would ordinarily cost at least $450 a day. Often the financial attraction is related to the wish to prevent admission to a state hospital.

The vast majority (99%) of private insurance policies in this nation limit payment for treatment of these illnesses, in many cases to a negligible level. Typically, lifetime spending on the treatment of such illnesses is capped at $50,000 or less. In other words, after one or two hospitalizations the patient is no longer eligible to receive private health insurance benefits. And although headway has been made recently on private health insurance discrimination, the progress is limited and incomplete.

The public safety net (or dumping ground) for such patients is strained and fraying as well. Federal and state budgets are being cut. Public responsibility has diminished. Hospitals are being torn down. Restrictive medication formularies form a one-size-fits-all pharmacological straitjacket and fly in the face of modern pharmacotherapy.

What is the result of these barriers? At least one-third of the homeless are people with severe brain disorders (Burt and Cohen 1989). Nearly 10% of our nation's prisoners have severe mental illness (Torrey et al. 1992). Suicide rates as high as 15% or more are common among individuals with severe brain illnesses (Pearson 1997–1998).

So why participate in research? Although the reasons may vary, it is important to keep in mind that participating in research may be the only path to treatment, as revealed in this statement by the mother of a daughter with severe schizophrenia (Becker 1994, p. 17):

> I learned of a research program that recruited patients who had a diagnosis of schizophrenia and who had not responded to several neuroleptics. Laura [my daughter] met these and the other requirements. After several interviews with

the inpatient staff . . . we thought their program seemed a way to alter the dismal course of her life. . . . At the time, Clozapine was only available for research purposes and I wanted this opportunity for Laura.

This statement raises questions about whether individual participation in research is truly uncoerced. It also should enlighten researchers about the realities faced by many patients with serious brain disorders and their families.

Informed Consent

Informed consent is the ethical mooring for biomedical research involving human subjects. The necessity of informed consent flows from the value of respect for persons first enumerated by the National Commission for the Protection of Human Subjects of Biomedical and Behavioral Research (1978). Respect allows people to make and pursue their own decisions in an informed and voluntary manner. Indeed, informed consent has been included in virtually every standard proposed to safeguard human subjects of experimental research, beginning with the Nuremberg Code published in 1949 in the aftermath of atrocities committed by Nazi physicians during World War II. U.S. Food and Drug Administration (FDA) regulations now permit the enrollment of patients in some medical research without their consent in carefully circumscribed situations. Patients must have a life-threatening condition and be unable to say whether they would want to be part of a study. They may be selected only if it is not feasible to obtain consent from a relative. The community in which the research is done must be notified about the study, and the research design must have been reviewed and approved by the FDA.

Federal regulations require that informed consent be obtained from each research subject. In the event that a person is found incompetent to provide informed consent, proxy consent by a legally authorized representative may be required. Under certain circumstances, requirements for informed consent may be waived. For an individual to provide informed consent, the anticipated benefits and potential risks associated with an experimental procedure must be explained to him or her; he or she (or his or her proxy) must understand these benefits and risks, rationally weigh them, and then make a voluntary decision about study participation.

The seemingly straightforward issue of informed consent can be a challenge to implement, especially in a world of complicated research designs and risks and benefits. In reality, the informed consent process is often reduced to the signing of a lengthy document packed with technical information and comprehensible only to an individual with specialized expertise. NAMI members have testified that informed consent, in practice, often focuses on getting a signature (U.S. Congress 1994; also see Sturges and Sternberg 1985), as indicated in the following statement of NAMI's executive director at a congressionally sponsored meeting (U.S. Congress 1994, p. 32):

> I'm not at all certain that we have done all that we can or the best job we could in terms of really thinking appropriately about informed consent. I appreciate the difficulties and understand the concerns that people have about informed consent in the research enterprise, but I also think that we have to respect what others are telling us about the increasing role that consumers are playing in their own lives and in shaping their own lives. My own information that we gather from talking to people in our office is that the work that's done is focused on getting a signature. Get the signature; get the paper signed. Sometimes there's a good description and discussion of what's going on and what may occur and what the research is pointing towards, and sometimes it's not so good and not so thorough.
>
> I think we need to realize, particularly in research of this type, that we may want to see it less as an event and more as a process. We may want to be sure as the research unfolds that those people most directly involved and affected continue to be updated and advised and that they understand what, in fact, is going on.

Findings from a research proposal review project conducted by the Advisory Committee on Human Radiation Experiments and published in October 1995 support these observations. The committee assessed documents related to 125 recently funded, federally supported research proposals (84 involving radiation and 41 not involving radiation research) from five federal agencies. Although this committee's work did not focus on research involving individuals with serious brain disorders, their findings confirm the prevalence of problems in informed consent noted by people with severe mental illnesses and their family members.

The committee reviewers found that some consent forms were difficult to read, uninformative, and even so misleading that committee reviewers regarded them as raising serious ethical issues. Reviewers found that investigators often drafted consent forms that were lengthy, highly technical, and generally unintelligible. A number of consent forms included standard "boilerplate" language, often in a smaller type and set off from the rest of the document. This format may have given prospective subjects the impression that the information was less important and easily skipped. Yet sometimes these sections contained the only discussion of critical topics such as the right to refuse participation, alternatives to participation, and confidentiality issues. A number of consent forms appeared to overstate the therapeutic potential of research, either explicitly or indirectly, especially to prospective research subjects with poor prognoses—a group particularly susceptible to false hope and vulnerable to confusion about the relationship of research to treatment. The disadvantages of participation were sometimes inadequately described or not presented at all. In several proposals that involved medications, the informed consent document described individually the hazards and side effects for each drug but did not list overall risks and possible harm to the research subject; in addition, how participation would affect the subject's ability to function in daily life and how ill a subject might be made to feel during the research were not mentioned.

Family members can be virtually excluded from the informed consent and research processes. Even if they are included, anxiety and lack of knowledge may prevent the family from asking questions (Sturges and Sternberg 1985). This situation presents problems because families may initiate the participation in research, may be the primary care providers of the individual with a serious brain disorder, or may be necessary for proxy consent or feedback on the status of the individual who is ill. Indeed, the individual with a serious brain disorder may be a late adolescent or young adult still residing at home.

NAMI staff testified at a congressionally sponsored panel on this issue (U.S. Congress 1994, p. 33):

> In mental illness the research subjects may be fairly young ... between the age of 18 and 21 ... with serious illnesses, and the families may be very involved in the individual's life. ... I would maintain in that type of situation ... that the ... ethical obligation (for informed consent and ongoing communication) extends to the family as well.
>
> Let me give you an example. Say a family has identified a particular research protocol at a particular university and has informed the individual who has the mental illness of that program and they've made a collective decision that that program is an appropriate one and the individual goes to the program and at some point sits down and is informed about the research protocol and risks of the research and the potential benefits of research, etc.
>
> In that type of situation where there is no apparent disagreement between the individual and his or her family, it would be my contention ... that the obligation on the part of the researchers to inform would extend to the family. ... This is something that we hear about a great deal, that families initiate a referral and then they're completely written out of the process.

Recognizing these problems in the process of gaining informed consent, a consensus is growing, among both experts and consumers, that authentic informed consent requires more than a one-time paper-signing event.

One-on-one, ongoing discussion is needed, and caregiving family members should be involved in the consent process, with all due respect for the subject's confidentiality. This involvement is particularly important for patients with a serious brain disorder who may become research subjects. When there is no apparent disagreement between the individual and his or her family, it is the researchers' obligation to extend information to the family.

NAMI's policies on the protection of individuals with serious brain disorders who participate as human subjects in research enunciate these principles. They mandate comprehensible, ongoing communication about consent with both the patient and the caregiving family member. These policies also note the importance of various kinds of information—the potential benefits and risks of research, the purpose of the study, and information about the IRB.

> Participants in research and their involved family members must be fully and continuously informed, orally and in writing, about all aspects of the research throughout the process. Research investigators must provide information in a clear, accessible manner to ensure that participants and their involved families fully understand the nature, risks, and benefits of the research.
>
> The consent protocol must provide information which is clear and understandable on an individual basis for participants and their family members. The consent protocol must provide information on the purposes and scale of the research, what is hoped to be learned and prospects for success, potential benefits and potential risks to the individual (including options for treatment other than participation in research, since research is not the same as treatment). The consent protocol should also contain information concerning the function of the Institutional Review Board (IRB), the identity of the IRB administrator, the address and telephone number of the IRB administrator and other information as appropriate.
>
> Whenever consent is given by someone other than the research participant, the participant and involved family members must receive information on the same basis as the person actually giving consent. (National Alliance for the Mentally Ill 1997, p. 22)

THE WITHHOLDING OF MEDICATION

Most scientists believe that studies involving the withdrawal of medication or the use of placebos provide the gold standard for testing the effectiveness of new drugs or make it possible to examine critical issues related to relapse.

However, discontinuation of medications presents a high risk of relapse, which may include psychotic, delusional, suicidal, or aggressive symptoms. It also presents a risk that a research subject who experiences exacerbated symptoms will quit the study, disappear, and/or refuse medications following the research project.

Because of the implications of medication withdrawal, the use of placebos in research and drug washout periods is controversial (Shamoo 1996). Many NAMI members now feel that a placebo is not acceptable, because we view schizophrenia and other psychotic disorders and affective illnesses as life-threatening diseases. In fact, 3 years ago NAMI asked for such a designation from the FDA for schizophrenia and bipolar disorder. This point of view reflects concern that the costs of medication withdrawal are too high, as illustrated by this mother's account (Becker 1994, p. 17):

> Laura, the third of my four children, was hospitalized at age eighteen. She had been on the honor roll at high school and had finished one semester at college when signs of schizophrenia began.
>
> Eight years and a succession of three hospitalizations later and she was indeed institutionalized. One drug after another and combinations of drugs were tried, but they did little to alleviate her symptoms. . . .
>
> During the summer of 1987 she was admitted [to a research program]. . . . After a few weeks, the time patients are given to adapt to the unit, medication weaning began. . . . For one year Laura remained drug free. . . . It was a terrible time, and if seeing her decompensate to a very psychotic state was distressful to me, imagine how tormenting her symptoms have been for her. . . .
>
> I am left with . . . questions. . . . Was Laura's condition aggravated by the suffering she endured through those repeated washouts?

Although NAMI has not adopted a policy concerning the removal of medication, this subject requires candid and comprehensive discussion involving clinicians, researchers, administrators, and, most importantly, patients and their families. Indeed, NAMI has serious questions about whether placebo-controlled studies are still necessary in this era. Researchers conducting such studies must be incredibly vigilant about these issues in their informed consent process, ongoing communication with families and patients, and follow-up to the research.

COMPETENCE TO CONSENT

A thorny issue for research involving human subjects with serious brain disorders arises in situations in which competence is in question or clearly lacking.

Some consumers and family members completely oppose involving patients with diminished capacity in research (Shamoo 1996). As an organization, NAMI believes that strong safeguards are necessary to protect research participants whose ability to understand the risks and benefits of research is compromised, whether consistently or intermittently. NAMI's policy reads as follows:

> Research participants should be carefully evaluated before and throughout the research for their capacity to comprehend information and their capacity to consent to continued participation in the research. The determination of competence shall be made by someone other than the principal investigator or others involved in the research. Except for research protocols approved by the Institutional Review Board (IRB) as minimal risk, whenever it is determined that the subject is not able to continue to provide consent, consent to continue participation in the research shall be sought from families or others legally entrusted to act in the participant's best interests.

NAMI has called for increased understanding of competence and its determination. We are heartened by recent research that sheds light on how competence can be determined and what competence research means for public policy (Appelbaum 1997).

No one questions that a brain disorder can affect competence. But NAMI is concerned that the view of patient competence is in fact far too dim. Even as we identify patients with brain disorders as vulnerable, it is vital to recognize that most patients are fully capable of consenting to research most of the time. These patients must be directly involved in decisions relating to research protocols for which they volunteer. Scientists must avoid paternalistic or stigmatizing views of patients with brain disorders.

We also know that many individuals with these illnesses need special protection to participate in research protocols. A consumer with a serious brain disorder has written poignantly about this issue (Frese 1994, p. 56):

> I write this . . . as a professional who has had more than two decades of experience serving seriously mentally ill persons. . . . I also write this article as a person who has been repeatedly diagnosed with and hospitalized myself for serious mental illness. Denial is a phenomenon that comes as part and parcel of the disorder of serious mental illness. No one wants to think of themselves as insane or crazy, but the nature of serious mental illness is such that it affects one's belief system. One actually believes that what one is thinking is real and true. Others can usually recognize that you have left the world of normality, but the nature of psychosis and other forms of serious mental illness tends to be such that the disorder blinds you to the fact that you have the disorder. As a

general rule, when you become seriously mentally ill, you do not initially believe that you are. For many of us this state of disbelief or denial may last for years, even a lifetime. . . . For those of us who tend to have periodic breakdowns, when we become rational or in remission, over the years, we may come to accept the fact that our brain functions in such a manner that we lose our ability to understand what is happening to us as we become ill. . . .

Allowing patients to make decisions while their minds are free from psychosis would seem to be a prudent approach to the informed consent issue. For patients who do not experience periods of rationality, having a designated, trusted family member or trusted "other" concur with the decision to become a subject in clinical research would seem advisable. Whether a patient who clearly lacks the capacity to make a rational decision concerning participation in clinical research can, in fact, ethically participate in such research—not being able to grasp the risks and benefits involved—remains a very serious question and forcefully raises the specter of possible exploitation.

Several key points are embedded in NAMI's policy statement on competence to consent. The first is an acknowledgment that capacity for consent may vary over time. The symptoms of serious brain disorders are not unchanging. And, as we have noted, clinical researchers must respect patients' periods of lucidity. So, as with informed consent, assessment of competence to consent must be repeated, and competence itself must be viewed as a variable that may change over time.

But because of the at least intermittent threat to competence, it is critical that a family member or other individual legally entrusted to act in a participant's best interest be involved in the consent process on an ongoing basis from the beginning of the project. Investigators should thus encourage research participants to designate a surrogate decision maker—family member, friend, or legal guardian—at the beginning of the research process when they are competent to do so to prepare for times of impaired capacity due to relapse. Specifically, people who are able to give informed consent but are at risk for developing impaired judgment during the course of their research participation should be encouraged to designate a surrogate by a durable power of attorney before or shortly after enrollment and to state in writing the conditions under which they would, and would not, want to participate in the present and future protocols in the event of impaired capacity. The surrogate—typically a family member—would then be responsible for deciding whether the research participant should continue in a research study if the person's judgment becomes impaired, making decisions based on the subject's known preferences. The caregiving family should not be excluded from discussions about the research until a crisis emerges. Family members should be fully involved in the informed consent process and kept abreast of the patient's status and the status of the research.

Another key issue NAMI addresses in this policy statement has to do with the involvement of a nonresearch clinician to evaluate the research participant's symptoms before and during the course of research and to determine whether the person is competent to initiate or continue participation in research activities. This separation of competence determination from the research itself would minimize the influence of a researcher, who desires to see the research proceed, from the competence determination, whose aim is solely to examine the status of the individual. Such a separation is an attempt to increase objectivity in the competence determination process to protect the patient and subject. Indeed, many patients, family members, and experts have suggested that a patient in a research protocol should have a care provider, independent from the research group, whose only concern is the patient's well-being. As stated by one father of an individual with a serious brain disorder (A. E. Shamoo, unpublished work, 1994):

> The patient should have a private physician, during the course of a research study, who will be concerned only with the welfare of his/her patient. The patient, with the assistance of the physician, should decide whether to withdraw or remain in the study. The physician should be independent of the research program and have no benefit from the results of the study such as publications that result from findings. [This is a major] flaw in the current system, in which the investigative researcher is also the physician of the subject in the study.

A related issue (not directly addressed by NAMI policy) concerns participation in research by people with serious brain disorders who are institutionalized in state hospitals or criminal justice facilities. Confinement to an institution is not equivalent to incompetence to consent, although the likelihood of incompetence may be greater among such individuals. However, confinement clearly diminishes personal freedom. The choices to participate in research may be made because of fear of reproach from institutional authorities or may be motivated by enticements such as better living conditions. The potential for coercion in institutional settings seems to directly violate a key value put forward by the National Commission for the Protection of Human Subjects of Biomedical and Behavioral Research (1978) in regard to the ethical conduct of research involving human subjects—justice, or the fair and uncoerced selection of human subjects for research, especially among vulnerable populations.

None of us likes to think that widespread abuses of institutional populations could occur in the United States, but it is appropriate to remember the not-so-distant past. A case in point is the intentional infection with hepatitis of residents of the Willowbrook State School for the Retarded. In a series of experiments begun in 1956 and spanning a decade, institutionalized children with mental disabilities were infected with live hepatitis virus in an effort to develop a vaccine. The scientists justified their procedures by noting that hepatitis was rampant in the institution and all of the children would eventually contract the disease. Further, they maintained that only children whose parents had given written consent were included in the experiments. Critics challenged these arguments, suggesting that parents may have been coerced into volunteering their children as a means of procuring placement at Willowbrook. Moreover, parents were misled into believing their children were to receive a vaccine against the virus, and they were not informed of the risk to their children of developing chronic hepatitis and the possible link to cirrhosis in later life. Clearly, abuses are possible; indeed, they have occurred. We cannot dismiss this fact and must continue to explore the ethical problems raised by research on institutionalized populations.

INSTITUTIONAL REVIEW BOARDS

The responsibility for ensuring that informed consent proceeds according to established principles and regulations and that other ethical issues in human subjects research are appropriately dealt with is left to the researcher and his or her IRB. Every institution in the United States involved in human research must establish an IRB or have access to an IRB to review and approve its human research projects before it can receive federal funding. IRBs are accountable to the Office of Protection of Human Subjects at the National Institutes of Health (NIH), which sets the boundaries of ethical conduct in research with human subjects.

The IRB, a multidisciplinary panel, considers the risks, benefits, subject selection, and consent issues for proposed studies involving human subjects. When an IRB reviews a research project, it must pay particular attention to the project's plan for obtaining research subjects' informed consent and to the documentation of informed consent. The IRB may require changes in the investigator's procedure for obtaining informed consent and in the consent documents. The IRB must also be allowed to observe the informed consent process if the board members consider such oversight important for ensuring that subjects are adequately protected by the process.

Many have raised questions about whether current IRB practices are adequate in general and in regard to individuals with serious brain disorders in particular. Some commentators have equated the typical IRB review process to a rubber-stamp exercise. Findings from a research proposal review conducted by the Advisory Committee on Human Radiation Experiments (1995) indicated that IRBs should not have approved a number of problematic consent forms in the condition in which they were submitted. The committee concluded that although IRBs serve important functions, they need to work to ensure that the informed consent process complies with current standards. Moreover, the committee concluded that IRBs do not have the capacity, if only by virtue of composition and lack of time, to either modify consent standards or, more generally, make any other decisions that could affect the fundamental constitutional rights and personal interests of subjects of research. The committee recommended that a national ethics board be created to discuss what constitutes acceptable research with human subjects, to develop guidelines to inform IRB deliberations, and to be available to offer advisory opinions whenever IRBs are confronted with new ethical problems. (In fact, such a board, the National Bioethics Advisory Commission, was created by President Clinton, and Laurie Flynn, NAMI's executive director, is a member of the commission.)

NAMI has questioned how well IRBs understand serious brain disorders and the issues of involving such individuals in research. Because IRBs are the cornerstone of the current process by which research involving human subjects is approved and overseen and the effectiveness of IRBs has been questioned, NAMI's policy contains two statements addressing this issue:

> Institutional Review Boards which regularly review research proposals on serious brain disorders must include consumers and family members who have direct and personal experience with serious brain disorders.
>
> Members of IRBs approving research on individuals with serious brain disorders must receive specialized training about mental illness and other cognitive impairments and the needs of individuals who experience these disorders. Persons with serious brain disorders and members of their families must be integrally involved in the development, provision, and evaluation of this training. (National Alliance for the Mentally Ill 1997, p. 23)

These policy statements about direct involvement of consumers and their family members in the IRB and education of IRBs about brain disorders will ensure that IRBs are more informed about the issues that arise from these illnesses. Federal regulations state only that "if an IRB regularly reviews research that involves a vulnerable category of subjects, including but not limited to subjects covered by other subparts of this part, the IRB shall include one or more individuals who are primarily concerned with the welfare of these subjects" (Department of Health and Human Services 1991, 45 *Code of Federal Regulations [CFR]* 46). More recently, the language has been shifted to "the inclusion of one or more individuals who are knowledgeable about and experienced in working with these subjects." However, no evidence indicates that NIH has required IRBs to include either persons with serious brain disorders, members of their families, NAMI, or any of the state affiliates to serve on these IRBs on a permanent basis (Shamoo and Irving 1993).

AFTER THE RESEARCH

When a research participant leaves a study or the study itself ends, a host of issues emerge that are critically important to patients and their family members. NAMI has therefore developed four policy statements about this part of the process:

> Without penalty, a research participant is free to withdraw consent at any time, with or without a stated reason. Any time a participant terminates participation, regardless of reason, investigators will make every effort to ensure that linkages to appropriate services occur, with follow-up to assist that participant to establish contact with appropriate service providers and/or care-givers. If a participant disappears or terminates his/her continued consent, the investigator shall contact his or her family or others designated to receive notification and information.
>
> When participation by an individual in a research protocol is completed, participants and/or their families are entitled to be informed of results as soon as this information is available, to have the opportunity to receive feedback concerning their individual participation in the protocol, to critique the protocol, and to provide input concerning possible additional research.
>
> All participants in research protocols involving the assessment of new medications will be provided with opportunities by the investigator for a trial on the medication being studied, so long as other research on the new medication has demonstrated potential safety and efficacy.
>
> All individuals who have benefited from the administration of experimental medications in research will be provided continual access to the medication by the investigator without cost until a source of third party payment is found. (National Alliance for the Mentally Ill 1997, pp. 23–24)

The issues discussed throughout this chapter in regard to true voluntary participation and the genuine involvement of family members are reflected in these policy statements. In studies that involve the use of placebos or in which patients are otherwise removed from medication, these issues are critical. An individual who relapses into psychosis may refuse medication or may even disappear. Because the consequences of such actions are potentially life threatening, the researcher must exercise great care in planning for such eventualities, provide good clinical care during research, and ensure good communication with families.

Because the care received during research trials is often superior to that available outside of the research setting, researchers must vigorously strive to ensure follow-up treatment for patients who have given their time and energy to the research. If medications used in the trial are not yet available outside of the research setting and they prove effective for the patient, then ongoing access to the medication is important. Effectively engaging the patient in the system of care in his or her community is also needed. Further, investigators should provide patients and their families with feedback on the results of the research. In short, the commitment to people with serious brain disorders and their families cannot end when the final data are collected. Respect for their contributions requires ongoing communication and linkage to clinical care.

CONCLUSION

People with serious brain disorders and their families look to research for a better tomorrow for themselves, their children and grandchildren, and others. The strength of this research depends on the positive treatment of participating individuals with brain disorders and their families. Some straightforward steps, enunciated by NAMI and others, can be taken to strengthen the ethical moorings of clinical research. Such guidelines boil down to communicating with patients and their families with respect and doing everything possible to ensure their well-being. Although some thorny issues remain unresolved and require continued consideration, true alliances among researchers, the consumers who participate in research, and their families can go a long way toward enhancing the strong research enterprise that exists today.

REFERENCES

Advisory Committee on Human Radiation Experiments: Final Report. Washington, DC, U.S. Government Printing Office, October 1995

Appelbaum P: Rethinking the conduct of psychiatric research. Arch Gen Psychiatry 54:117–120, 1997

Becker JC: A mother's testimony (letter). Journal of the California Alliance for the Mentally Ill 5:17, 1994

Berg JW: Legal and ethical complexities of consent with cognitively impaired research subjects: proposed guidelines. Journal of Law, Medicine, and Ethics 24:18–35, 1996

Bonnie RJ: Research with cognitively impaired subjects: unfinished business in the regulation of human research. Arch Gen Psychiatry 54:105–111, 1997

Burt MR, Cohen BE: America's Homeless: Numbers, Characteristics, and Programs That Serve Them. Washington, DC, Urban Institute Press, 1989

Cassileth BR, Lusk EJ, Miller DS, et al: Attitudes toward clinical trials among patients and the public. JAMA 248:968–970, 1982

Daugherty C, Ratain MJ, Grochowski E, et al: Perceptions of cancer patients and their physicians involved in phase I trials. J Clin Oncol 13:1062–1072, 1995

Department of Health and Human Services: Rules and Regulations for the Protection of Human Research Subjects, 45 Code of Federal Regulations 46 (1991)

Dresser R: Mentally disabled research subjects: the enduring policy issues. JAMA 276:67–72, 1996

Frese F: Informed consent and the right to refuse or participate (letter). Journal of the California Alliance for the Mentally Ill 5:56, 1994

Hall LL, Mark TL: The Efficacy of Schizophrenia Treatment. Arlington, VA, National Alliance for the Mentally Ill, 1995

Lehman AF, Steinwachs DM, Survey Co-Investigators of the PORT Project: Patterns of usual care for schizophrenia: initial results from the schizophrenia patient outcomes research team (PORT) client survey. Schizophr Bull 24:11–20, 1998

National Alliance for the Mentally Ill, Public Policy Platform, 2nd Edition, March, 1997

National Commission for the Protection of Human Subjects of Biomedical and Behavioral Research: The Belmont Report: ethical principles and guidelines for the protection of human subjects of research (DHEW Publ No OS-78-0012). Washington, DC, U.S. Government Printing Office, 1978

Newburg SM, Holland AE, Pearce LA: Motivation of subjects to participate in a research trial. Appl Nurs Res 5:89–104, 1992

Pearson J: Suicide in the United States. Decade of the Brain 8:1–2, 1997–1998

Penman DT, Holland JC, Bahna GF, et al: Informed consent for investigational chemotherapy: patients' and physicians' perceptions. J Clin Oncol 2:849–855, 1984

Shamoo AE: Human rights in reference to persons with mental illness. Accountability in Research 4:207–216, 1996

Shamoo AE, Irving DN: Accountability in research using persons with mental illness. Accountability in Research 1:12–15, 1993

Sturges JS, Sternberg DE: Family concerns about hospitalizing a patient in a psychiatric research unit. Hosp Community Psychiatry 36:1187–1191, 1985

Torrey EF, Stieber J, Ezekiel J, et al: Criminalizing the Seriously Mentally Ill: The Abuse of Jails as Mental Hospitals. Arlington, VA, National Alliance for the Mentally Ill, 1992

U.S. Congress, Office of Technology, Assessment, Mental Disorders, and Genetics: Bridging the gap between research and society (Publ No OTA-BP-H-133). Washington, DC, U.S. Government Printing Office, 1994

National Alliance for the Mentally Ill Public Policy Platform,

Revised, Second Edition, Research Section 6

[Reprinted with permission from the National Alliance for the Mentally Ill (NAMI).]

---

6. RESEARCH

6.1 Neuroscience research, behavioral research, pharmaceutical research, clinical research, as well as service system research are some of the initiatives supported by NAMI. To this end, NAMI endorses the Presidential proclamation of the 1990s as the Decade of the Brain, which calls upon Congress and the Executive Branch to focus more attention on research, treatment, education, and rehabilitation related to brain disorders and to appropriate funds sufficient to make that promise a reality. NAMI expects the rigor and pace of the field of services research to be equal to that of biomedical research.

6.2 *Standards for Protecting the Well-being of Individuals Participating in Research*

(6.2.1)   NAMI accepts the critical necessity for research using human subjects, acknowledges the important contribution of persons who become human subjects, and affirms that all such research should be conducted in accordance with the highest medical, ethical, and scientific standards.

(6.2.2)   National standards to govern voluntary consent, comprehensive exchange of information, and related protections of persons with cognitive impairments who become research subjects must be developed and they must include the interests of persons who become human subjects, families, and other caregivers.

(6.2.3)   Participants in research and their involved family members must be fully and continuously informed, orally and in writing, about all aspects of the research throughout the process. Research investigators must provide information in a clear, accessible manner to ensure that participants and their involved families fully understand the nature, risks, and benefits of the research.

(6.2.4)   The consent protocol must provide information that is clear and understandable on an individual basis for each participant and his or her family members. The consent protocol must provide information about the purposes and scale of the research, what is hoped to be learned, prospects for success, and potential benefits and risks to the individual (including options for treatment other than participation in research, since research is not the same as treatment). The consent protocol should also contain information about the function of the institutional review board (IRB), the identity of the IRB administrator, the address and telephone number of the IRB administrator and other information, as appropriate.

(6.2.5)   Whenever consent is given by someone other than the research participant, the participant and involved family members must receive information on the same basis as the person actually giving consent.

(6.2.6)   Research participants should be carefully evaluated before and throughout the research for their capacity to comprehend information and their capacity to consent to continued participation in the research. The determination of competence shall be made by someone other than the principal investigator or others involved in the research. Except for research protocols approved by the institutional review board (IRB) as minimal risk, whenever it is determined that the subject is not able to continue to provide consent, consent to continue participation in the research shall be sought from families or others legally entrusted to act in the participant's best interests.

(6.2.7)   Institutional review boards that regularly review research proposals for brain disorders must include consumers and family members who have direct and personal experience with brain disorders.

(6.2.8)   Members of IRBs approving research on individuals with brain disorders must receive specialized training about brain disorders and other cognitive impairments and the needs of individuals who experience these disorders. Persons with brain disorders and members of their families must be integrally involved in the development, provision, and evaluation of this training.

(6.2.9)   Without penalty, a research participant must be free to withdraw consent at any time, with or without a stated reason. Any time a participant terminates participation, regardless of the reason, investigators will make every effort to ensure that linkages to appropriate services occur with follow-up to assist that participant to establish contact with appropriate service providers and/or care-givers. If a participant disappears or terminates his or her continued consent, the investigator shall contact his or her family or others designated to receive notification and information.

(6.2.10)   When participation by an individual in a research protocol is completed, participants and/or their families are entitled to be informed of results as soon as this information is available, to have the opportunity to receive feedback concerning their individual participation in the protocol, to critique the protocol, and to provide input concerning possible additional research.

(6.2.11)   All participants in research protocols involving the assessment of new medications will be provided with opportunities by the investigator for a trial on the medication being studied, so long as other research on the new medication has demonstrated potential safety and efficacy.

(6.2.12) All individuals who have benefited from the administration of experimental medications in research will be provided continual access to the medication by the investigator without cost until a source of third-party payment is found.

(6.2.13) NAMI endorses the development of a uniform, standard definition of "brain disorders" to help all states obtain priority funding and services for the population that suffers the most severe disabilities.

6.3 Biomedical Research

(6.3.1) NAMI strongly encourages the donation of human organs and other tissue for transplant, research, and education, and the donation of tissue samples to developing gene banks. NAMI recognizes the severe shortage for research purposes of postmortem human brain tissue of persons who were afflicted with brain disorders and members of their immediate families with their clinical records.

(6.3.2) NAMI believes that the careful, responsible use of animals is indispensable in research on brain disorders. At the same time, NAMI advocates the use of non-animal systems whenever feasible and urges researchers to observe the traditional, compassionate standards of animal experimentation; and to comply fully with the Federal Animal Welfare Act.

6.4 Psychopharmacological Research

(6.4.1) *FDA Drug Approval*
NAMI urges the Food and Drug Administration (FDA) to categorize brain disorders as "life-threatening," which would make drugs for the treatment of these disorders eligible for special expeditious evaluation and approval by the FDA.

(6.4.2) *Patent Protection*
NAMI supports patent protection for pharmaceutical manufacturers as a legitimate and worthwhile incentive to stimulate research into and development of new products. However, when a patent is combined with restrictive business practices to maintain exorbitant prices, NAMI may seek antitrust action through the attorney general or may initiate or participate in civil actions.

(6.4.3) With Board review, NAMI may support legislation to place reasonable caps on product liability awards to encourage greater research and development.

CHAPTER 10

Administrative Issues and Informed Consent

DAVID SHORE, M.D., AND JANE A. STEINBERG, PH.D.

A dministrative issues in the protection of human subjects focus on documentation of the investigator's ability to develop an ethical experimental
design and a process for obtaining informed consent. To ensure robust protections, before beginning the project the investigator needs to interact with all of
the constituencies involved in the research enterprise, including the applicant
institution (e.g., the investigator's university), the funding institution (e.g., a
National Institutes of Health [NIH] institute, a foundation, or another organization), the research team, and the community of potential subjects and their
family members. In this chapter we provide an overview of the processes involved in working with these entities, along with some useful tips for navigating
the administrative hurdles in dealing with funding agencies or the university.

Requirements for informed consent are fairly straightforward, but informed
consent is an ongoing process, not a one-time event. Potential participants must
be told that their participation is voluntary and that they can withdraw at any
time. Investigators must also inform subjects about the purpose of the study
and which procedures involve research, how long they will be asked to participate, what the anticipated benefits are, and what appropriate alternatives might
be of value. Researchers must also disclose whether and how subjects' confidentiality will be maintained and reasonably foreseeable risks or discomforts.
All such information must be provided in understandable language, with adequate opportunity for subjects to decide voluntarily whether to participate, and
include whom to contact with questions or complaints. Depending on the type
of study, additional information, such as the availability of treatment and/or
compensation for any research-related injuries incurred, may also be required.

239

SOME IMPORTANT STARTING POINTS

Before submitting a protocol for review, applicants should prepare by reading the relevant regulations, policies, and/or texts (Levine 1988). Although most investigators already have a working understanding of ethical considerations in research, reading the regulations and policies can be enlightening. These Department of Health and Human Services regulations can be found at Title 45, *Code of Federal Regulations*, part 46, usually referred to as 45 *CFR* 46 (see Appendix C). Although federal rules and regulations have a reputation for not being particularly user-friendly, in this case they are quite straightforward and brief. The code (45 *CFR* 46) describes the elements of informed consent (46.116) and the procedures by which the local institutional review board (IRB) is to be constituted (46.107) and to go about the review of research proposals (46.109, 46.111).

Subpart A describes several requirements for informed consent and delegates the primary review of human subjects research to local IRBs. These IRBs must include researchers; experts in clinical, legal, and ethical issues; and at least one nonscientist and one individual not otherwise affiliated with the institution. Most research facilities (e.g., universities and hospitals) have their own or share IRBs, but independent IRBs can be contracted with to cover clinical sites for research.

The IRB system is under local institutional control and authorized to review proposals, evaluate potential risks and benefits, and consider the adequacy of protections for human subjects. Federally conducted or supported research (and research regulated by the U.S. Food and Drug Administration [FDA]) cannot be undertaken without IRB approval. The university or other institution must certify that it has a properly constituted IRB and obtain an assurance through the NIH Office for Protection From Research Risks (OPRR). Grant applications for NIH funding generally require an assurance number and date of IRB review on the first page of the grant application. This document must be signed by both the principal investigator and the institutional business official.

The material in 45 *CFR* 46 (presented in Appendix C) makes it clear that some research is exempt from certain administrative procedures, if the IRB concurs. The regulations contain a list of possible exemptions (46.101), which include, for example, secondary analysis of data and certain record reviews. The IRB decides what research is exempt. However, many hospitals and universities consider IRB review so useful that they mandate it for studies even when approval is not required by law. The rules for organizing and running the IRB, also presented in these regulations, show what the IRB is looking for in application materials and help investigators avoid the time requirements and aggravation of revisions and resubmission. Also, if an investigator has problems with the IRB, the regulations provide insight into possible sources of the problems.

Some individuals, including pregnant women, prisoners, and children, require additional protections when they participate in studies (see 45 *CFR* 46, subparts B, C, and D). These additional considerations are all clearly presented in the regulations.

Investigators may also find it helpful to familiarize themselves with provisions that protect the confidentiality of research subjects. Such provisions include federal regulations concerning issuance of certificates of confidentiality that can be granted for research projects (regardless of whether they are federally supported); such certificates can prevent a court from compelling an investigator to divulge information about a subject. This protection is available only if the research is of a sensitive nature in which the protection is judged necessary to achieve the research objectives. Examples of such research data include the following:

1. Information relating to sexual attitudes, preferences, or practices
2. Information relating to the use of alcohol, drugs, or other addictive products
3. Information pertaining to illegal conduct
4. Information that if released could reasonably be damaging to an individual's financial standing, employability, or reputation within the community
5. Information that would normally be recorded in a patient's medical record and the disclosure of which could reasonably lead to social stigmatization or discrimination
6. Information pertaining to an individual's psychological well-being or mental health
7. Information relating to genetics

In clinical psychiatric research, such protection may be considered useful. Because the certificate does not protect against voluntary or consented-to disclosures, however, it is important that subjects do not reveal their participation to insurers, who might then require the subject's consent to such disclosure. Also, researchers are not excluded from the requirement to disclose matters such as ongoing child abuse or a subject's threatened violence to self or others. The consent form should clearly indicate whether a researcher intends to report such information. Knowing about certificates of confidentiality and indicating whether you are considering applying for one may help you in dealing with your IRB, but to obtain the certificate, you first need approval from your local IRB. The regulations also describe the general issues of confidentiality and the specifics of obtaining a certificate (42 *CFR* part 2a).

Reading through the local institution's guidelines for IRB operations and learning who serves on the IRB are also essential steps. If no one on the panel understands mental health research, investigators may want to ask for additional representation from the mental health field (e.g., researchers, family members, or consumers) to inform the IRB's decision process. Obviously, checking IRB membership and offering suggestions before the review is more effective than waiting for a denial and then suggesting that an expert be added to the board for the second attempt.

The time required to obtain IRB approval varies. Some institutions are generous about emergency reviews, but many are not. Do not count on the willingness of IRB members to expedite your particular project; estimate the proper time for clearance, and in preparing these complex materials, allow yourself some leeway. It is especially important to allow sufficient time to obtain feedback from family members or consumers to ensure that you have thought through the relevant issues from their perspectives. Also, asking a colleague to review and edit your materials can make them clearer. Remember, IRB members are making complex decisions, and they must have clear, thoughtful documents on which to base valid conclusions.

The temptation to simply follow the example of a colleague whose application materials and consent documents have been approved by the IRB is understandable, but this approach is not recommended. Although a model can be helpful, each research project is different, and standards change over time. Carefully reviewing the regulations and considering your design are the best ways to develop rigorous consent procedures.

REVIEWING YOUR DESIGN AND INFORMED CONSENT ISSUES

Reading the regulations and policies of the entities that judge the adequacy of a study's protection procedures helps investigators ensure that a particular study reflects the principles of ethical research. Taking a step back from the design and questioning issues can also be worthwhile. For example, consider confidentiality: although certificates of confidentiality are available, more useful procedures may exist. To illustrate, if you do not need the name of an individual, do not keep it. If knowing a particular bit of information (e.g., substance abuse or criminal behavior) is not relevant to your hypothesis, do not ask about it. These approaches may provide the strongest protection for participants in your study and will save you the time and effort of applying for a certificate of confidentiality that you really do not need.

Also, consider participants' time as the rare commodity it is. Have you done your best to reduce procedures to those critical for the study? Shaving off minimally useful or duplicative procedures will increase your chances of IRB approval, as well as your recruitment and retention rates. More important, you will be demonstrating appropriate respect for your volunteers.

If you consult with the National Institute of Mental Health (NIMH) or other federal funding officials on the scientific aspects of your application, remember to ask them about ethical considerations. Program staff can help refine your design based on their considerable experience in reviewing protocols and their understanding of current regulations on human subjects protections.

The presentation of a given study's risks and benefits is an especially sensitive issue (Office for Protection From Research Risks 1994). For example, during the course of the study, a participant's symptoms may improve, remain stable, or worsen. If the experimental intervention involves discontinuing effective treatments and the probability of these outcomes is known, telling subjects that they may get worse or better is not considered adequate. If three patients are expected to deteriorate for every one who remains stable or improves, this information must be provided in the consent documents. And if it is reasonably expected (or so far observed) that some subjects will worsen significantly, this likelihood should be stated clearly and the consequences noted explicitly, along with an explanation of what procedures exist to protect subjects. Consent documents may need to be revised or amended in collaboration with the IRB as new information becomes available on the benefits or risks of participating in a study.

Consent documents are expected to present *anticipated benefits* and *foreseeable risks,* and in this documentation the threshold for risks must differ from that for benefits. Only reasonably expected benefits for the subject or others should be presented; those that might (but probably will not) occur should not be presented. In contrast, when it comes to risks, *foreseeable* is a very imprecise term. Exceptionally rare events are not generally considered foreseeable, but those within the range for which forecasts are possible may be. Legally effective informed consent also requires disclosure of appropriate alternative procedures or courses of treatment, if any, that might be advantageous to the subject. For mental disorders, of course, it can be difficult or impossible to predict which alternative will be most useful for which patient.

In formal treatment protocol studies it is particularly important to inform potential research subjects that referral for individualized treatment is an alternative to participating in the research. Sometimes, researchers have argued that the treatments in their protocols are standard or within the range of acceptable clinical practice. However, using only one specific drug (or one specific route of administration), a fixed dose of medication, or intervention(s) based on randomized assignment would generally be considered a research procedure, not clinical practice. The clinician who provides a patient with whatever treatment, in whatever form, at whatever dosage is considered most likely to be beneficial for that individual at that time is providing clinical treatment. The use of standardized procedures to create or expand generalizable knowledge is by definition research. Thus, if a protocol involves a fixed dose, a specific route of administration, or the use of one particular medication (rather than a choice of any drug that might be best for a given individual), then this information must be clearly described in consent documents, and individualized treatment must be presented as an alternative to participating in the protocol (Office for Protection From Research Risks 1994).

Those who wish to design acceptable clinical research protocols also encounter several other difficult issues. For instance, if an investigator in a research protocol is also a subject's clinician, confusion about the investigator's role may result. Some have even argued that a person in the dual role of investigator and clinician creates a conflict of interest in which the goals of the research may compromise the clinician's judgment such that subjects may be disadvantaged. For instance, individuals in a research protocol often require a clinical evaluation to determine whether they should remain in the study or whether their symptoms are so severe as to require therapeutic intervention. If it is possible to designate an independent clinician (rather than an investigator who might benefit from the research project) to make such a decision, this evaluation is less likely to be seen as a conflict of interest.

Sometimes, however, the most appropriate clinicians available are those affiliated with research endeavors. One could argue that it would not make sense (and could even be detrimental) to disqualify such expert clinicians from the decision-making process. Certainly being an investigator (whether funded as such or not) does not override a physician's oath. The primacy of the clinical role is indicated by the routine termination of subjects' participation in a study that appears to be detrimental to their well-being. Nevertheless, clinical researchers in this dual role should be aware of the possibility that involvement in research might bias their judgment. If possible, they should build in a safeguard or independent clinical override, which is a process by which assessments of potential clinical deterioration, when needed, can be conducted by another clinician who is not part of the research team but who has the authority to overrule research decisions to ensure an individual subject's welfare.

Clinical investigators should also be aware that states vary in their definitions of legally effective informed consent. Researchers should know the state laws that apply to competence and consent, including substituted judgment, durable powers of attorney, and the like. A related and important concern is the competence of patients with severe mental disorders to consent to research.

Although IRBs can waive some elements of informed consent for certain projects that do not exceed minimal risk, most psychiatric research requires informed consent. Thus, subjects must be competent to judge risks and benefits or have a legally authorized representative to consent on their behalf. It has traditionally been the responsibility of the investigators to determine the competence of subjects to consent, although some now claim that this role also causes a potential conflict of interest and competence should be assessed independently.

Those conducting clinical research with patients experiencing severe mental disorders (such as acute psychotic conditions or chronic and recurrent disorders) are encouraged to involve immediate family members in the consent process with the patient's permission. Also, again with the patient's permission, researchers should keep the family informed on an ongoing basis and be available to listen to the views of family members on the progress, clinical symptoms, and functioning of the patient. Involving the family in the informed consent process can be invaluable to the patient and the researcher (Shore 1996; Skirboll et al. 1997). If a patient has a conservator or legal guardian, that patient cannot participate in most types of research without the guardian's consent.

Unfortunately, no gold standard or objective test clearly and reliably measures competence. Although competence includes a patient's ability to articulate the risks, benefits, and experimental procedures involved in a given study, truly informed consent should include a determination of whether the potential subject understands these matters, can discuss them rationally, and can determine how they apply to that individual. For instance, if an individual denies having an illness, it is unlikely that that person can give informed consent to experimental therapeutic measures that may affect the course of the illness.

Grisso and Appelbaum (1995) have reviewed the literature on competence to consent and conducted well-designed studies with control subjects matched on socioeconomic status and education. Focusing on inpatients with depression or schizophrenia, they have found that a significant number of patients with acute schizophrenia have impaired capacity to consent. The finding may not surprise researchers in this area, but it should make us reevaluate our views on competence. As Grisso and Appelbaum note, subjects may appear to be competent on one measure but incompetent when judged by another; thus, a broad and multifaceted assessment of competence to consent is needed. It should also be noted that under the stress of making medical treatment decisions, even individuals without a mental disorder may have problems in evaluating information and making decisions.

Research involving people with mental disorders clearly requires a process of informed consent that ensures that all relevant information about risks, benefits, and alternatives is clearly presented. Research on competence and consent is needed, and the development of valid tests for competence should be a top priority.

THE ROUTE AT NIH

On receipt of a grant application by an NIH institute, a peer review for scientific merit is undertaken. If the protocol involves human subjects, the study section or initial review group (IRG) will also review the adequacy of human subjects protections. This procedure often involves a request for consent documents and sometimes additional documentation from the applicant institution or principal investigator. The IRG reviews the contents of the grant application and the description of human subjects protections and risk-benefit considerations and may critique the wording of informed consent documents. If the peer reviewers are satisfied with human subjects protections and the adequacy of the informed consent process, then the application is coded as having no human subjects concerns or comments.

If the IRG perceives significant problems with the protection of human subjects, the competence of subjects to consent, or the adequacy of the presentation of risks and benefits, then reviewers may code the application as having a human subjects concern. For example, researchers might label a study with a human subjects concern because the application does not adequately describe risks, precautions, or exclusion criteria or because consent documents do not fully describe the study. Even though a local IRB may have approved a protocol and consent document, the IRG may be concerned about risk-benefit issues, the information given to subjects, or other factors related to human subjects. If a concern is designated, the application cannot be funded until that concern is resolved to the satisfaction of the NIH program staff and OPRR.

Resolving such issues generally involves communication among NIH program staff, and perhaps OPRR staff, the principal investigator, and the applicant's institution or IRB. Some problems may be so serious that they diminish the scientific merit of the application and therefore lead to a poorer priority score for funding the study.

Communication of a human subjects concern to the applicant institution will occur regardless of the likelihood of a grant application's approval. Generally, the IRG's concern is described in a letter sent to the institution. The rationale for this procedure is that a local IRB may not have properly reviewed a protocol or consent process in light of 45 *CFR* 46 or may not have provided adequate documentation. If the IRG (or study section) notes deficiencies in this process, it must notify the local IRB of the concern. Such notification is necessary because if a project is not funded by NIH but is perhaps carried out with local funding, the human subjects concern identified by peer reviewers can be conveyed to, and taken into account by, the applicant institution.

The IRG may also code an application with a human subjects comment, which is a less serious problem and not likely to result in substantially increased risks for subjects. A human subjects comment does not constitute a bar to funding or ordinarily require the IRG to contact the institution. If a study is to be funded by the NIH, and a human subjects comment is coded, then program staff may want to obtain a letter from the investigator responding to the human subjects comment to satisfactorily resolve the issue raised. In many cases, this response is largely a matter of clarifying some aspect of human subjects participation.

The NIH program staff or the project officer guides applicants through the federal process to ensure that applicants follow grant-related regulations and policies and may advise the investigators about scientific and administrative matters. As mentioned previously, human subjects concerns or comments identified by the IRG are generally resolved by the project officer working in conjunction with the investigator, the applicant institution, and OPRR. Sometimes, subject protection issues may arise after the review process, through questions raised by researchers, review of progress reports, or the like. Program staff have an obligation to investigate these matters, consult with colleagues and/or OPRR staff, and attempt to resolve the issues satisfactorily. If human subjects problems cannot be resolved, program staff working with OPRR have the authority to require a second IRB review or changes in consent documents. In certain situations, funding of a grant might be discontinued because of human subjects problems.

Should OPRR conclude that a local IRB is not adequately reviewing human subjects research, it can restrict or even cancel the institution's multiple project assurance (MPA). Any institution without an MPA must obtain a single project assurance (SPA) for each federally funded protocol it wishes to have approved. SPAs are negotiated by OPRR on a project-by-project basis. An SPA must be obtained from any non-MPA institution before it is awarded support for U.S. Department of Health and Human Services–backed human subjects research. OPRR reviews the grant application and the IRB-approved informed consent document as part of the SPA approval process.

Because many investigators are unfamiliar with these assurances, it may be useful to describe them briefly. Federal regulations state that any institution engaged in research supported (or conducted) by the U.S. Department of Health and Human Services (e.g., NIH) must provide OPRR with an "assurance of compliance" with the regulations (45 *CFR* 46). The assurance details each institution's procedures for implementing the regulatory protections required for its human subjects research. An assurance number is simply the number assigned by OPRR to the approved assurance. MPA numbers begin with an *M* (e.g., M-1000), and SPA numbers begin with an *S*. MPAs cover all of an institution's federally supported research for a period of 5 years, and most major clinical research facilities in the United States have MPAs. About 95% of MPA institutions voluntarily extend the regulatory protections to all of their human subjects research, regardless of funding source. OPRR does not routinely review the protocols and informed consent documents approved by an MPA IRB unless noncompliance is alleged.

Some NIH institutes sponsor multi-institutional cooperative studies and may prepare a sample consent document and distribute it to the participating institutions. In such a case, an institute can stipulate that none of the information about risks or alternative approaches can be modified without approval of the institute.

If an NIH institute has serious concerns about a specific type of research, it may work with OPRR to set up specific consent oversight procedures, even for investigator-initiated grant applications. Or an NIH institute could determine that a particular type of research is so dangerous that such an application warrants an automatic human subjects concern. This designation mandates that, regardless of local IRB or peer review, program staff and OPRR are responsible for assuring that consent documents and other relevant information are obtained and reviewed.

THE ROUTE AT THE FDA

The FDA's regulatory authority for research focuses on studies involving drugs, biological products, and devices. An investigational new drug (IND) application is required for all human research involving drugs that are not the subject of an approved new drug application (NDA), and the application may be required for certain approved drugs as well, depending on the nature and intended uses in the proposed studies. However, most research involving approved drugs is exempt from FDA review, and the details of such exemptions from the IND requirement are provided under 21 *CFR* 312.2. Generally, drug studies that involve approved products; that are not intended to support a new indication or important labeling or advertising change; and that do not involve a route of administration, dose, or patient population that would significantly increase the risks associated with the product are exempt. An important point, however, is that these studies, although exempt from FDA review, are not exempt from the

FDA's IRB and informed consent regulations. General information about when an IND is required, and what sections within the FDA will be involved in the review, can be obtained from the Division of Communication Management in the Office of Training and Communications at the FDA (301-594-1012).

For drug studies that do require an IND, the sponsor must submit a signed form FDA 1571, and all investigators must submit a signed form FDA 1572. By signing these documents, the sponsor and any other investigators commit 1) to having an IRB, in compliance with the requirements stated in part 56 of the FDA's regulations, that will take responsibility for the initial and continuing review of each study to be conducted under the IND and 2) to abiding by the informed consent requirements detailed in part 50 of the FDA's regulations. In their general provisions for IRB membership, functions, and operations, the FDA's IRB regulations (21 *CFR* 56) are very similar to those described earlier under 45 *CFR* 46. Included among an IRB's responsibilities is the requirement for informed consent, and the FDA has regulations pertinent to informed consent (21 *CFR* 50) that are also similar to those described under 45 *CFR* 46.

The procedures for reviewing consent documents within the FDA are specific to each center. For instance, the Center for Drug Evaluation and Research (CDER) does not routinely require submission of the actual consent document for review as part of the IND application process. However, CDER may, if it is felt necessary, request this document and make specific recommendations for its wording. When such reviews occur, one element often found missing is an acknowledgment that the FDA has the authority to inspect patient records. The Center for Devices and Radiological Health, on the other hand, requires submission and approval of all consent forms for studies conducted under an investigational device exemption (IDE).

The FDA has a program for both routine and for-cause inspection of IRBs to ensure compliance with parts 50 and 56 of the regulations and protection of human subjects. It has a number of administrative options available for addressing IRB deficiencies, including disqualification.

THE INVESTIGATOR AS ADMINISTRATOR

Although investigators are primarily scientists, they are also to some extent administrators (Burke et al. 1986). As an administrator, the investigator assumes responsibility for documentation of human subjects protections, revision of protection procedures when required, and supervision of staff to promote the appropriate treatment of participants.

The expectation is that every research laboratory will have a zeitgeist that promotes the ethical treatment of subjects. Administrators should not assume this climate to be inherent but rather encourage the ethical treatment of subjects by staff. First, consider the common language in the laboratory. References to "getting the data or else" are clearly jokes among peers, but to subordinates, they may sound like expectations. As pressure within a laboratory mounts to obtain a sample, research assistants may feel pressure to take shortcuts to achieve the recruitment goals of the study, be tempted to minimize a potential subject's concern, or try to make due without all of the materials required. The investigator can avert misinterpretation of priorities by explicitly conveying concern for the protection of subjects. Administrators should tell staff that they would rather not have the data than to shortcut any of the safety procedures and that this concern extends to the safety of staff as well.

CONCLUSION

It is the responsibility first of the local IRB, and second of the IRG (study section), to review human subjects issues, including risk-benefit considerations and the informed consent process and documents. NIH program staff, in consultation with OPRR, may help investigators resolve questions or problems with human subjects protocols. Although federal regulations concerning informed consent have undergone little modification during the past 15 years, the standards by which research protocols and consent documents are judged have changed considerably. Research protocols and explanations of risks and benefits that were considered appropriate 5 or 10 years ago may be considered unacceptable now. Results of recent studies may provide additional data relevant to research risk assessments, but many questions remain unresolved. With changing perspectives about informed consent, the NIMH has recommended that each investigator reevaluate the consent process for clinical research protocols involving human volunteers.

REFERENCES

Burke J, Pincus HA, Pardes H: The clinician researcher in psychiatry. Am J Psychiatry 143:968–975, 1986

Department of Health and Human Services: Protection of Identity— Research Subjects. 42 Code of Federal Regulations, part 2[a] (1991)

Department of Health and Human Services: Rules and Regulations for the Protection of Human Research Subjects, 45 Code of Federal Regulations, part 46[a] (1991)

Grisso T, Appelbaum PS: A comparison of standards for assessing patients' capacities to make treatment decisions. Am J Psychiatry 152:1033–1037, 1995

Levine RJ: Ethics and Regulation of Clinical Research, 2nd Edition. New Haven, CT, Yale University Press, 1988

Office for Protection From Research Risks (Division of Human Subject Protection, National Institutes of Health): Evaluation of Human Subjects Protections in Schizophrenia Research Conducted by the University of California, Los Angeles. Washington, DC, U.S. Government Printing Office, May 11, 1994

Shore D: Ethical principles and informed consent: an NIMH perspective. Psychopharmacol Bull 32:7–10, 1996

Skirboll L, Shore D, Baruchin A, et al: National Institute of Mental Health human subject activities, in The Baltimore Conference on Ethics: Ethics in Neurobiological Research With Human Subjects. Edited by Shamoo AE. New York, Gordon & Breach, 1997

Appendixes

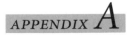

World Medical Association Declaration of Helsinki

Recommendations Guiding Physicians in Biomedical Research Involving Human Subjects

Adopted by the 18th World Medical Assembly, Helsinki, Finland, June 1964,

and amended by the 29th World Medical Assembly, Tokyo, Japan, October 1975; the 35th World Medical Assembly, Venice, Italy, October 1983; the 41st World Medical Assembly, Hong Kong, September 1989; and the 48th General Assembly, Somerset West, Republic of South Africa, October 1996

[Reprinted with permission from the World Medical Association.]

INTRODUCTION

It is the mission of the physician to safeguard the health of the people. His or her knowledge and conscience are dedicated to the fulfillment of this mission.

The Declaration of Geneva of the World Medical Association binds the physician with the words, "The Health of my patient will be my first consideration," and the International Code of Medical Ethics declares that, "A physician shall act only in the patient's interest when providing medical care which might have the effect of weakening the physical and mental condition of the patient."

The purpose of biomedical research involving human subjects must be to improve diagnostic, therapeutic, and prophylactic procedures and the understanding of the aetiology and pathogenesis of disease.

In current medical practice most diagnostic, therapeutic or prophylactic procedures involve hazards. This applies especially to biomedical research.

Medical progress is based on research which ultimately must rest in part on experimentation involving human subjects.

In the field of biomedical research a fundamental distinction must be recognized between medical research in which the aim is essentially diagnostic or therapeutic for a patient, and medical research, the essential object of which is purely scientific and without implying direct diagnostic or therapeutic value to the person subjected to the research.

Special caution must be exercised in the conduct of research which may affect the environment, and the welfare of animals used for research must be respected.

Because it is essential that the results of laboratory experiments be applied to human beings to further scientific knowledge and to help suffering humanity, the World Medical Association has prepared the following recommendations as a guide to every physician in biomedical research involving human subjects. They should be kept under review in the future. It must be stressed that the standards as drafted are only a guide to physicians all over the world. Physicians are not relieved from criminal, civil and ethical responsibilities under the laws of their own countries.

I. Basic Principles

1. Biomedical research involving human subjects must conform to generally accepted scientific principles and should be based on adequately performed laboratory and animal experimentation and on a thorough knowledge of the scientific literature.

2. The design and performance of each experimental procedure involving human subjects should be clearly formulated in an experimental protocol which should be transmitted for consideration, comment and guidance to a specially appointed committee independent of the investigator and the sponsor provided that this independent committee is in conformity with the laws and regulations of the country in which the research experiment is performed.

3. Biomedical research involving human subjects should be conducted only by scientifically qualified persons and under the supervision of a clinically competent medical person. The responsibility for the human subject must always rest with a medically qualified person and never rest on the subject of the research, even though the subject has given his or her consent.

4. Biomedical research involving human subjects cannot legitimately be carried out unless the importance of the objective is in proportion to the inherent risk to the subject.

5. Every biomedical research project involving human subjects should be preceded by careful assessment of predictable risks in comparison with foreseeable benefits to the subject or to others. Concern for the interests of the subject must always prevail over the interests of science and society.

6. The right of the research subject to safeguard his or her integrity must always be respected. Every precaution should be taken to respect the privacy of the subject and to minimize the impact of the study on the subject's physical and mental integrity and on the personality of the subject.

7. Physicians should abstain from engaging in research projects involving human subjects unless they are satisfied that the hazards involved are believed to be predictable. Physicians should cease any investigation if the hazards are found to outweigh the potential benefits.

8. In publication of the results of his or her research, the physician is obliged to preserve the accuracy of the results. Reports of experimentation not in accordance with the principles laid down in this Declaration should not be accepted for publication.

9. In any research on human beings, each potential subject must be adequately informed of the aims, methods, anticipated benefits and potential hazards of the study and the discomfort it may entail. He or she should be informed that he or she is at liberty to abstain from participation in the study and that he or she is free to withdraw his or her consent to participation at any time. The physician should then obtain the subject's freely-given informed consent, preferably in writing.

10. When obtaining informed consent for the research project the physician should be particularly cautious if the subject is in a dependent relationship to him or her or may consent under duress. In that case the informed consent should be obtained by a physician who is not engaged in the investigation and who is completely independent of this official relationship.

11. In case of legal incompetence, informed consent should be obtained from the legal guardian in accordance with national legislation. Where physical or mental incapacity makes it impossible to obtain informed consent, or when the subject is a minor, permission from the responsible relative replaces that of the subject in accordance with national legislation.

    Whenever the minor child is in fact able to give a consent, the minor's consent must be obtained in addition to the consent of the minor's legal guardian.

12. The research protocol should always contain a statement of the ethical considerations involved and should indicate that the principles enunciated in the present Declaration are complied with.

II. Medical Research Combined With Professional Care (Clinical Research)

1. In the treatment of the sick person, the physician must be free to use a new diagnostic and therapeutic measure, if in his or her judgment it offers hope of saving life, reestablishing health or alleviating suffering.

2. The potential benefits, hazards, and discomfort of a new method should be weighed against the advantages of the best current diagnostic and therapeutic methods.

3. In any medical study, every patient—including those of a control group, if any—should be assured of the best proven diagnostic and therapeutic method. This does not exclude the use of inert placebo in studies where no proven diagnostic or therapeutic method exists.

4. The refusal of the patient to participate in a study must never interfere with the physician-patient relationship.

5. If the physician considers it essential not to obtain informed consent, the specific reasons for this proposal should be stated in the experimental protocol for transmission to the independent committee (I, 2).

6. The physician can combine medical research with professional care, the objective being the acquisition of new medical knowledge, only to the extent that medical research is justified by its potential diagnostic or therapeutic value for the patient.

III. Non-Therapeutic Biomedical Research Involving Human Subjects (Non-Clinical Biomedical Research)

1. In the purely scientific application of medical research carried out on a human being, it is the duty of the physician to remain the protector of the life and health of that person on whom biomedical research is being carried out.

2. The subjects should be volunteers—either healthy persons or patients for whom the experimental design is not related to the patient's illness.

3. The investigator or the investigating team should discontinue the research if in his/her or their judgment it may, if continued, be harmful to the individual.

4. In research on man, the interest of science and society should never take precedence over considerations related to the wellbeing of the subject.

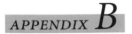

The Belmont Report

Office of the Secretary

Ethical Principles and Guidelines for the Protection of Human Subjects of Research

The National Commission for the Protection of Human Subjects of Biomedical and Behavioral Research

April 18, 1979

AGENCY: Department of Health, Education, and Welfare.

ACTION: Notice of Report for Public Comment.

SUMMARY: On July 12, 1974, the National Research Act (Pub. L. 93-348) was signed into law, there-by creating the National Commission for the Protection of Human Subjects of Biomedical and Behavioral Research. One of the charges to the Commission was to identify the basic ethical principles that should underlie the conduct of biomedical and behavioral research involving human subjects and to develop guidelines which should be followed to assure that such research is conducted in accordance with those principles. In carrying out the above, the Commission was directed to consider: (i) the boundaries between biomedical and behavioral research and the accepted and routine practice of medicine, (ii) the role of assessment of risk-benefit criteria in the determination of the appropriateness of research involving human subjects, (iii) appropriate guidelines for the selection of human subjects for participation in such research and (iv) the nature and definition of informed consent in various research settings.

The Belmont Report attempts to summarize the basic ethical principles identified by the Commission in the course of its deliberations. It is the outgrowth of an intensive four-day period of discussions that were held in February 1976 at the Smithsonian Institution's Belmont Conference Center supplemented by the monthly deliberations of the Commission that were held over a period of nearly four years. It is a statement of basic ethical principles and guidelines that should assist in resolving the ethical problems that surround the conduct of research with human subjects. By publishing the Report in the Federal Register, and providing reprints upon request, the Secretary intends that it may be made readily available to scientists, members of Institutional Review Boards, and Federal employees. The two-volume Appendix, containing the lengthy reports of experts and specialists who assisted the Commission in fulfilling this part of its charge, is available as DHEW Publication No. (OS) 78–0013 and No. (OS) 78–0014, for sale by the Superintendent of Documents, U.S. Government Printing Office, Washington, D.C. 20402.

Unlike most other reports of the Commission, the Belmont Report does not make specific recommendations for administrative action by the Secretary of Health, Education, and Welfare. Rather, the Commission recommended that the Belmont Report be adopted in its entirety, as a statement of the Department's policy. The Department requests public comment on this recommendation.

National Commission for the Protection of Human Subjects of Biomedical and Behavioral Research

Members of the Commission

Kenneth John Ryan, M.D., Chairman, Chief of Staff, Boston Hospital for Women.
Joseph V. Brady, Ph.D., Professor of Behavioral Biology, Johns Hopkins University.
Robert E. Cooke, M.D., President, Medical College of Pennsylvania.
Dorothy I. Height, President, National Council of Negro Women, Inc.
Albert R. Jonsen, Ph.D., Associate Professor of Bioethics, University of California at San Francisco.
Patricia King, J.D., Associate Professor of Law, Georgetown University Law Center.
Karen Lebacqz, Ph.D., Associate Professor of Christian Ethics, Pacific School of Religion.
*** David W. Louisell, J.D., Professor of Law, University of California at Berkeley.
Donald W. Seldin, M.D., Professor and Chairman, Department of Internal Medicine, University of Texas at Dallas.
***Eliot Stellar, Ph.D., Provost of the University and Professor of Physiological Psychology, University of Pennsylvania.
*** Robert H. Turtle, LL.B., Attorney, VomBaur, Coburn, Simmons & Turtle, Washington, D.C.

*** Deceased.

Table of Contents

Ethical Principles and Guidelines for Research Involving Human Subjects

A. Boundaries Between Practice and Research

B. Basic Ethical Principles

1. Respect for Persons
2. Beneficence
3. Justice

C. Applications

1. Informed Consent
2. Assessment of Risk and Benefits
3. Selection of Subjects

Ethical Principles and Guidelines for Research Involving Human Subjects

Scientific research has produced substantial social benefits. It has also posed some troubling ethical questions. Public attention was drawn to these questions by reported abuses of human subjects in biomedical experiments, especially during the Second World War. During the Nuremberg War Crime Trials, the Nuremberg code was drafted as a set of standards for judging physicians and scientists who had conducted biomedical experiments on concentration camp prisoners. This code became the prototype of many later codes[1] intended to assure that research involving human subjects would be carried out in an ethical manner.

The codes consist of rules, some general, others specific, that guide the investigators or the reviewers of research in their work. Such rules often are inadequate to cover complex situations; at times they come into conflict, and they are frequently difficult to interpret or apply. Broader ethical principles will provide a basis on which specific rules may be formulated, criticized and interpreted.

Three principles, or general prescriptive judgments, that are relevant to research involving human subjects are identified in this statement. Other principles may also be relevant. These three are comprehensive, however, and are stated at a level of generalization that should assist scientists, subjects, reviewers and interested citizens to understand the ethical issues inherent in research involving human subjects. These principles cannot always be applied so as to resolve beyond dispute particular ethical problems. The objective is to provide an analytical framework that will guide the resolution of ethical problems arising from research involving human subjects.

This statement consists of a distinction between research and practice, a discussion of the three basic ethical principles, and remarks about the application of these principles.

A. Boundaries Between Practice and Research

It is important to distinguish between biomedical and behavioral research, on the one hand, and the practice of accepted therapy on the other, in order to know what activities ought to undergo review for the protection of human subjects of research. The distinction between research and practice is blurred partly because both often occur together (as in research designed to evaluate a therapy) and partly because notable departures from standard practice are often called "experimental" when the terms "experimental" and "research" are not carefully defined.

For the most part, the term *practice* refers to interventions that are designed solely to enhance the well-being of an individual patient or client and that have a reasonable expectation of success. The purpose of medical or behavioral practice is to provide diagnosis, preventive treatment or therapy to particular individuals.[2] By contrast, the term *research* designates an activity designed to test an hypothesis, permit conclusions to be drawn, and thereby to develop or contribute to generalizable knowledge (expressed, for example, in theories, principles, and statements of relationships). Research is usually described in a formal protocol that sets forth an objective and a set of procedures designed to reach that objective.

When a clinician departs in a significant way from standard or accepted practice, the innovation does not, in and of itself, constitute research. The fact that a procedure is "experimental," in the sense of new, untested, or different, does not automatically place it in the category of research. Radically new procedures of this description should, however, be made the object of formal research at an early stage in order to determine whether they are safe and effective. Thus, it is the responsibility of medical practice committees, for example, to insist that a major innovation be incorporated into a formal research project.[3]

Research and practice may be carried on together when research is designed to evaluate the safety and efficacy of a therapy. This need not cause any confusion regarding whether or not the activity requires review; the general rule is that if there is any element of research in an activity, that activity should undergo review for the protection of human subjects.

B. Basic Ethical Principles

The expression "basic ethical principles" refers to those general judgments that serve as a basic justification for the many particular ethical prescriptions and evaluations of human actions. Three basic principles, among those generally accepted in our cultural tradition, are particularly relevant to the ethics of research involving human subjects: the principles of respect of persons, beneficence and justice.

1. Respect for Persons.   Respect for persons incorporates at least two ethical convictions: first, that individuals should be treated as autonomous agents, and second, that persons with diminished autonomy are entitled to protection. The principle of respect for persons thus divides into two separate moral requirements: the requirement to acknowledge autonomy and the requirement to protect those with diminished autonomy.

An autonomous person is an individual capable of deliberation about personal goals and of acting under the direction of such deliberation. To respect autonomy is to give weight to autonomous persons' considered opinions and choices while refraining from obstructing their actions unless they are clearly detrimental to others.

To show lack of respect for an autonomous agent is to repudiate that person's considered judgments, to deny an individual the freedom to act on those considered judgments, or to withhold information necessary to make a considered judgment, when there are no compelling reasons to do so.

However, not every human being is capable of self-determination. The capacity for self-determination matures during an individual's life, and some individuals lose this capacity wholly or in part because of illness, mental disability, or circumstances that severely restrict liberty. Respect for the immature and the incapacitated may require protecting them as they mature or while they are incapacitated.

Some persons are in need of extensive protection, even to the point of excluding them from activities which may harm them; other persons require little protection beyond making sure they undertake activities freely and with awareness of possible adverse consequence. The extent of protection afforded should depend upon the risk of harm and the likelihood of benefit. The judgment that any individual lacks autonomy should be periodically reevaluated and will vary in different situations.

In most cases of research involving human subjects, respect for persons demands that subjects enter into the research voluntarily and with adequate information. In some situations, however, application of the principle is not obvious. The involvement of prisoners as subjects of research provides an instructive example. On the one hand, it would seem that the principle of respect for persons requires that prisoners not be deprived of the opportunity to volunteer for research. On the other hand, under prison conditions they may be subtly coerced or unduly influenced to engage in research activities for which they would not otherwise volunteer. Respect for persons would then dictate that prisoners be protected. Whether to allow prisoners to "volunteer" or to "protect" them presents a dilemma. Respecting persons, in most hard cases, is often a matter of balancing competing claims urged by the principle of respect itself.

2. Beneficence.   Persons are treated in an ethical manner not only by respecting their decisions and protecting them from harm, but also by making efforts to secure their well-being. Such treatment falls under the principle of beneficence. The term "beneficence" is often understood to cover acts of kindness or charity that go beyond strict obligation. In this document, beneficence is understood in a stronger sense, as an obligation. Two general rules have been formulated as complementary expressions of beneficent actions in this sense: (1) do not harm and (2) maximize possible benefits and minimize possible harms.

The Hippocratic maxim "do no harm" has long been a fundamental principle of medical ethics. Claude Bernard extended it to the realm of research, saying that one should not injure one person regardless of the benefits that might come to others. However, even avoiding harm requires learning what is harmful; and, in the process of obtaining this information, persons may be exposed to risk of harm. Further, the Hippocratic Oath requires physicians to benefit their patients "according to their best judgment." Learning what will in fact benefit may require exposing persons to risk. The problem posed by these imperatives is to decide when it is justifiable to seek certain benefits despite the risks involved, and when the benefits should be foregone because of the risks.

The obligations of beneficence affect both individual investigators and society at large, because they extend both to particular research projects and to the entire enterprise of research. In the case of particular projects, investigators and members of their institutions are obliged to give forethought to the maximization of benefits and the reduction of risk that might occur from the research investigation. In the case of scientific research in general, members of the larger society are obliged to recognize the longer term benefits and risks that may result from the improvement of knowledge and from the development of novel medical, psychotherapeutic, and social procedures.

The principle of beneficence often occupies a well-defined justifying role in many areas of research involving human subjects. An example is found in research involving children. Effective ways of treating childhood diseases and fostering healthy development are benefits that serve to justify research involving children— even when individual research subjects are not direct beneficiaries. Research also makes it possible to avoid the harm that may result from the application of previously accepted routine practices that on closer investigation turn out to be dangerous. But the role of the principle of beneficence is not always so unambiguous. A difficult ethical problem remains, for example, about research that presents more than minimal risk without immediate prospect of direct benefit to the children involved. Some have argued that such research is inadmissible, while others have pointed out that this limit would rule out much research promising great benefit to children in the future. Here again, as with all hard cases, the different claims covered by the principle of beneficence may come into conflict and force difficult choices.

3. Justice. Who ought to receive the benefits of research and bear its burdens? This is a question of justice, in the sense of "fairness in distribution" or "what is deserved." An injustice occurs when some benefit to which a person is entitled is denied without good reason or when some burden is imposed unduly. Another way of conceiving the principle of justice is that equals ought to be treated equally. However, this statement requires explication. Who is equal and who is unequal? What considerations justify departure from equal distribution? Almost all commentators allow that distinctions based on experience, age, deprivation, competence, merit and position do sometimes constitute criteria justifying differential treatment for certain purposes. It is necessary, then, to explain in what respects people should be treated equally. There are several widely accepted formulations of just ways to distribute burdens and benefits. Each formulation mentions some relevant property on the basis of which burdens and benefits should be distributed. These formulations are (1) to each person an equal share, (2) to each person according to individual need, (3) to each person according to individual effort, (4) to each person according to societal contribution, and (5) to each person according to merit.

Questions of justice have long been associated with social practices such as punishment, taxation and political representation. Until recently these questions have not generally been associated with scientific research. However, they are fore-shadowed even in the earliest reflections on the ethics of research involving human subjects. For example, during the 19th and early 20th centuries the burdens of serving as research subjects fell largely upon poor ward patients, while the benefits of improved medical care flowed primarily to private patients. Subsequently, the exploitation of unwilling prisoners as research subjects in Nazi concentration camps was condemned as a particularly flagrant injustice. In this country, in the 1940s, the Tuskegee syphilis study used disadvantaged, rural black men to study the untreated course of a disease that is by no means confined to that population. These subjects were deprived of demonstrably effective treatment in order not to interrupt the project, long after such treatment became generally available.

Against this historical background, it can be seen how conceptions of justice are relevant to research involving human subjects. For example, the selection of research subjects needs to be scrutinized in order to determine whether some classes (e.g., welfare patients, particular racial and ethnic minorities, or persons confined to institutions) are being systematically selected simply because of their easy availability, their compromised position, or their manipulability, rather than for reasons directly related to the problem being studied. Finally, whenever research supported by public funds leads to the development of therapeutic devices and procedures, justice demands both that these not provide advantages only to those who can afford them and that such research should not unduly involve persons from groups unlikely to be among the beneficiaries of subsequent applications of the research.

C. Applications

Applications of the general principles to the conduct of research leads to consideration of the following requirements: informed consent, risk/benefit assessment, and the selection of subjects of research.

1. Informed Consent. Respect for persons requires that subjects, to the degree that they are capable, be given the opportunity to choose what shall or shall not happen to them. This opportunity is provided when adequate standards for informed consent are satisfied.

While the importance of informed consent is unquestioned, controversy prevails over the nature and possibility of an informed consent. Nonetheless, there is widespread agreement that the consent process can be analyzed as containing three elements: information, comprehension and voluntariness.

Information. Most codes of research establish specific items for disclosure intended to assure that subjects are given sufficient information. These items generally include: the research procedure, their purposes, risks and anticipated benefits, alternative procedures (where therapy is involved), and a statement offering the subject the opportunity to ask questions and to withdraw at any time from the research. Additional items have been proposed, including how subjects are selected, the person responsible for the research, etc.

However, a simple listing of items does not answer the question of what the standard should be for judging how much and what sort of information should be provided. One standard frequently invoked in medical practice, namely the information commonly provided by practitioners in the field or in the locale, is inadequate since research takes place precisely when a common understanding does not exist. Another standard, currently popular in malpractice law, requires the practitioner to reveal the information that reasonable persons would wish to know in order to make a decision regarding their care. This, too, seems insufficient since the research subject, being in essence a volunteer, may wish to know considerably more about risks gratuitously undertaken than do patients who deliver themselves into the hand of a clinician for needed care. It may be that a standard of "the reasonable volunteer" should be proposed: the extent and nature of information should be such that persons, knowing that the procedure is neither necessary for their care nor perhaps fully understood, can decide whether they wish to participate in the furthering of knowledge. Even when some direct benefit to them is anticipated, the subjects should understand clearly the range of risk and the voluntary nature of participation.

A special problem of consent arises where informing subjects of some pertinent aspect of the research is likely to impair the validity of the research. In many cases, it is sufficient to indicate to subjects that they are being invited to participate in research of which some features will not be revealed until the research is concluded. In all cases of research involving incomplete disclosure, such research is justified only if it is clear that (1) incomplete disclosure is truly necessary to accomplish the goals of the research, (2) there are no undisclosed risks to subjects that are more than minimal, and (3) there is an adequate plan for debriefing subjects, when appropriate, and for dissemination of research results to them. Information about risks should never be withheld for the purpose of eliciting the cooperation of subjects, and truthful answers should always be given to direct questions about the research. Care should be taken to distinguish cases in which disclosure would destroy or invalidate the research from cases in which disclosure would simply inconvenience the investigator.

Comprehension. The manner and context in which information is conveyed is as important as the information itself. For example, presenting information in a disorganized and rapid fashion, allowing too little time for consideration or curtailing opportunities for questioning, all may adversely affect a subject's ability to make an informed choice.

Because the subject's ability to understand is a function of intelligence, rationality, maturity and language, it is necessary to adapt the presentation of the information to the subject's capacities. Investigators are responsible for ascertaining that the subject has comprehended the information. While there is always an obligation to ascertain that the information about risk to subjects is complete and adequately comprehended, when the risks are more serious, that obligation increases. On occasion, it may be suitable to give some oral or written tests of comprehension.

Special provision may need to be made when comprehension is severely limited—for example, by conditions of immaturity or mental disability. Each class of subjects that one might consider as incompetent (e.g., infants and young children, mentally disabled patients, the terminally ill and the comatose) should be considered on its own terms. Even for these persons, however, respect requires giving them the opportunity to choose to the extent they are able, whether or not to participate in research. The objections of these subjects to involvement should be honored, unless the research entails providing them a therapy unavailable elsewhere. Respect for persons also requires seeking the permission of other parties in order to protect the subjects from harm. Such persons are thus respected both by acknowledging their own wishes and by the use of third parties to protect them from harm.

The third parties chosen should be those who are most likely to understand the incompetent subject's situation and to act in that person's best interest. The person authorized to act on behalf of the subject should be given an opportunity to observe the research as it proceeds in order to be able to withdraw the subject from the research, if such action appears in the subject's best interest.

Voluntariness. An agreement to participate in research constitutes a valid consent only if voluntarily given. This element of informed consent requires conditions free of coercion and undue influence. Coercion occurs when an overt threat of harm is intentionally presented by one person to another in order to obtain compliance. Undue influence, by contrast, occurs through an offer of an excessive, unwarranted, inappropriate or improper reward or other overture in order to obtain compliance. Also, inducements that would ordinarily be acceptable may become undue influences if the subject is especially vulnerable.

Unjustifiable pressures usually occur when persons in positions of authority or commanding influence—especially where possible sanctions are involved—urge a course of action for a subject. A continuum of such influencing factors exists, however, and it is impossible to state precisely where justifiable persuasion ends and undue influence begins. But undue influence would include actions such as manipulating a person's choice through the controlling influence of a close relative and threatening to withdraw health services to which an individual would otherwise be entitled.

2. Assessment of Risks and Benefits. The assessment of risks and benefits requires a careful arrayal of relevant data, including, in some cases, alternative ways of obtaining the benefits sought in the research. Thus, the assessment presents both an opportunity and a responsibility to gather systematic and comprehensive information about proposed research. For the investigator, it is a means to examine whether the proposed research is properly designed. For a review committee, it is a method for determining whether the risks that will be presented to subjects are justified. For prospective subjects, the assessment will assist the determination whether or not to participate.

The Nature and Scope of Risks and Benefits. The requirement that research be justified on the basis of a favorable risk/benefit assessment bears a close relation to the principle of beneficence, just as the moral requirement that informed consent be obtained is derived primarily from the principle of respect for persons. The term "risk" refers to a possibility that harm may occur. However, when expressions such as "small risk" or "high risk" are used, they usually refer (often ambiguously) both to the chance (probability) of experiencing a harm and the severity (magnitude) of the envisioned harm.

The term *benefit* is used in the research context to refer to something of positive value related to health or welfare. Unlike *risk, benefit* is not a term that expresses probabilities. Risk is properly contrasted to probability of benefits, and benefits are properly contrasted with harms rather than risks of harm. Accordingly, so-called risk/benefit assessments are concerned with the probabilities and magnitudes of possible harm and anticipated benefits. Many kinds of possible harms and benefits need to be taken into account. There are, for example, risks of psychological harm, physical harm, legal harm, social harm and economic harm and the corresponding benefits. While the most likely types of harms to research subjects are those of psychological or physical pain or injury, other possible kinds should not be over-looked.

Risks and benefits of research may affect the individual subjects, the families of the individual subjects, and society at large (or special groups of subjects in society). Previous codes and Federal regulations have required that risks to subjects be out-weighed by the sum of both the anticipated benefit to the subject, if any, and the anticipated benefit to society in the form of knowledge to be gained from the research. In balancing these different elements, the risks and benefits affecting the immediate research subject will normally carry special weight. On the other hand, interests other than those of the subject may on some occasions be sufficient by themselves to justify the risks involved in the research, so long as the subjects' rights have been protected. Beneficence thus requires that we protect against risk of harm to subjects and also that we be concerned about the loss of the substantial benefits that might be gained from research.

The Systematic Assessment of Risks and Benefits. It is commonly said that benefits and risks must be "balanced" and shown to be "in a favorable ratio." The metaphorical character of these terms draws attention to the difficulty of making precise judgments. Only on rare occasions will quantitative techniques be available for the scrutiny of research protocols. However, the idea of systematic, nonarbitrary analysis of risks and benefits should be emulated insofar as possible. This ideal requires those making decisions about the justifiability of research to be thorough in the accumulation and assessment of information about all aspects of the research, and to consider alternatives systematically. This procedure renders the assessment of research more rigorous and precise, while making communication between review board members and investigators less subject to misinterpretation, misinformation and conflicting judgments. Thus, there should first be a determination of the validity of the presuppositions of the research; then the nature, probability and magnitude of risk should be distinguished with as much clarity as possible. The method of ascertaining risks should be explicit, especially where there is no alternative to the use of such vague categories as small or slight risk. It should also be determined whether an investigator's estimates of the probability of harm or benefits are reasonable, as judged by known facts or other available studies.

Finally, assessment of the justifiability of research should reflect at least the following considerations: (i) Brutal or inhumane treatment of human subjects is never morally justified. (ii) Risks should be reduced to those necessary to achieve the research objective. It should be determined whether it is in fact necessary to use human subjects at all. Risk can perhaps never be entirely eliminated, but it can often be reduced by careful attention to alternative procedures. (iii) When research involves significant risk of serious impairment, review committees should be extraordinarily insistent on the justification of the risk (looking usually to the likelihood of benefit to the subject—or, in some rare cases, to the manifest voluntariness of the participation). (iv) When vulnerable populations are involved in research, the appropriateness of involving them should itself be demonstrated. A number of variables go into such judgments, including the nature and degree of risk, the condition of the particular population involved, and the nature and level of the anticipated benefits. (v) Relevant risks and benefits must be thoroughly arrayed in documents and procedures used in the informed consent process.

3. Selection of Subjects. Just as the principle of respect for persons finds expression in the requirements for consent, and the principle of beneficence in risk/benefit assessment, the principle of justice gives rise to moral requirements that there be fair procedures and outcomes in the selection of research subjects.

Justice is relevant to the selection of subjects of research at two levels: the social and the individual. Individual justice in the selection of subjects would require that researchers exhibit fairness: thus, they should not offer potentially beneficial research only to some patients who are in their favor or select only "undesirable" persons for risky research. Social justice requires that distinction be drawn between classes of subjects that ought, and ought not, to participate in any particular kind of research, based on the ability of members of that class to bear burdens and on the appropriateness of placing further burdens on already burdened persons. Thus, it can be considered a matter of social justice that there is an order of preference in the selection of classes of subjects (e.g., adults before children) and that some classes of potential subjects (e.g., the institutionalized mentally infirm or prisoners) may be involved as research subjects, if at all, only on certain conditions.

Injustice may appear in the selection of subjects, even if individual subjects are selected fairly by investigators and treated fairly in the course of research. Thus injustice arises from social, racial, sexual and cultural biases institutionalized in society. Thus, even if individual researchers are treating their research subjects fairly, and even if IRBs are taking care to assure that subjects are selected fairly within a particular institution, unjust social patterns may nevertheless appear in the overall distribution of the burdens and benefits of research. Although individual institutions or investigators may not be able to resolve a problem that is pervasive in their social setting, they can consider distributive justice in selecting research subjects.

Some populations, especially institutionalized ones, are already burdened in many ways by their infirmities and environments. When research is proposed that involves risks and does not include a therapeutic component, other less burdened classes of persons should be called upon first to accept these risks of research, except where the research is directly related to the specific conditions of the class involved. Also, even though public funds for research may often flow in the same directions as public funds for health care, it seems unfair that populations dependent on public health care constitute a pool of preferred research subjects if more advantaged populations are likely to be the recipients of the benefits.

One special instance of injustice results from the involvement of vulnerable subjects. Certain groups, such as racial minorities, the economically disadvantaged, the very sick, and the institutionalized may continually be sought as research subjects, owing to their ready availability in settings where research is conducted. Given their dependent status and their frequently compromised capacity for free consent, they should be protected against the danger of being involved in research solely for administrative convenience, or because they are easy to manipulate as a result of their illness or socioeconomic condition.

Notes:

1. Since 1945, various codes for the proper and responsible conduct of human experimentation in medical research have been adopted by different organizations. The best known of these codes are the Nuremberg Code of 1947, the Helsinki Declaration of 1964 (revised in 1975), and the 1971 Guidelines (codified into Federal Regulations in 1974) issued by the U.S. Department of Health, Education, and Welfare. Codes for the conduct of social and behavioral research have also been adopted, the best known being that of the American Psychological Association, published in 1973.

2. Although practice usually involves interventions designed solely to enhance the well-being of a particular individual, interventions are sometimes applied to one individual for the enhancement of the well-being of another (e.g., blood donation, skin grafts, organ transplants) or an intervention may have the dual purpose of enhancing the well-being of a particular individual, and, at the same time, providing some benefit to others (e.g., vaccination, which protects both the person who is vaccinated and society generally). The fact that some forms of practice have elements other than immediate benefit to the individual receiving an intervention, however, should not confuse the general distinction between research and practice. Even when a procedure applied in practice may benefit some other person, it remains an intervention designed to enhance the well-being of a particular individual or groups of individuals; thus, it is practice and need not be reviewed as research.

3. Because the problems related to social experimentation may differ substantially from those of biomedical and behavioral research, the Commission specifically declines to make any policy determination regarding such research at this time. Rather, the Commission believes that the problem ought to be addressed by one of its successor bodies.

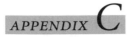

Protection of Human Subjects

CODE OF FEDERAL REGULATIONS
TITLE 45
PART 46

PUBLIC WELFARE
DEPARTMENT OF HEALTH AND HUMAN SERVICES
(45 CFR 46)

Revised June 18, 1991
(Effective August 19, 1991)

Edition October 1, 1994

[Authority: 5 U.S.C. 301; Section 474(a) 88 Stat. 352 (42 U.S.C. 2891–3(a))]

[Editorial Note: The Department of Health and Human Services issued a notice of waiver regarding the requirements set forth in part 46, relating to protection of human subjects, as they pertain to demonstration projects approved under section 1115 of the Social Security Act, which test the use of cost-sharing, such as deductibles, copayment and coinsurance, in the Medicaid program. For further information see 47 FR 9208, March 4, 1982.]

PART 46—PROTECTION OF HUMAN SUBJECTS

Subpart A—Federal Policy for the Protection of Human Subjects (Basic DHHS Policy for Protection of Human Research Subjects)

[Authority: 5 U.S.C. 301; 42 U.S.C. 289, 42 U.S.C. 300v–1(b).]

[Source: 58 FR 28012, 28022, June 18, 1991, unless otherwise noted.]

§46.101 To what does this policy apply?

a. Except as provided in paragraph (b) of this section, this policy applies to all research involving human subjects conducted, supported or otherwise subject to regulation by any federal department or agency which takes appropriate administrative action to make the policy applicable to such research. This includes research conducted by federal civilian employees or military personnel, except that each department or agency head may adopt such procedural modifications as may be appropriate from an administrative standpoint. It also includes research conducted, supported, or otherwise subject to regulation by the federal government outside the United States.

 1. Research that is conducted or supported by a federal department or agency, whether or not it is regulated as defined in §46.102(e), must comply with all sections of this policy.

 2. Research that is neither conducted nor supported by a federal department or agency, but is subject to regulation as defined in §46.102(e) must be reviewed and approved, in compliance with §46.101, §46.102, and §46.107 through §46.117 of this policy, by an institutional review board (IRB) that operates in accordance with the pertinent requirements of this policy.

b. Unless otherwise required by department or agency heads, research activities in which the only involvement of human subjects will be in one or more of the following categories are exempt from this policy:

 1. Research conducted in established or commonly accepted educational settings, involving normal educational practices, such as (i) research on regular and special education instructional strategies, or (ii) research on the effectiveness of or the comparison among instructional techniques, curricula, or classroom management methods.

 2. Research involving the use of educational tests (cognitive, diagnostic, aptitude, achievement), survey procedures, interview procedures or observation of public behavior, unless: (i) information obtained is recorded in such a manner that human subjects can be identified, directly or through identifiers linked to the subjects; and (ii) any disclosure of the human subjects' responses outside the research could reasonably place the subjects at risk of criminal or civil liability, or be damaging to the subjects' financial standing, employability, or reputation.

 3. Research involving the use of educational tests (cognitive, diagnostic, aptitude, achievement), survey procedures, interview procedures, or observation of public behavior that is not exempt under paragraph (b)(2) of this section, if: (i) the human subjects are elected or appointed public officials or candidates for public office; or (ii) federal statute(s) require(s) without exception that the confidentiality of the personally identifiable information will be maintained throughout the research and thereafter.

 4. Research involving the collection or study of existing data, documents, records, pathological specimens, or diagnostic specimens, if these sources

are publicly available, or if the information is recorded by the investigator in such a manner that subjects cannot be identified, directly or through identifiers linked to the subjects.

5. Research and demonstration projects which are conducted by or subject to the approval of department or agency heads, and which are designed to study, evaluate, or otherwise examine: (i) public benefit or service programs; (ii) procedures for obtaining benefits or services under those programs; (iii) possible changes in or alternatives to those programs or procedures; or (iv) possible changes in methods or levels of payment for benefits or services under those programs.

6. Taste and food quality evaluation and consumer acceptance studies, (i) if wholesome foods without additives are consumed, or (ii) if a food is consumed that contains a food ingredient at or below the level and for a use found to be safe, or agricultural chemical or environmental contaminant at or below the level found to be safe, by the Food and Drug Administration, or approved by the Environmental Protection Agency, or the Food Safety and Inspection Service of the U.S. Department of Agriculture.

c. Department or agency heads retain final judgment as to whether a particular activity is covered by this policy.

d. Department or agency heads may require that specific research activities or classes of research activities conducted, supported, or otherwise subject to regulation by the department or agency but not otherwise covered by this policy, comply with some or all of the requirements of this policy.

e. Compliance with this policy requires compliance with pertinent federal laws or regulations which provide additional protections for human subjects.

f. This policy does not affect any state or local laws or regulations which may otherwise be applicable and which provide additional protections for human subjects.

g. This policy does not affect any foreign laws or regulations which may otherwise be applicable and which provide additional protections to human subjects of research.

h. When research covered by this policy takes place in foreign countries, procedures normally followed in the foreign countries to protect human subjects may differ from those set forth in this policy. [An example is a foreign institution, which complies with guidelines consistent with the World Medical Assembly Declaration (Declaration of Helsinki, amended 1989) issued either by sovereign states or by an organization whose function for the protection of human research subjects is internationally recognized.] In these circumstances, if a department or agency head determines that the procedures prescribed by the institution afford protections that are at least equivalent to those provided in this policy, the department or agency head may approve the substitution of the foreign procedures in lieu of the procedural requirements provided in this policy. Except when otherwise required by statute, Executive Order, or the department or agency head, notices of these actions, as they occur, will be published in the *Federal Register*, or will be otherwise published, as provided in department or agency procedures.

i. Unless otherwise required by law, department or agency heads may waive the applicability of some or all of the provisions of this policy to specific research activities or classes of research activities otherwise covered by this policy. Except when otherwise required by statute or Executive Order, the department or agency head shall forward advance notices of these actions to the Office for Protection from Research Risks, Department of Health and Human Services (HHS), and shall also publish them in the *Federal Register* or in such other manner as provided in department or agency procedures.
[56 FR 28012, 28022, June 18, 1991; 56 FR 29756, June 28, 1991]

§46.102 Definitions.

a. *Department or agency head* means the head of any federal department or agency, and any other officer or employee of any department or agency to whom authority has been delegated.

b. *Institution* means any public or private entity or agency (including federal, state, and other agencies).

c. *Legally authorized representative* means an individual or judicial or other body authorized under applicable law to consent on behalf of a prospective subject to the subject's participation in the procedure(s) involved in the research.

d. *Research* means a systematic investigation, including research development, testing and evaluation, designed to develop or contribute to generalizable knowledge. Activities which meet this definition constitute research for purposes of this policy, whether or not they are conducted or supported under a program which is considered research for other purposes. For example, some demonstration and service programs may include research activities.

e. *Research subject to regulation* and similar terms are intended to encompass those research activities for which a federal department or agency has specific responsibility for regulating as a research activity (for example, Investigational New Drug requirements administered by the Food and Drug Administration). It does not include research activities which are incidentally regulated by a federal department or agency solely as part of the department's or agency's broader responsibility to regulate certain types of activities, whether research or non-research in nature (for example, Wage and Hour requirements administered by the Department of Labor).

f. *Human subject* means a living individual about whom an investigator (whether professional or student) conducting research obtains
1. data through intervention or interaction with the individual, or
2. identifiable private information.
   Intervention includes both physical procedures, by which data are gathered (for example, venipuncture), and manipulations of the subject or the subject's environment that are performed for research purposes. *Interaction* includes communication or interpersonal contact between investigator and

subject. *Private information* includes information about behavior that occurs in a context in which an individual can reasonably expect that no observation or recording is taking place, and information which has been provided for specific purposes by an individual and which the individual can reasonably expect will not be made public (for example, a medical record). Private information must be individually identifiable (i.e., the identity of the subject is or may readily be ascertained by the investigator or associated with the information), in order for obtaining the information to constitute research involving human subjects.

g. *IRB* means an Institutional Review Board, established in accord with and for the purposes expressed in this policy.

h. *IRB approval* means the determination of the IRB that the research has been reviewed and may be conducted at an institution within the constraints set forth by the IRB and by other institutional and federal requirements.

i. *Minimal risk* means that the probability and magnitude of harm or discomfort anticipated in the research are not greater in and of themselves than those ordinarily encountered in daily life or during the performance of routine physical or psychological examinations or tests.

j. *Certification* means the official notification by the institution to the supporting department or agency, in accordance with the requirements of this policy, that a research project or activity involving human subjects has been reviewed and approved by an IRB in accordance with an approved assurance.

§46.103 Assuring compliance with this policy—research conducted or supported by any Federal Department or Agency.

a. Each institution engaged in research which is covered by this policy, and which is conducted or supported by a federal department or agency, shall provide written assurance, satisfactory to the department or agency head, that it will comply with the requirements set forth in this policy. In lieu of requiring submission of an assurance, individual department or agency heads shall accept the existence of a current assurance, appropriate for the research in question, on file with the Office for Protection from Research Risks, HHS, and approved for federal-wide use by that office. When the existence of an approved assurance is accepted in lieu of requiring submission of an assurance, reports (except certification) required by this policy to be made to department and agency heads, shall also be made to the Office for Protection from Research Risks, HHS.

b. Departments and agencies will conduct or support research covered by this policy only if the institution has assurance approved as provided in this section, and only if the institution has certified to the department or agency head that the research has been reviewed and approved by an IRB provided for in the assurance, and will be subject to continuing review by the IRB. Assurances applicable to federally supported or conducted research shall at a minimum include:

1. A statement of principles governing the institution in the discharge of its responsibilities for protecting the rights and welfare of human subjects of research conducted at or sponsored by the institution, regardless of whether the research is subject to federal regulation. This may include an appropriate existing code, declaration, or statement of ethical principles, or a statement formulated by the institution itself. This requirement does not preempt provisions of this policy applicable to department- or agency-supported or regulated research, and need not be applicable to any research exempted or waived under §46.101 (b) or (i).

2. Designation of one or more IRBs established in accordance with the requirements of this policy, and for which provisions are made for meeting space and sufficient staff to support the IRBs' review and recordkeeping duties.

3. A list of IRB members identified by name; earned degrees; representative capacity; indications of experience such as board certifications, licenses, etc., sufficient to describe each member's chief anticipated contributions to IRB deliberations; and any employment or other relationship between each member and the institution (for example: full-time employee, part-time employee, member of governing panel or board, stockholder, paid or unpaid consultant). Changes in IRB membership shall be reported to the department or agency head, unless in accord with §46.103(a) of this policy, the existence of an HHS-approved assurance is accepted. In this case, change in IRB membership shall be reported to the Office for Protection from Research Risks, HHS.

4. Written procedures which the IRB will follow (i) for conducting its initial and continuing review of research and for reporting its findings and actions to the investigator and the institution; (ii) for determining which projects require review more often than annually and which projects need verification from sources other than the investigators that no material changes have occurred since previous IRB review; and (iii) for ensuring prompt reporting to the IRB of proposed changes in a research activity, and for ensuring that such changes in approved research, during the period for which IRB approval has already been given, may not be initiated without IRB review and approval except when necessary to eliminate apparent immediate hazards to the subject.

5. Written procedures for ensuring prompt reporting to the IRB, appropriate institutional officials, and the department or agency head, of (i) any unanticipated problems involving risks to subjects or others or any serious or continuing noncompliance with this policy or the requirements or determinations of the IRB; and (ii) any suspension or termination of IRB approval.

c. The assurance shall be executed by an individual authorized to act for the institution and to assume on behalf of the institution the obligations imposed by this policy and shall be filed in such form and manner as the department or agency head prescribes.

d. The department or agency head will evaluate all assurances submitted in accordance with this policy through such officers and employees of the department or agency and such experts or consultants engaged for this purpose as the department or agency head determines to be appropriate. The department or agency head's evaluation will take into consideration the adequacy of the proposed IRB in light of the anticipated scope of the institution's research activities and the types of subject populations likely to be involved, the appropriateness of the proposed initial and continuing review procedures in light of the probable risks, and the size and complexity of the institution.

e. On the basis of this evaluation, the department or agency head may approve or disapprove the assurance, or enter into negotiations to develop an approvable one. The department or agency head may limit the period during which any particular approved assurance or class of approved assurances shall remain effective or otherwise condition or restrict approval.

f. Certification is required when the research is supported by a federal department or agency, and not otherwise exempted or waived under §46.101 (b) or (i). An institution with an approved assurance shall certify that each application or proposal for research covered by the assurance and by §46.103 of this policy has been reviewed and approved by the IRB. Such certification must be submitted with the application or proposal or by such later date as may be prescribed by the department or agency to which the application or proposal is submitted. Under no condition shall research covered by §46.103 of the policy be supported prior to receipt of the certification that the research has been reviewed and approved by the IRB. Institutions without an approved assurance covering the research shall certify within 30 days after receipt of a request for such a certification from the department or agency, that the application or proposal has been approved by the IRB. If the certification is not submitted within these time limits, the application or proposal may be returned to the institution.

(Approved by the Office of Management and Budget, under control number 9999-0020.)

[56 FR 28012, 28022, June 18, 1991; 56 FR 29756, June 28, 1991]

§§46.104–106 [Reserved]

§46.107 IRB membership.

a. Each IRB shall have at least five members, with varying backgrounds to promote complete and adequate review of research activities commonly conducted by the institution. The IRB shall be sufficiently qualified through the experience and expertise of its members, and the diversity of the members, including consideration of race, gender, and cultural backgrounds, and sensitivity to such issues as community attitudes, to promote respect for its advice and counsel in safeguarding the rights and welfare of human subjects. In addition to possessing the professional competence necessary to review specific research activities, the IRB shall be able to ascertain the acceptability of proposed research in terms of institutional commitments and regulations, applicable law, and standards of professional conduct and practice. The IRB shall therefore include persons knowledgeable in these areas. If an IRB regularly reviews research that involves a vulnerable category of subjects, such as children, prisoners, pregnant women, or handicapped or mentally disabled persons, consideration shall be given to the inclusion of one or more individuals who are knowledgeable about and experienced in working with these subjects.

b. Every nondiscriminatory effort will be made to ensure that no IRB consists entirely of men or entirely of women, including the institution's consideration of qualified persons of both sexes, so long as no selection is made to the IRB on the basis of gender. No IRB may consist entirely of members of one profession.

c. Each IRB shall include at least one member whose primary concerns are in scientific areas and at least one member whose primary concerns are in nonscientific areas.

d. Each IRB shall include at least one member, who is not otherwise affiliated with the institution, and who is not part of the immediate family of a person who is affiliated with the institution.

e. No IRB may have a member participate in the IRB's initial or continuing review of any project in which the member has a conflicting interest, except to provide information requested by the IRB.

f. An IRB may, in its discretion, invite individuals with competence in special areas to assist in the review of issues which require expertise beyond or in addition to that available on the IRB. These individuals may not vote with the IRB.

§46.108 IRB functions and operations.

In order to fulfill the requirements of this policy, each IRB shall:

a. Follow written procedures in the same detail as described in §46.103(b)(4) and to the extent required by §46.103(b)(5).

b. Except when an expedited review procedure is used (see §46.110), review proposed research at convened meetings, at which a majority of the members of the IRB are present, including at least one member whose primary concerns are in nonscientific areas. In order for the research to be approved, it shall receive the approval of a majority of those members present at the meeting.

§46.109 IRB review of research.

a. An IRB shall review, and have authority to approve, require modifications in (to secure approval), or disapprove all research activities covered by this policy.

b. An IRB shall require that information given to subjects as part of informed consent is in accordance with §46.116. The IRB may require that information, in addition to that specifically mentioned in §46.116, be given to the subjects when, in the IRB's judgment, the information would meaningfully add to the protection of the rights and welfare of subjects.

c. An IRB shall require documentation of informed consent, or may waive documentation in accordance with §46.117.

d. An IRB shall notify investigators and the institution in writing of its decision to approve or disapprove the proposed research activity, or of modifications required to secure IRB approval of the research activity. If the IRB decides to disapprove a research activity, it shall include in its written notification a statement of the reasons for its decision, and give the investigator an opportunity to respond in person or in writing.

e. An IRB shall conduct continuing review of research covered by this policy at intervals appropriate to the degree of risk, but not less than once per year, and shall have authority to observe or have a third party observe the consent process and the research.

(Approved by the Office of Management and Budget, under control number 9999-0020.)

§46.110 Expedited review procedures for certain kinds of research involving no more than minimal risk, and for minor changes in approved research.

a. The Secretary, HHS, has established, and published as a Notice in the *Federal Register,* a list of categories of research that may be reviewed by the IRB through an expedited review procedure. The list will be amended, as appropriate, after consultation with other departments and agencies, through periodic republication by the Secretary, HHS, in the *Federal Register.* A copy of the list is available from the Office for Protection from Research Risks, National Institutes of Health, HHS, Bethesda, Maryland 20892.

[Editor: See Addendum 46 FR 8392 at the end of this document.]

b. An IRB may use the expedited review procedure to review either or both of the following:

1. some or all of the research appearing on the list and found by the reviewer(s) to involve no more than minimal risk,

2. minor changes in previously approved research during the period (of one year or less) for which approval is authorized.

Under an expedited review procedure, the review may be carried out by the IRB chairperson or by one or more experienced reviewers designated by the chairperson from among members of the IRB. In reviewing the research, the reviewers may exercise all of the authorities of the IRB, except that the reviewers may not disapprove the research. A research activity may be disapproved only after review in accordance with the non-expedited procedure set forth in §46.108(b).

c. Each IRB which uses an expedited review procedure shall adopt a method for keeping all members advised of research proposals which have been approved under the procedure.

d. The department or agency head may restrict, suspend, terminate, or choose not to authorize an institution's or IRB's use of the expedited review procedure.

§46.111 Criteria for IRB approval of research.

a. In order to approve research covered by this policy, the IRB shall determine that all of the following requirements are satisfied:

1. Risks to subjects are minimized: (i) by using procedures which are consistent with sound research design and which do not unnecessarily expose subjects to risk, and (ii) whenever appropriate, by using procedures already being performed on the subjects for diagnostic or treatment purposes.

2. Risks to subjects are reasonable in relation to anticipated benefits, if any, to subjects, and the importance of the knowledge that may reasonably be expected to result. In evaluating risks and benefits, the IRB should consider only those risks and benefits that may result from the research (as distinguished from risks and benefits of therapies subjects would receive even if not participating in the research). The IRB should not consider possible long-range effects of applying knowledge gained in the research (for example, the possible effects of the research on public policy) as among those research risks that fall within the purview of its responsibility.

3. Selection of subjects is equitable. In making this assessment the IRB should take into account the purposes of the research, and the setting in which the research will be conducted, and should be particularly cognizant of the special problems of research involving vulnerable populations, such as children, prisoners, pregnant women, mentally disabled persons, or economically or educationally disadvantaged persons.

4. Informed consent will be sought from each prospective subject or the subject's legally authorized representative, in accordance with, and to the extent required by §46.116.

5. Informed consent will be appropriately documented, in accordance with, and to the extent required by §46.117.

6. When appropriate, the research plan makes adequate provision for monitoring the data collected to ensure the safety of subjects.

7. When appropriate, there are adequate provisions to protect the privacy of subjects and to maintain the confidentiality of data.

b. When some or all of the subjects are likely to be vulnerable to coercion or undue influence, such as children, prisoners, pregnant women, mentally disabled persons, or economically or educationally disadvantaged persons, additional safeguards have been included in the study to protect the rights and welfare of these subjects.

§46.112 Review by institution.

Research covered by this policy that has been approved by an IRB may be subject to further appropriate review and approval or disapproval by officials of the institution. However, those officials may not approve the research if it has not been approved by an IRB.

§46.113 Suspension or termination of IRB approval of research.

An IRB shall have authority to suspend or terminate approval of research that is not being conducted in accordance with the IRB's requirements or that has been associated with unexpected serious harm to subjects. Any suspension or termination of approval shall include a statement of the reasons for the IRB's action and shall be reported promptly to the investigator, appropriate institutional officials, and the department or agency head.

(Approved by the Office of Management and Budget, under control number 9999-0020.)

§46.114 Cooperative research.

Cooperative research projects are those projects covered by this policy which involve more than one institution. In the conduct of cooperative research projects, each institution is responsible for safeguarding the rights and welfare of human subjects and for complying with this policy. With the approval of the department or agency head, an institution participating in a cooperative project may enter into a joint review arrangement, rely upon the review of another qualified IRB, or make similar arrangements for avoiding duplication of effort.

§46.115 IRB records.

a. An institution, or when appropriate an IRB, shall prepare and maintain adequate documentation of IRB activities, including the following:
1. Copies of all research proposals reviewed, scientific evaluations, if any, that accompany the proposals, approved sample consent documents, progress reports submitted by investigators, and reports of injuries to subjects.
2. Minutes of IRB meetings, which shall be in sufficient detail to show attendance at the meetings; actions taken by the IRB; the vote on these actions, including the number of members voting for, against, and abstaining; the basis for requiring changes in or disapproving research; and a written summary of the discussion of controverted issues and their resolution.
3. Records of continuing review activities.
4. Copies of all correspondence between the IRB and the investigators.
5. A list of IRB members, in the same detail as described in §46.103(b)(3).
6. Written procedures for the IRB, in the same detail as described in §46.103(b)(4) and §46.103(b)(5).

7. Statements of significant new findings provided to subjects, as required by §46.116(b)(5).

b. The records required by this policy shall be retained for at least 3 years, and records relating to research which is conducted shall be retained for at least 3 years after completion of the research. All records shall be accessible for inspection and copying by authorized representatives of the department or agency at reasonable times and in a reasonable manner.

(Approved by the Office of Management and Budget, under control number 9999-0020.)

§46.116 General requirements for informed consent.

Except as provided elsewhere in this policy, no investigator may involve a human being as a subject in research covered by this policy unless the investigator has obtained the legally effective informed consent of the subject or the subject's legally authorized representative. An investigator shall seek such consent only under circumstances that provide the prospective subject or the representative sufficient opportunity to consider whether or not to participate and that minimize the possibility of coercion or undue influence. The information that is given to the subject or the representative shall be in language understandable to the subject or the representative. No informed consent, whether oral or written, may include any exculpatory language through which the subject or the representative is made to waive or appear to waive any of the subject's legal rights, or releases or appears to release the investigator, the sponsor, the institution or its agents from liability for negligence.

a. Basic elements of informed consent. Except as provided in paragraph (c) or (d) of this section, in seeking informed consent the following information shall be provided to each subject:
   1. A statement that the study involves research, an explanation of the purposes of the research and the expected duration of the subject's participation, a description of the procedures to be followed, and identification of any procedures which are experimental;
   2. A description of any reasonably foreseeable risks or discomforts to the subject;
   3. A description of any benefits to the subject or to others which may reasonably be expected from the research;
   4. A disclosure of appropriate alternative procedures or courses of treatment, if any, that might be advantageous to the subject;
   5. A statement describing the extent, if any, to which confidentiality of records identifying the subject will be maintained;
   6. For research involving more than minimal risk, an explanation as to whether any compensation and an explanation as to whether any medical treatments are available if injury occurs and, if so, what they consist of, or where further information may be obtained;

7. An explanation of whom to contact for answers to pertinent questions about the research and research subjects' rights, and whom to contact in the event of a research-related injury to the subject; and

8. A statement that participation is voluntary, refusal to participate will involve no penalty or loss of benefits to which the subject is otherwise entitled, and the subject may discontinue participation at any time without penalty or loss of benefits to which the subject is otherwise entitled.

b. Additional elements of informed consent. When appropriate, one or more of the following elements of information shall also be provided to each subject:

1. A statement that the particular treatment or procedure may involve risks to the subject (or to the embryo or fetus, if the subject is or may become pregnant) which are currently unforeseeable;

2. Anticipated circumstances under which the subject's participation may be terminated by the investigator without regard to the subject's consent;

3. Any additional costs to the subject that may result from participation in the research;

4. The consequences of a subject's decision to withdraw from the research and procedures for orderly termination of participation by the subject;

5. A statement that significant new findings developed during the course of the research which may relate to the subject's willingness to continue participation will be provided to the subject; and

6. The approximate number of subjects involved in the study.

c. An IRB may approve a consent procedure, which does not include, or which alters, some or all of the elements of informed consent set forth above, or waive the requirement to obtain informed consent, provided the IRB finds and documents that:

1. The research or demonstration project is to be conducted by, or subject to the approval of, state or local government officials, and is designed to study, evaluate, or otherwise examine: (i) public benefit or service programs; (ii) procedures for obtaining benefits or services under those programs; (iii) possible changes in or alternatives to those programs or procedures; or (iv) possible changes in methods or levels of payment for benefits or services under those programs; and

2. The research could not practicably be carried out without the waiver or alteration.

d. An IRB may approve a consent procedure which does not include, or which alters, some or all of the elements of informed consent set forth in this section, or waive the requirements to obtain informed consent provided the IRB finds and documents that:

1. the research involves no more than minimal risk to the subjects;

2. the waiver or alteration will not adversely affect the rights and welfare of the subjects;

3. the research could not practicably be carried out without the waiver or alteration; and

4. whenever appropriate, the subjects will be provided with additional pertinent information after participation.

e. The informed consent requirements in this policy are not intended to preempt any applicable federal, state, or local laws which require additional information to be disclosed, in order for informed consent to be legally effective.

f. Nothing in this policy is intended to limit the authority of a physician to provide emergency medical care, to the extent the physician is permitted to do so under applicable federal, state, or local law.

(Approved by the Office of Management and Budget, under control number 9999-0020.)

§46.117 Documentation of informed consent.

a. Except as provided in paragraph (c) of this section, informed consent shall be documented by the use of a written consent form approved by the IRB and signed by the subject or the subject's legally authorized representative. A copy shall be given to the person signing the form.

b. Except as provided in paragraph (c) of this section, the consent form may be either of the following:

1. A written consent document that embodies the elements of informed consent required by §46.116. This form may be read to the subject or the subject's legally authorized representative, but in any event, the investigator should give either the subject or the representative adequate opportunity to read it before it is signed.

2. A short form written consent document stating that the elements of informed consent required by §46.116 have been presented orally to the subject or the subject's legally authorized representative. When this method is used, there shall be a witness to the oral presentation. Also, the IRB shall approve a written summary of what is to be said to the subject or the representative. Only the short form itself is to be signed by the subject or the representative. However, the witness shall sign both the short form and a copy of the summary, and the person actually obtaining consent shall sign a copy of the summary. A copy of the summary shall be given to the subject or the representative, in addition to a copy of the short form.

c. An IRB may waive the requirement for the investigator to obtain a signed consent form for some or all subjects, if it finds either:

1. That the only record linking the subject and the research would be the consent document and the principal risk would be potential harm resulting from a breach of confidentiality. Each subject will be asked whether the subject wants documentation linking the subject with the research, and the subject's wishes will govern; or

2. That the research presents no more than minimal risk of harm to subjects and involves no procedures for which written consent is normally required outside of the research context.

In cases in which the documentation requirement is waived, the IRB may require the investigator to provide subjects with a written statement regarding the research.

(Approved by the Office of Management and Budget, under control number 9999-0020.)

§46.118 Applications and proposals lacking definite plans for involvement of human subjects.

Certain types of applications for grants, cooperative agreements, or contracts are submitted to departments or agencies with the knowledge that subjects may be involved within the period of support, but definite plans would not normally be set forth in the application or proposal. These include activities such as institutional-type grants when selection of specific projects is the institution's responsibility; research training grants in which the activities involving subjects remain to be selected; and projects in which human subjects' involvement will depend upon completion of instruments, prior animal studies, or purification of compounds. These applications need not be reviewed by an IRB before an award may be made. However, except for research exempted or waived under §46.101 (b) or (i), no human subjects may be involved in any project supported by these awards until the project has been reviewed and approved by the IRB, as provided in this policy, and certification submitted, by the institution, to the department or agency.

§46.119 Research undertaken without the intention of involving human subjects.

In the event research is undertaken without the intention of involving human subjects, but it is later proposed to involve human subjects in the research, the research shall first be reviewed and approved by an IRB, as provided in this policy, a certification submitted, by the institution, to the department or agency, and final approval given to the proposed change by the department or agency.

§46.120 Evaluation and disposition of application and proposals for research to be conducted or supported by a Federal Department or Agency.

a. The department or agency head will evaluate all applications and proposals involving human subjects submitted to the department or agency through such officers and employees of the department or agency and such experts and consultants as the department or agency head determines to be appropriate. This evaluation will take into consideration the risks to the subjects, the adequacy of protection against these risks, the potential benefits of the research to the subjects and others, and the importance of the knowledge gained or to be gained.

b. On the basis of this evaluation, the department or agency head may approve or disapprove the application or proposal, or enter into negotiations to develop an approvable one.

§46.121 [Reserved]

§46.122 Use of Federal funds.

Federal funds administered by a department or agency may not be expended for research involving human subjects unless the requirements of this policy have been satisfied.

§46.123 Early termination of research support: Evaluation of applications and proposals.

a. The department or agency head may require that department or agency support for any project be terminated or suspended, in the manner prescribed in applicable program requirements, when the department or agency head finds an institution has materially failed to comply with the terms of this policy.

b. In making decisions about supporting or approving applications or proposals covered by this policy, the department or agency head may take into account, in addition to all other eligibility requirements and program criteria, factors such as whether the applicant has been subject to a termination or suspension under paragraph (a) of this section, and whether the applicant or the person or persons who would direct or has or have directed the scientific and technical aspects of an activity, has or have, in the judgment of the department or agency head, materially failed to discharge responsibility for the protection of the rights and welfare of human subjects (whether or not the research was subject to federal regulation).

§46.124 Conditions.

With respect to any research project or any class of research projects, the department or agency head may impose additional conditions prior to or at the time of approval when, in the judgment of the department or agency head, additional conditions are necessary for the protection of human subjects.

Subpart B—Additional DHHS Protections Pertaining to Research, Development, and Related Activities Involving Fetuses, Pregnant Women, and Human In Vitro Fertilization

[Source: 40 FR 33528, August 8, 1975, unless otherwise noted.]

§46.201 Applicability.

a. The regulations in this subpart are applicable to all Department of Health and Human Services grants and contracts supporting research, development, and related activities involving: (1) the fetus, (2) pregnant women, and (3) human *in vitro* fertilization.

b. Nothing in this subpart shall be construed as indicating that compliance with the procedures set forth herein will in any way render inapplicable pertinent State or local laws bearing upon activities covered by this subpart.

c. The requirements of this subpart are in addition to those imposed under the other subparts of this part.

§46.202 Purpose.

It is the purpose of this subpart to provide additional safeguards in reviewing activities to which this subpart is applicable to assure that they conform to appropriate ethical standards and relate to important societal needs.

§46.203 Definitions.

As used in this subpart:

a. *Secretary* means the Secretary of Health and Human Services and any other officer or employee of the Department of Health and Human Services to whom authority has been delegated.

b. *Pregnancy* encompasses the period of time from confirmation of implantation (through any of the presumptive signs of pregnancy, such as missed menses, or by a medically acceptable pregnancy test), until expulsion or extraction of the fetus.

c. *Fetus* means the product of conception from the time of implantation (as evidenced by any of the presumptive signs of pregnancy, such as missed menses, or a medically acceptable pregnancy test), until a determination is made, following expulsion or extraction of the fetus, that it is viable.

d. *Viable* as it pertains to the fetus means being able, after either spontaneous or induced delivery, to survive (given the benefit of available medical therapy) to the point of independently maintaining heart beat and respiration. The Secretary may from time to time, taking into account medical advances, publish in the *Federal Register* guidelines to assist in determining whether a fetus is viable for purposes of this subpart. If a fetus is viable after delivery, it is a premature infant.

e. *Nonviable fetus* means a fetus *ex utero* which, although living, is not viable.

f. *Dead fetus* means a fetus *ex utero* which exhibits neither heartbeat, spontaneous respiratory activity, spontaneous movement of voluntary muscles, nor pulsation of the umbilical cord (if still attached).

g. *In vitro fertilization* means any fertilization of human ova, which occurs outside the body of a female, either through admixture of donor human sperm and ova or by any other means.

[40 FR 33528, August 8, 1975, as amended at 43 FR 1759, January 11, 1978]

§46.204 Ethical Advisory Boards.

a. One or more Ethical Advisory Boards shall be established by the Secretary. Members of these board(s) shall be so selected that the board(s) will be competent to deal with medical, legal, social, ethical, and related issues and may include, for example, research scientists, physicians, psychologists, sociologists, educators, lawyers, and ethicists, as well as representatives of the general public.

No board member may be a regular, full-time employee of the Department of Health and Human Services.

b. At the request of the Secretary, the Ethical Advisory Board shall render advice consistent with the policies and requirements of this part as to ethical issues, involving activities covered by this subpart, raised by individual applications or proposals. In addition, upon request by the Secretary, the Board shall render advice as to classes of applications or proposals and general policies, guidelines, and procedures.

c. A Board may establish, with the approval of the Secretary, classes of applications or proposals which: (1) must be submitted to the Board, or (2) need not be submitted to the Board. Where the Board so establishes a class of applications or proposals, which must be submitted, no application or proposal within the class may be funded by the Department or any component thereof until the application or proposal has been reviewed by the Board, and the Board has rendered advice as to its acceptability from an ethical standpoint.

[40 FR 33528, August 8, 1975, as amended at 43 FR 1759, January 11, 1978; 59 FR 28276, June 1, 1994]

§46.205 Additional duties of the Institutional Review Boards in connection with activities involving fetuses, pregnant women, or human in vitro fertilization.

a. In addition to the responsibilities prescribed for Institutional Review Boards under Subpart A of this part, the applicant's or offeror's Board shall, with respect to activities covered by this subpart, carry out the following additional duties:

1. Determine that all aspects of the activity meet the requirements of this subpart;

2. Determine that adequate consideration has been given to the manner in which potential subjects will be selected, and adequate provision has been made by the applicant or offeror for monitoring the actual informed consent process (e.g., through such mechanisms, when appropriate, as participation by the Institutional Review Board or subject advocates in: (i) overseeing the actual process by which individual consents required by this subpart are secured either by approving induction of each individual into the activity or verifying, perhaps through sampling, that approved procedures for induction of individuals into the activity are being followed, and (ii) monitoring the progress of the activity and intervening as necessary through such steps as visits to the activity site, and continuing evaluation to determine if any unanticipated risks have arisen);

3. Carry out such other responsibilities, as may be assigned by the Secretary.

b. No award may be issued until the applicant or offeror has certified to the Secretary that the Institutional Review Board has made the determinations required under paragraph (a) of this section, and the Secretary has approved these determinations, as provided in §46.120 of Subpart A of this part.

c. Applicants or offerors seeking support for activities covered by this subpart must provide for the designation of an Institutional Review Board, subject to approval by the Secretary, where no such Board has been established under Subpart A of this part.

[40 FR 33628, August 8, 1975, as amended at 46 FR 8386, January 26, 1981]

§46.206 General limitations.

a. No activity to which this subpart is applicable may be undertaken, unless:
1. Appropriate studies on animals and nonpregnant individuals have been completed;
2. Except where the purpose of the activity is to meet the health needs of the mother or the particular fetus, the risk to the fetus is minimal and, in all cases, is the least possible risk for achieving the objectives of the activity;
3. Individuals engaged in the activity will have no part in (i) any decisions as to the timing, method, and procedures used to terminate the pregnancy, and (ii) determining the viability of the fetus at the termination of the pregnancy; and
4. No procedural changes which may cause greater than minimal risk to the fetus or the pregnant woman will be introduced into the procedure for terminating the pregnancy, solely in the interest of the activity.
b. No inducements, monetary or otherwise, may be offered to terminate pregnancy for purposes of the activity.

[40 FR 33628, August 8, 1975, as amended at 40 FR 51638, November 6, 1975]

§46.207 Activities directed toward pregnant women as subjects.

a. No pregnant woman may be involved as a subject in an activity covered by this subpart, unless: (1) the purpose of the activity is to meet the health needs of the mother and the fetus will be placed at risk only to the minimum extent necessary to meet such needs, or (2) the risk to the fetus is minimal.
b. An activity permitted under paragraph (a) of this section may be conducted only if the mother and father are legally competent and have given their informed consent after having been fully informed regarding possible impact on the fetus, except that the father's informed consent need not be secured, if: (1) the purpose of the activity is to meet the health needs of the mother; (2) his identity or whereabouts cannot reasonably be ascertained; (3) he is not reasonably available; or (4) the pregnancy resulted from rape.

§46.208 Activities directed toward fetuses in utero as subjects.

a. No fetus in utero may be involved as a subject in any activity covered by this subpart unless: (1) the purpose of the activity is to meet the health needs of the particular fetus and the fetus will be placed at risk only to the minimum extent necessary to meet such needs, or (2) the risk to the fetus imposed by the research is minimal, and the purpose of the activity is the development of important biomedical knowledge which cannot be obtained by other means.

b. An activity permitted under paragraph (a) of this section may be conducted only if the mother and father are legally competent and have given their informed consent, except that the father's consent need not be secured, if: (1) his identity or whereabouts cannot reasonably be ascertained, (2) he is not reasonably available, or (3) the pregnancy resulted from rape.

§46.209 Activities directed toward fetuses *ex utero,* including nonviable fetuses as subjects.

a. Until it has been ascertained whether or not a fetus *ex utero* is viable, a fetus *ex utero* may not be involved as a subject in an activity covered by this subpart, unless:

1. there will be no added risk to the fetus resulting from the activity, and the purpose of the activity is the development of important biomedical knowledge, which cannot be obtained by other means, or

2. the purpose of the activity is to enhance the possibility of survival of the particular fetus to the point of viability.

b. No nonviable fetus may be involved as a subject in an activity covered by this subpart, unless:

1. vital functions of the fetus will not be artificially maintained;

2. experimental activities, which of themselves would terminate the heartbeat or respiration of the fetus, will not be employed; and

3. the purpose of the activity is the development of important biomedical knowledge, which cannot be obtained by other means.

c. In the event the fetus *ex utero* is found to be viable, it may be included as a subject in the activity only to the extent permitted by and in accordance with the requirements of other subparts of this part.

d. An activity permitted under paragraph (a) or (b) of this section may be conducted only if the mother and father are legally competent and have given their informed consent, except that the father's informed consent need not be secured, if: (1) his identity or whereabouts cannot reasonably be ascertained; (2) he is not reasonably available; or (3) the pregnancy resulted from rape.

[40 FR 33528, August 8, 1975, as amended at 43 FR 1759, January 11, 1978]

§46.210 Activities involving the dead fetus, fetal material, or the placenta.

Activities involving the dead fetus, macerated fetal material, or cells, tissue, or organs excised from a dead fetus shall be conducted only in accordance with any applicable State or local laws regarding such activities.

§46.211 Modification or waiver of specific requirements.

Upon the request of an applicant or offeror (with the approval of its Institutional Review Board), the Secretary may modify or waive specific requirements of this subpart, with the approval of the Ethical Advisory Board after such opportunity for public comment as the Ethical Advisory Board considers appropriate in the particular instance. In making such decisions, the Secretary will consider whether the risks to the subject are so outweighed by the sum of the benefit to the subject and the importance of the knowledge to be gained as to warrant such modification or waiver and that such benefits cannot be gained except through a modification or waiver. Any such modifications or waivers will be published as notices in the *Federal Register*.

Subpart C—Additional DHHS Protections Pertaining to Biomedical and Behavioral Research Involving Prisoners as Subjects

[Source: 43 FR 53655, November 16, 1978, unless otherwise noted.]

§46.301 Applicability.

a. The regulations in this subpart are applicable to all biomedical and behavioral research conducted or supported by the Department of Health and Human Services involving prisoners as subjects.
b. Nothing in this subpart shall be construed as indicating that compliance with the procedures set forth herein will authorize research involving prisoners as subjects, to the extent such research is limited or barred by applicable State or local law.
c. The requirements of this subpart are in addition to those imposed under the other subparts of this part.

§46.302 Purpose.

Inasmuch as prisoners may be under constraints because of their incarceration which could affect their ability to make a truly voluntary and uncoerced decision whether or not to participate as subjects in research, it is the purpose of this subpart to provide additional safeguards for the protection of prisoners involved in activities to which this subpart is applicable.

§46.303 Definitions.

As used in this subpart:
a. *Secretary* means the Secretary of Health and Human Services and any other officer or employee of the Department of Health and Human Services to whom authority has been delegated.
b. *DHHS* means the Department of Health and Human Services.
c. *Prisoner* means any individual involuntarily confined or detained in a penal institution. The term is intended to encompass individuals sentenced to such

an institution under a criminal or civil statute, individuals detained in other facilities by virtue of statutes or commitment procedures which provide alternatives to criminal prosecution or incarceration in a penal institution, and individuals detained pending arraignment, trial, or sentencing.

d. *Minimal risk* is the probability and magnitude of physical or psychological harm that is normally encountered in the daily lives, or in the routine medical, dental, or psychological examination of healthy persons.

§46.304 Composition of Institutional Review Boards where prisoners are involved.

In addition to satisfying the requirements in §46.107 of this part, an Institutional Review Board, carrying out responsibilities under this part with respect to research covered by this subpart, shall also meet the following specific requirements:

a. A majority of the Board (exclusive of prisoner members) shall have no association with the prison(s) involved, apart from their membership on the Board.

b. At least one member of the Board shall be a prisoner, or a prisoner representative with appropriate background and experience to serve in that capacity, except that, where a particular research project is reviewed by more than one Board, only one Board need satisfy this requirement.

[43 FR 53655, November 16, 1978, as amended at 46 FR 8386, January 26, 1981]

§46.305 Additional duties of the Institutional Review Boards where prisoners are involved.

a. In addition to all other responsibilities prescribed for Institutional Review Boards under this part, the Board shall review research covered by this subpart and approve such research only if it finds that:

1. the research under review represents one of the categories of research permissible under §46.306(a)(2);

2. any possible advantages accruing to the prisoner through his or her participation in the research, when compared to the general living conditions, medical care, quality of food, amenities and opportunity for earnings in the prison, are not of such a magnitude that his or her ability to weigh the risks of the research against the value of such advantages in the limited choice environment of the prison is impaired;

3. the risks involved in the research are commensurate with risks that would be accepted by nonprisoner volunteers;

4. procedures for the selection of subjects within the prison are fair to all prisoners and immune from arbitrary intervention by prison authorities or prisoners. Unless the principal investigator provides to the Board justification in writing for following some other procedures, control subjects must be selected randomly from the group of available prisoners who meet the characteristics needed for that particular research project;

5. the information is presented in language which is understandable to the subject population;

6. adequate assurance exists that parole boards will not take into account a prisoner's participation in the research in making decisions regarding parole, and each prisoner is clearly informed in advance that participation in the research will have no effect on his or her parole; and

7. where the Board finds there may be a need for follow-up examination or care of participants after the end of their participation, adequate provision has been made for such examination or care, taking into account the varying lengths of individual prisoner's sentences, and for informing participants of this fact.

b. The Board shall carry out such other duties as may be assigned by the Secretary.

c. The institution shall certify to the Secretary, in such form and manner as the Secretary may require, that the duties of the Board under this section have been fulfilled.

§46.306 Permitted research involving prisoners.

a. Biomedical or behavioral research conducted or supported by DHHS may involve prisoners as subjects, only if:

1. the institution responsible for the conduct of the research has certified to the Secretary that the Institutional Review Board has approved the research under §46.305 of this subpart; and

2. in the judgment of the Secretary the proposed research involves solely the following: (i) study of the possible causes, effects, and processes of incarceration and of criminal behavior, provided that the study presents no more than minimal risk and no more than inconvenience to the subjects; (ii) study of prisons as institutional structures or of prisoners as incarcerated persons, provided that the study presents no more than minimal risk and no more than inconvenience to the subjects; (iii) research on conditions particularly affecting prisoners as a class (for example, vaccine trials and other research on hepatitis, which is much more prevalent in prisons than elsewhere; and research on social and psychological problems, such as alcoholism, drug addiction and sexual assaults), provided that the study may proceed only after the Secretary has consulted with appropriate experts, including experts in penology medicine and ethics, and published notice in the *Federal Register,* of his intent to approve such research; or (iv) research on practices, both innovative and accepted, which have the intent and reasonable probability of improving the health or well-being of the subject. In cases in which those studies require the assignment of prisoners in a manner consistent with protocols approved by the IRB to control groups which may not benefit from the research, the study may proceed only after the Secretary has consulted with appropriate experts, including experts in penology medicine and ethics, and published notice, in the *Federal Register,* of his intent to approve such research.

b. Except as provided in paragraph (a) of this section, biomedical or behavioral research conducted or supported by DHHS shall not involve prisoners as subjects.

Subpart D—Additional DHHS Protections for Children Involved as Subjects in Research

[Source: 48 FR 9818, March 8, 1983, unless otherwise noted.]

§46.401 To what do these regulations apply?

a. This subpart applies to all research involving children as subjects, conducted or supported by the Department of Health and Human Services.

    1. This includes research conducted by Department employees, except that each head of an Operating Division of the Department may adopt such nonsubstantive, procedural modifications as may be appropriate from an administrative standpoint.

    2. It also includes research conducted or supported by the Department of Health and Human Services outside the United States, but in appropriate circumstances, the Secretary may, under paragraph (e) of §46.101 of Subpart A, waive the applicability of some or all of the requirements of these regulations for research of this type.

b. Exemptions at §46.101(b)(1) and (b)(3) through (b)(6) are applicable to this subpart. The exemption at §46.101(b)(2) regarding educational tests is also applicable to this subpart. However, the exemption at §46.101(b)(2) for research involving survey or interview procedures or observations of public behavior does not apply to research covered by this subpart, except for research involving observation of public behavior, when the investigator(s) do not participate in the activities being observed.

c. The exceptions, additions, and provisions for waiver, as they appear in paragraphs (c) through (i) of §46.101 of Subpart A, are applicable to this subpart.

[48 FR 9818, March 8, 1983; 56 FR 28032, June 18, 1991; 56 FR 29757, June 28, 1991]

§46.402 Definitions.

The definitions in §46.102 of Subpart A shall be applicable to this subpart as well. In addition, as used in this subpart:

a. *Children* are persons who have not attained the legal age for consent to treatments or procedures involved in the research, under the applicable law of the jurisdiction in which the research will be conducted.

b. *Assent* means a child's affirmative agreement to participate in research. Mere failure to object should not, absent affirmative agreement, be construed as assent.

c. *Permission* means the agreement of parent(s) or guardian to the participation of their child or ward in research.

d. *Parent* means a child's biological or adoptive parent.

e. *Guardian* means an individual who is authorized under applicable State or local law to consent on behalf of a child to general medical care.

§46.403 IRB duties.

In addition to other responsibilities assigned to IRBs under this part, each IRB shall review research covered by this subpart, and approve only research which satisfies the conditions of all applicable sections of this subpart.

§46.404 Research not involving greater than minimal risk.

DHHS will conduct or fund research in which the IRB finds that no greater than minimal risk to children is presented, only if the IRB finds that adequate provisions are made for soliciting the assent of the children and the permission of their parents or guardians, as set forth in §46.408.

§46.405 Research involving greater than minimal risk, but presenting the prospect of direct benefit to the individual subjects.

DHHS will conduct or fund research in which the IRB finds that more than minimal risk to children is presented by an intervention or procedure that holds out the prospect of direct benefit for the individual subject, or by a monitoring procedure that is likely to contribute to the subject's well-being, only if the IRB finds that:

a. the risk is justified by the anticipated benefit to the subjects;

b. the relation of the anticipated benefit to the risk is at least as favorable to the subjects as that presented by available alternative approaches; and

c. adequate provisions are made for soliciting the assent of the children and permission of their parents or guardians, as set forth in §46.408.

§46.406 Research involving greater than minimal risk and no prospect of direct benefit to individual subjects, but likely to yield generalizable knowledge about the subject's disorder or condition.

DHHS will conduct or fund research in which the IRB finds that more than minimal risk to children is presented by an intervention or procedure that does not hold out the prospect of direct benefit for the individual subject, or by a monitoring procedure which is not likely to contribute to the well-being of the subject, only if the IRB finds that:

a. the risk represents a minor increase over minimal risk;

b. the intervention or procedure presents experiences to subjects that are reasonably commensurate with those inherent in their actual or expected medical, dental, psychological, social or educational situations;

c. the intervention or procedure is likely to yield generalizable knowledge about the subjects' disorder or condition which is of vital importance for the understanding or amelioration of the subjects' disorder or condition; and

d. adequate provisions are made for soliciting assent of the children and permission of their parents or guardians, as set forth in §46.408.

§46.407 Research not otherwise approvable which presents an opportunity to understand, prevent, or alleviate a serious problem affecting the health or welfare of children.

DHHS will conduct or fund research that the IRB does not believe meets the requirements of §46.404, §46.405, or §46.406, only if:

a. the IRB finds that the research presents a reasonable opportunity to further the understanding, prevention, or alleviation of a serious problem affecting the health or welfare of children, and

b. the Secretary, after consultation with a panel of experts in pertinent disciplines (for example: science, medicine, education, ethics, law), and following opportunity for public review and comment, has determined either:

  1. that the research in fact satisfies the conditions of §46.404, §46.405, or §46.406, as applicable, or

  2. the following: (i) the research presents a reasonable opportunity to further the understanding, prevention, or alleviation of a serious problem affecting the health or welfare of children; (ii) the research will be conducted in accordance with sound ethical principles; (iii) adequate provisions are made for soliciting the assent of children and the permission of their parents or guardians, as set forth in §46.408.

§46.408 Requirements for permission by parents or guardians and for assent by children.

a. In addition to the determinations required under other applicable sections of this subpart, the IRB shall determine that adequate provisions are made for soliciting the assent of the children, when in the judgment of the IRB the children are capable of providing assent. In determining whether children are capable of assenting, the IRB shall take into account the ages, maturity, and psychological state of the children involved. This judgment may be made for all children to be involved in research under a particular protocol, or for each child, as the IRB deems appropriate. If the IRB determines that the capability of some or all of the children is so limited that they cannot reasonably be consulted, or that the intervention or procedure involved in the research holds out a prospect of direct benefit that is important to the health or well-being of the children, and is available only in the context of the research, the assent of the children is not a necessary condition for proceeding with the research. Even where the IRB determines that the subjects are capable of assenting, the IRB may still waive the assent requirement under circumstances, in which consent may be waived in accord with §46.116 of Subpart A.

b. In addition to the determinations required under other applicable sections of this subpart, the IRB shall determine, in accordance with and to the extent that consent is required by §46.116 of Subpart A, that adequate provisions are made for soliciting the permission of each child's parents or guardian. Where parental permission is to be obtained, the IRB may find that the permission of one parent is sufficient for research to be conducted under §46.404 or §46.405. Where research is covered by §46.406 and §46.407, and permission is to be obtained from parents, both parents must give their permission, unless one parent is deceased, unknown, incompetent, or not reasonably available, or when only one parent has legal responsibility for the care and custody of the child.

c. In addition to the provisions for waiver contained in §46.116 of Subpart A, if the IRB determines that a research protocol is designed for conditions or for a subject population for which parental or guardian permission is not a reasonable requirement to protect the subjects (for example, neglected or abused children), it may waive the consent requirements in Subpart A of this part and paragraph (b) of this section, provided an appropriate mechanism for protecting the children who will participate as subjects in the research is substituted, and provided further that the waiver is not inconsistent with Federal, state or local law. The choice of an appropriate mechanism would depend upon the nature and purpose of the activities described in the protocol, the risk and anticipated benefit to the research subjects, and their age, maturity, status, and condition.

d. Permission by parents or guardians shall be documented in accordance with and to the extent required by §46.117 of Subpart A.

e. When the IRB determines that assent is required, it shall also determine whether and how assent must be documented.

§46.409 Wards

a. Children, who are wards of the state or any other agency, institution, or entity can be included in research approved under §46.406 or §46.407, only if such research is:

1. related to their status as wards; or
2. conducted in schools, camps, hospitals, institutions, or similar settings, in which the majority of children involved as subjects are not wards.

b. If the research is approved under paragraph (a) of this section, the IRB shall require appointment of an advocate for each child who is a ward, in addition to any other individual acting on behalf of the child as guardian or in loco parentis. One individual may serve as advocate for more than one child. The advocate shall be an individual, who has the background and experience to act in, and agrees to act in, the best interests of the child for the duration of the child's participation in the research, and who is not associated in any way (except in the role as advocate or member of the IRB) with the research, the investigator(s), or the guardian organization.

Addendum 46 FR 8392

Research Activities Which May Be Reviewed Through Expedited Review

Research activities involving no more than minimal risk *and* in which the only involvement of human subjects will be in one or more of the following categories (carried out through standard methods) may be reviewed by the Institutional Review Board through the expedited review procedure, authorized in §46.110 of 45 CFR Part 46.

1. Collection of: hair and nail clippings, in a nondisfiguring manner; deciduous teeth, and permanent teeth if patient care indicates a need for extraction.

2. Collection of excreta and external secretions, including sweat, uncannulated saliva, placenta removed at delivery, and amniotic fluid at the time of rupture of the membrane prior to or during labor.

3. Recording of data from subjects 18 years of age or older, using noninvasive procedures routinely employed in clinical practice. This includes the use of physical sensors that are applied either to the surface of the body or at a distance and do not involve input of matter or significant amounts of energy into the subject or an invasion of the subject's privacy. It also includes such procedures as weighing, testing sensory acuity, electrocardiography, electroencephalography, thermography, detection of naturally occurring radioactivity, diagnostic echography, and electroretinography. It does not include exposure to electromagnetic radiation outside the visible range (for example, x-rays, microwaves).

4. Collection of blood samples by venipuncture, in amounts not exceeding 450 milliliters in an eight-week period, and no more often than two times per week, from subjects 18 years of age or older and who are in good health and not pregnant.

5. Collection of both supra- and sub-gingival dental plaque and calculus, provided the procedure is not more invasive than routine prophylactic sealing of the teeth and the process is accomplished in accordance with accepted prophylactic techniques.

6. Voice recordings made for research purposes, such as investigations of speech defects.

7. Moderate exercise by healthy volunteers.

8. The study of existing data, documents, records, pathological specimens, or diagnostic specimens.

9. Research on individual or group behavior or characteristics of individuals, such as studies of perception, cognition, game theory, or test development, where the investigator does not manipulate subjects' behavior and the research will not involve stress to subjects.

10. Research on drugs or devices for which an investigational new drug exemption or an investigational device exemption is not required.

[Source: 46 FR 8392; January 26, 1981.]

Code of Federal Regulations
Title 42, Public Health
Chapter 1, Subchapter A

PART 2a—PROTECTION OF IDENTITY—RESEARCH SUBJECTS

(Revised as of October 1, 1995)

AUTHORITY: Sec. 3(a), Pub. L. 91-513 as amended by sec. 122(b), Pub. L. 93-282; 84 Stat. 1241 (42 U.S.C. 242a(a)), as amended by 88 Stat. 132.

SOURCE: 44 FR 20384, Apr. 4, 1979, unless otherwise noted.

Sec. 2a.1 Applicability.

(a) Section 303(a) of the Public Health Service Act (42 U.S.C. 242a(a)) provides that '(t)he Secretary (of Health and Human Services) may authorize persons engaged in research on mental health, including research on the use and effect of alcohol and other psychoactive drugs, to protect the privacy of individuals who are the subject of such research by withholding from all persons not connected with the conduct of such research the names or other identifying characteristics of such individuals. Persons so authorized to protect the privacy of such individuals may not be compelled in any Federal, State, or local civil, criminal, administrative, legislative, or other proceedings to identify such individuals.' The regulations in this part establish procedures under which any person engaged in research on mental health including research on the use and effect of alcohol and other psychoactive drugs (whether or not the research is federally funded) may, subject to the exceptions set forth in paragraph (b) of this section, apply for such an authorization of confidentiality.

(b) These regulations do not apply to:

(1) Authorizations of confidentiality for research requiring an Investigational New Drug exemption under section 505(I) of the Federal Food, Drug, and Cosmetic Act (21 U.S.C. 355(I)) or to approved new drugs, such as methadone, requiring continuation of long-term studies, records, and reports. Attention is called to 21 CFR 291.505(g) relating to authorizations of confidentiality for patient records maintained by methadone treatment programs.

(2) Authorizations of confidentiality for research which are related to law enforcement activities or otherwise within the purview of the Attorney General's authority to issue authorization of confidentiality pursuant to section 502 (c) of the Controlled Substances Act (21 U.S.C. 872(c)) and 21 CFR 1316.21.

(c) The Secretary's regulations on confidentiality of alcohol and drug abuse patient records (42 CFR part 2) and the regulations of this part may, in some instances, concurrently cover the same transaction. As explained in 42 CFR 2.24 and 2.24–1, 42 CFR part 2 restricts voluntary disclosures of information from applicable patient records while a Confidentiality Certificate issued pursuant to the regulations of this part protects a person engaged in applicable research from being compelled to disclose identifying characteristics of individuals who are the subject of such research.

Sec. 2a.2 Definitions.

(a) *Secretary* means the Secretary of Health and Human Services and any other officer or employee of the Department of Health and Human Services to whom the authority involved has been delegated.

(b) *Person* means any individual, corporation, government, or governmental subdivision or agency, business trust, partnership, association, or other legal entity.

(c) *Research* means systematic study directed toward new or fuller knowledge and understanding of the subject studied. The term includes, but is not limited to, behavioral science studies, surveys, evaluations, and clinical investigations.

(d) *Drug* has the meaning given that term by section 201(g)(1) of the Federal Food, Drug, and Cosmetic Act (21 U.S.C. 321(g)(1)).

(e) *Controlled drug* means a drug which is included in schedule I, II, III, IV, or V of part B of the Controlled Substances Act (21 U.S.C. 811–812).

(f) *Administer* refers to the direct application of a drug to the body of a human research subject, whether such application be by injection, inhalation, ingestion, or any other means, by (1) a qualified person engaged in research (or, in his or her presence, by his or her authorized agent), or (2) a research subject in accordance with instructions of a qualified person engaged in research, whether or not in the presence of a qualified person engaged in research.

(g) *Identifying characteristics* refers to the name, address, any identifying number, fingerprints, voiceprints, photographs or any other item or combination of data about a research subject which could reasonably lead directly or indirectly by reference to other information to identification of that research subject.

(h) *Psychoactive drug* means, in addition to alcohol, any drug which has as its principal action an effect on thought, mood, or behavior.

Sec. 2a.3 Application; coordination.

(a) Any person engaged in (or who intends to engage in) the research to which this part applies, who desires authorization to withhold the names and other identifying characteristics of individuals who are the subject of such research from any person or authority not connected with the conduct of such research may apply to the Office of the Director, National Institute on Drug Abuse, the Office of the Director, National Institute of Mental Health, or the Office of the Director, National Institute on Alcohol Abuse and Alcoholism, 5600 Fishers Lane, Rockville, Maryland 20857 for an authorization of confidentiality.

(b) If there is uncertainty with regard to which Institute is appropriate or if the research project falls within the purview of more than one Institute, an application need be submitted only to one Institute. Persons who are uncertain with regard to the applicability of these regulations to a particular type of research may apply for an authorization of confidentiality under the regulations of this part to one of the Institutes. Requests which are within the scope of the authorities described in Sec. 2a.1(b) will be forwarded to the appropriate agency for consideration and the person will be advised accordingly.

(c) An application may accompany, precede, or follow the submission of a request for DHHS grant or contract assistance, though it is not necessary to request DHHS grant or contract assistance in order to apply for a Confidentiality Certificate. If a person has previously submitted any information required in this part in connection with a DHHS grant or contract, he or she may substitute a copy of information thus submitted, if the information is current and accurate. If a person requests a Confidentiality Certificate at the same time he or she submits an application for DHHS grant or contract assistance, the application for a Confidentiality Certificate may refer to the pertinent section(s) of the DHHS grant or contract application which provide(s) the information required to be submitted under this part. (See Sec. 2a.4 and 2a.5.)

(d) A separate application is required for each research project for which an authorization of confidentiality is requested.

Sec. 2a.4 Contents of application; in general.

In addition to any other pertinent information which the Secretary may require, each application for an authorization of confidentiality for a research project shall contain:

(a) The name and address of the individual primarily responsible for the conduct of the research and the sponsor or institution with which he or she is affiliated, if any. Any application from a person affiliated with an institution will be considered only if it contains or is accompanied by documentation of institutional approval. This documentation may consist of a written statement signed by a responsible official of the institution or of a copy of or reference to a valid certification submitted in accordance with 45 CFR Part 46.

(b) The location of the research project and a description of the facilities available for conducting the research, including the name and address of any hospital, institution, or clinical laboratory facility to be utilized in connection with the research.

(c) The names, addresses, and summaries of the scientific or other appropriate training and experience of all personnel having major responsibilities in the research project and the training and experience requirements for major positions not yet filled.

(d) An outline of the research protocol for the project including a clear and concise statement of the purpose and rationale of the research project and the general research methods to be used.

(e) The date on which research will begin or has begun and the estimated date for completion of the project.

(f) A specific request, signed by the individual primarily responsible for the conduct of the research, for authority to withhold the names and other identifying characteristics of the research subjects and the reasons supporting such request.

(g) An assurance (1) From persons making application for a Confidentiality Certificate for a research project for which DHHS grant or contract support is received or sought that they will comply with all the requirements of 45 CFR Part 46, 'Protection of Human Subjects,' or (2) From all other persons making application that they will comply with the informed consent requirements of 45 CFR 46.103(c) and document legally effective informed consent in a manner consistent with the principles stated in 45 CFR 46.110, if it is determined by the Secretary, on the basis of information submitted by the person making application, that subjects will be placed at risk. If a modification of paragraphs (a) or (b) of 45 CFR 46.110 is to be used, as permitted under paragraph (c) of that section, the applicant will describe the proposed modification and submit it for approval by the Secretary.

(h) An assurance that if an authorization of confidentiality is given it will not be represented as an endorsement of the research project by the Secretary or used to coerce individuals to participate in the research project.

(i) An assurance that any person who is authorized by the Secretary to protect the privacy of research subjects will use that authority to refuse to disclose identifying characteristics of research subjects in any Federal, State, or local civil, criminal, administrative, legislative, or other proceedings to compel disclosure of the identifying characteristics of research subjects.

(j) An assurance that all research subjects who participate in the project during the period the Confidentiality Certificate is in effect will be informed that:

(1) A Confidentiality Certificate has been issued;

(2) The persons authorized by the Confidentiality Certificate to protect the identity of research subjects may not be compelled to identify research subjects in any civil, criminal, administrative, legislative, or other proceedings whether Federal, State, or local;

(3) If any of the following conditions exist the Confidentiality Certificate does not authorize any person to which it applies to refuse to reveal identifying information concerning research subjects: (i) The subject consents in writing to disclosure of identifying information, (ii) Release is required by the Federal Food, Drug, and Cosmetic Act (21 U.S.C. 301) or regulations promulgated thereunder (title 21, Code of Federal Regulations), or (iii) Authorized personnel of DHHS request identifying information for audit or program evaluation of a research project funded by DHHS or for investigation of DHHS grantees or contractors and their employees or agents carrying out such a project. (See Sec. 2a.7(b));

(4) The Confidentiality Certificate does not govern the voluntary disclosure of identifying characteristics of research subjects;

(5) The Confidentiality Certificate does not represent an endorsement of the research project by the Secretary.

(k) An assurance that all research subjects who enter the project after the termination of the Confidentiality Certificate will be informed that the authorization of confidentiality has ended and that the persons authorized to protect the identity of research subjects by the Confidentiality Certificate may not rely on the Certificate to refuse to disclose identifying characteristics of research subjects who were not participants in the project during the period the Certificate was in effect. (See Sec. 2a.8(c)).

Sec. 2a.5 Contents of application; research projects in which drugs will be administered.

(a) In addition to the information required by Sec. 2a.4 and any other pertinent information which the Secretary may require, each application for an authorization of confidentiality for a research project which involves the administering of a drug shall contain:

(1) Identification of the drugs to be administered in the research project and a description of the methods for such administration, which shall include a statement of the dosages to be administered to the research subjects;

(2) Evidence that individuals who administer drugs are authorized to do so under applicable Federal and State law; and

(3) In the case of a controlled drug, a copy of the Drug Enforcement Administration Certificate of Registration (BND Form 223) under which the research project will be conducted.

(b) An application for an authorization of confidentiality with respect to a research project which involves the administering of a controlled drug may include a request for exemption of persons engaged in the research from State or Federal prosecution for possession, distribution, and dispensing of controlled drugs as authorized under section 502(d) of the Controlled Substances Act (21 U.S.C. 872(d)) and 21 CFR 1316.22. If the request is in such form, and is supported by such information, as is required by 21 CFR 1316.22, the Secretary will forward it, together with his or her recommendation that such request be approved or disapproved, for the consideration of the Administrator of the Drug Enforcement Administration.

Sec. 2a.6 Issuance of Confidentiality Certificates; single project limitation.

(a) In reviewing the information provided in the application for a Confidentiality Certificate, the Secretary will take into account:

(1) The scientific or other appropriate training and experience of all personnel having major responsibilities in the research project;

(2) Whether the project constitutes bona fide 'research' which is within the scope of the regulations of this part; and

(3) Such other factors as he or she may consider necessary and appropriate. All applications for Confidentiality Certificates shall be evaluated by the Secretary through such officers and employees of the Department and such experts or consultants engaged for this purpose as he or she determines to be appropriate.

(b) After consideration and evaluation of an application for an authorization of confidentiality, the Secretary will either issue a Confidentiality Certificate or a letter denying a Confidentiality Certificate, which will set forth the reasons for such denial, or will request additional information from the person making application. The Confidentiality Certificate will include:

(1) The name and address of the person making application;

(2) The name and address of the individual primarily responsible for conducting the research, if such individual is not the person making application;

(3) The location of the research project;

(4) A brief description of the research project;

(5) A statement that the Certificate does not represent an endorsement of the research project by the Secretary;

(6) The Drug Enforcement Administration registration number for the project, if any; and

(7) The date or event upon which the Confidentiality Certificate becomes effective, which shall not be before the later of either the commencement of the research project or the date of issuance of the Certificate, and the date or event upon which the Certificate will expire.

(c) A Confidentiality Certificate is not transferable and is effective only with respect to the names and other identifying characteristics of those individuals who are the subjects of the single research project specified in the Confidentiality Certificate. The recipient of a Confidentiality Certificate shall, within 15 days of any completion or discontinuance of the research project which occurs prior to the expiration date set forth in the Certificate, provide written notification to the Director of the Institute to which application was made. If the recipient determines that the research project will not be completed by the expiration date set forth in the Confidentiality Certificate he or she may submit a written request for an extension of the expiration date which shall include a justification for such extension and a revised estimate of the date for completion of the project. Upon approval of such a request, the Secretary will issue an amended Confidentiality Certificate.

(d) The protection afforded by a Confidentiality Certificate does not extend to significant changes in the research project as it is described in the application for such Certificate (e.g., changes in the personnel having major responsibilities in the research project, major changes in the scope or direction of the research protocol, or changes in the drugs to be administered and the persons who will administer them). The recipient of a Confidentiality Certificate shall notify the Director of the Institute to which application was made of any proposal for such a significant change by submitting an amended application for a Confidentiality Certificate in the same form and manner as an original application. On the basis of such application and other pertinent information the Secretary will either:

(1) Approve the amended application and issue an amended Confidentiality Certificate together with a Notice of Cancellation terminating the original Confidentiality Certificate in accordance with Sec. 2a.8; or

(2) Disapprove the amended application and notify the applicant in writing that adoption of the proposed significant changes will result in the issuance of a Notice of Cancellation terminating the original Confidentiality Certificate in accordance with Sec. 2a.8.

Sec. 2a.7 Effect of Confidentiality Certificate.

(a) A Confidentiality Certificate authorizes the withholding of the names and other identifying characteristics of individuals who participate as subjects in the research project specified in the Certificate while the Certificate is in effect. The authorization applies to all persons who, in the performance of their duties in connection with the research project, have access to information which would identify the subjects of the research. Persons so authorized may not, at any time, be compelled in any Federal, State, or local civil, criminal, administrative, legislative, or other proceedings to identify the research subjects encompassed by the Certificate, except in those circumstances specified in paragraph (b) of this section.

(b) A Confidentiality Certificate granted under this part does not authorize any person to refuse to reveal the name or other identifying characteristics of any research subject in the following circumstances: (1) The subject (or, if he or she is legally incompetent, his or her guardian) consents, in writing, to the disclosure of such information, (2) Authorized personnel of DHHS request such information for audit or program evaluation of a research project funded by DHHS or for investigation of DHHS grantees or contractors and their employees or agents carrying out such a project. (See 45 CFR 5.71 for confidentiality standards imposed on such DHHS personnel), or (3) Release of such information is required by the Federal Food, Drug, and Cosmetic Act (21 U.S.C. 301) or the regulations promulgated thereunder (title 21, Code of Federal Regulations).

(c) Neither a Confidentiality Certificate nor the regulations of this part govern the voluntary disclosure of identifying characteristics of research subjects.

Sec. 2a.8 Termination.

(a) A Confidentiality Certificate is in effect from the date of its issuance until the effective date of its termination. The effective date of termination shall be the earlier of:

(1) The expiration date set forth in the Confidentiality Certificate; or

(2) Ten days from the date of mailing a Notice of Cancellation to the applicant, pursuant to a determination by the Secretary that the research project has been completed or discontinued or that retention of the Confidentiality Certificate is otherwise no longer necessary or desirable.

(b) A Notice of Cancellation shall include: an identification of the Confidentiality Certificate to which it applies; the effective date of its termination; and the grounds for cancellation. Upon receipt of a Notice of Cancellation the applicant shall return the Confidentiality Certificate to the Secretary.

(c) Any termination of a Confidentiality Certificate pursuant to this section is operative only with respect to the names and other identifying characteristics of individuals who begin their participation as research subjects after the effective date of such termination. (See Sec. 2a.4(k) requiring researchers to notify subjects who enter the project after the termination of the Confidentiality Certificate of termination of the Certificate). The protection afforded by a Confidentiality Certificate is permanent with respect to subjects who participated in research during any time the authorization was in effect.

The Nuremberg Code

From "Trials of War Criminals Before the Nuremberg Military Tribunals Under Control Council Law No. 10", Vol. 2, Nuremberg, October 1946– April 1949 (Washington, DC: US Government Printing Office, 1949), pp 181–182.

The great weight of the evidence before us is to the effect that certain types of medical experiments on human beings, when kept within reasonably well-defined bounds, conform to the ethics of the medical profession generally. The protagonists of the practice of human experimentation justify their views on the basis that such experiments yield results for the good of society that are unprocurable by other methods or means of study. All agree, however, that certain basic principles must be observed in order to satisfy moral, ethical and legal concepts.

1. The voluntary consent of the human subject is absolutely essential.

   This means that the person involved should have legal capacity to give consent; should be so situated as to be able to exercise free power of choice, without the intervention of any element of force, fraud, deceit, duress, overreaching, or other ulterior form of constraint or coercion; and should have sufficient knowledge and comprehension of the elements of the subject matter involved as to enable him to make an understanding and enlightened decision.

   This latter element requires that before the acceptance of an affirmative decision by the experimental subject there should be made known to him the nature, duration, and purpose of the experiment; the method and means by which it is to be conducted; all inconveniences and hazards reasonably to be expected; and the effects upon his health or person which may possibly come from his participation in the experiment.

   The duty and responsibility for ascertaining the quality of the consent rests upon each individual who initiates, directs or engages in the experiment. It is a personal duty and responsibility which may not be delegated to another with impunity.

2. The experiment should be such as to yield fruitful results for the good of society, unprocurable by other methods or means of study, and not random and unnecessary in nature.

3. The experiment should be so designed and based on the results of animal experimentation and a knowledge of the natural history of the disease or other problems under study that the anticipated results will justify the performance of the experiment.
4. The experiment should be so conducted as to avoid all unnecessary physical and mental suffering and injury.
5. No experiment should be conducted where there is an a priori reason to believe that death or disabling injury will occur; except perhaps, in those experiments where the experimental physicians also serve as subjects.
6. The degree of risk to be taken should never exceed that determined by the humanitarian importance of the problem to be solved by the experiment.
7. Proper preparations should be made and adequate facilities provided to protect the experimental subject against even remote possibilities of injury, disability, or death.
8. The experiment should be conducted only by scientifically qualified persons. The highest degree of skill and care should be required through all stages of the experiment of those who conduct or engage in the experiment.
9. During the course of the experiment the human subject should be at liberty to bring the experiment to an end if he has reached the physical or mental state where continuation of the experiment seems to him to be impossible.
10. During the course of the experiment the scientist in charge must be prepared to terminate the experiment at any stage, if he has probable cause to believe in the exercise of the good faith, superior skill and careful judgement required of him that a continuation of the experiment is likely to result in injury, disability, or death to the experimental subject.

A Statement of Principles of Ethical Conduct for Neuropsychopharmacologic Research in Human Subjects

[Reprinted with permission from the American College of Neuropsycho-pharmacology.]

This Statement of Principles *is an edited version of the statement approved by Council and the membership in February 1996. Because it does not deal with studies on alcoholism and drug abuse, a revision of this statement is currently underway.*

INTRODUCTION

The purpose of this *Statement of Principles* is to serve as an ethical guide for neuropsychopharmacologic research with human subjects performed by the members of the American College of Neuropsychopharmacology (ACNP). This *Statement* defines neuropsychopharmacologic research as the evaluation of the effects of synthetic compounds or natural products employed as investigational agents that affect the brain, the peripheral nervous system, and/or behavior. While the principles provided below may be relevant to other areas of research with human subjects, this *Statement of Principles* was not designed with that broad goal in mind. The *Statement* is intended to be a framework for meeting existing as well as evolving concepts, and therefore, it should not be used retrospectively to judge research conducted prior to its adoption by the ACNP.

    The purpose of scientific research is to generate new knowledge and the subject who agrees to participate in a research study cooperates in advancing this goal. Ethical guidelines are required because the subject may be placed at risk during the research. Risk must be evaluated both within the context of a given study and within the context of the risks ordinarily borne by such subjects. Although minimizing risk relative to benefit is a goal of research, the uncertainty regarding the outcome of the research makes the precise estimation of the risk difficult at the outset of a research study. Despite this limitation, risk can and should be minimized by safeguards in study design, by the informed consent process for enrolling research subjects, and by the timely notification of research subjects when new information changes the risks involved in their continued participation.

The first consideration, therefore, is whether the study design itself incorporates reasonable safeguards to minimize anticipated risks. This is an appropriate subject for ethical review.

The second issue is whether the subject has been appropriately informed of the foreseeable risks of the study and the degree to which current knowledge may limit the accuracy of an estimate of future risks.

Since the purpose of informed consent is to allow potential subjects to rationally judge the risk that they may incur, the degree of informed consent can vary. Informed consent does not mean that the subject must be fully acquainted with every aspect of the study, but only those aspects that are pertinent to evaluating risk. For instance, in certain studies it is possible to deceive the subject concerning the nature of the experimental interventions if such deception does not alter objective risk.

A particular problem for neuropsychopharmacologic research in humans is that some subjects will be patients. Research involving patients is necessary for the advance of medical science. However, such research exposes a patient-subject to certain risks and influences that would not exist if he/she were not a patient. These risks and influences must also be evaluated in the context of the specific experiment. For instance, a patient at extremely high risk from disease may reasonably volunteer to participate in an experiment whose degree of risk might deter a non-patient. This may be the case even though there is no prospect of direct therapeutic benefit from the experiment because the patient views the experiment as not significantly affecting his overall degree of risk.

TERMS

This *Statement of Principles* employs the following terms:

1. Subject—An encompassing term that refers to all persons who are being scientifically studied.
2. Patient—A person who is being diagnosed or treated for an illness.

BACKGROUND

Neuropsychopharmacologic research has made significant contributions to human welfare. For example, as a result of the discovery and development of new drugs, patients with severe psychiatric and neurological illnesses, who were once considered untreatable and relegated to overcrowded institutions, have been able to return to their families and communities, often as productive persons. Others have been able to avoid institutionalization or to reduce its duration substantially as a result of drug therapy. However, the imperfections of existing treatment methods require continued scientific efforts to decrease the pain and suffering of patients and their families.

Scientific research does not exist in a vacuum. All persons living in society have a moral responsibility to participate in efforts to promote and contribute to the present and future welfare of that society. Research is one of these obligations. However, researchers have a responsibility to society to protect the welfare of each subject. These principles are designed to reconcile society's need for advancing knowledge and for conducting research in an ethically informed and regulated manner. It should be emphasized that advances in medical research with subsequent benefit to society are impossible without individual risks, yet society and researchers should strive to minimize these risks.

This *Statement of Principles* is independent of standards currently contained in law or governmental regulations. This independence has significant implications: (1) Although law and ethics interrelate, they are by no means identical, for ethical requirements may affect behavior not within legal control. (2) This *Statement of Principles* applies to all neuropsychopharmacologic research in human subjects. (3) Standards of governmental regulations may vary, and there is no assurance that present standards will prevail in the future. (4) Finally, the existence of a *Statement of Principles* provides a reference point for the conduct of neuropsychopharmacologic research in human subjects.

This *Statement of Principles* affirms the consideration of risks versus benefits, the requirement of voluntary informed competent consent, the avoidance of unnecessary pain or disabling long-term effects, and the evaluation of potential benefits to both the individual and society.

PRINCIPLE 1: *Qualifications of the Scientific Investigator*

A scientific investigator, before assuming full responsibility for conducting neuropsychopharmacologic research studies with human subjects, shall have had adequate training and experience to conduct the research study proposed. Any research undertaken by an unqualified investigator is unethical behavior.

Commentary

The scientific investigator's prior experience in neuropsychopharmacologic studies with human subjects shall be given weight in assessing scientific expertise. The adequacy of the investigator's experience should be confirmed by the Institutional Review Board (IRB) or its equivalent.

PRINCIPLE 2: *Design and Methodology of Research Studies*

A neuropsychopharmacologic research study with human subjects shall be designed and carried out in accordance with generally accepted scientific principles and must reasonably anticipate increasing knowledge. Expert understanding of design and statistical analysis is essential. Independent replication of findings and cross validation is usually necessary.

Commentary

The following examples are some of the many considerations that should be taken into account in the preparation of research protocols:

1. Subjects should be selected only if they appear suitable to test the specific hypotheses proposed in the research.
2. Whenever feasible, studies should be planned so that the number of subjects in the study is consistent with the statistical requirements necessary to assure that conclusions are likely to be valid.
3. When appropriate, provision should be made for control or comparison groups (including placebo controls), or for subjects who serve as their own controls, to assure that information gathered has potential utility.
4. The investigator should have access to appropriate statistical expertise to assure that the results of the experiment will be meaningful to the scientific community.
5. In the research designs of studies whose subjects are also patients, randomization of assignment to treatment may be required. The relative merits of randomization versus other approaches should be considered.

PRINCIPLE 3: *Review and Approval of Human Research Studies*

A scientific investigator shall undertake a neuropsychopharmacologic research study involving human subjects only after the approval of an appropriate, qualified reviewing body. Once having secured initial approval, the investigator shall obtain subsequent approval for any substantial modification to the protocol. Annual review of continuing studies is required.

Commentary

Scientific investigators advocate and the United States Department of Health and Human Services (DHHS) requires the organization of IRBs for review and approval of research with human subjects.[1] Guidelines were published by the Department of Health, Education and Welfare in 1971, and the policy was codified into federal regulation in 1974.[2,3] The National Research Act (Pub. L. 93-348) enacted in 1974 established the National Commission for the Protection of Human Subjects of Biomedical and Behavioral Research (NCPHSBBR). The Commission's influential Belmont Report was published in 1979.[4] The most recent regulations were issued in 1994.[5] The Food and Drug Administration (FDA) published regulations in 1981 for protection of human subjects that included standards for IRBs for clinical investigation and a list of research activities that IRBs may review.[6] The most recent FDA regulations were issued in 1994.[7] According to these regulations and this *Statement,* the IRB has the primary responsibility for protecting the rights and welfare of research participants.

A scientific investigator who is not affiliated with an institution that has an IRB shall not undertake a neuropsychopharmacologic research study unless it is initially approved and reviewed annually by an independent review body that is the functional equivalent of an IRB.

In the event that DHHS should abandon or substantially restrict its requirements for IRBs, the approval and review of research studies by appropriate review bodies will continue to be required by this *Statement of Principles.* The intent of this principle is that all human research, regardless of the source of funds, should be subject to review.

Scientific investigators have the responsibility to serve on an IRB or its equivalent, when requested, in order to maintain the necessary principle of review of research by peers. If a scientific investigator is a member of an IRB that is considering the investigator's own project, the investigator should not participate in the review of that research project.

Because IRBs may be fallible, a procedure for the appeal and independent review of their decisions is necessary.

Research papers submitted for publication shall include a clear statement that IRB approval for the protocol was obtained.

PRINCIPLE 4: *Responsibilities of the Scientific Investigator and the Application of This Statement of Principles*

General Responsibilities

The scientific investigator engaged in neuropsychopharmacologic research with human subjects should take all reasonable precautions to preserve the autonomy, rights, and safety of all subjects. Studies differ in their goals and entail different degrees of risk. For instance, experimental studies of treatment may entail more risk than studies of the course and nature of psychiatric illness. Therefore, the degree of precaution taken by the investigator must correspond to the degree of risk expected.

Individual Responsibility

Each scientific investigator shall ascertain and consider the current ethical standards applicable to neuropsychopharmacologic research studies with human subjects in substantial accordance with the ethical principles contained in this *Statement of Principles* with respect for subjects and with concern for their dignity, welfare, and rights. In addition, these *Principles* impose this responsibility on all associates, employees, or students who assist the scientific investigator.

1. The scientific investigator shall take reasonable precautions to assure that the principles contained in this *Statement* are observed by all persons who assist in the research study.
2. The ethical responsibilities imposed by this *Statement of Principles* shall become applicable when the scientific investigator makes the initial decision to undertake a neuropsychopharmacologic research study with human subjects and shall continue through the conclusion of the research study, including all necessary steps to protect any privileged or confidential material pertaining to subjects in the study.
3. The scientific investigator shall make a reasonable effort to become acquainted with regulations that are relevant to the research study proposed, and shall take reasonable precautions to follow these regulations.

PRINCIPLE 5: *Considerations in Determining Who May Be a Proper Subject in a Research Study*

Studies of Treatment Intervention

In neuropsychopharmacologic research in which the subjects are patients, the scientific investigator should evaluate the research regimen with a view toward doing no harm to the patient. If there is a treatment that has a high probability of improving the patient's condition significantly, that treatment should not be withheld indefinitely. However, potential research subjects may accept the possibility of deferring a specific treatment for a specified time by enrolling in studies in which treatment is randomly assigned rather than determined on the basis of individualized clinical judgment. Randomization to treatments may include marketed medications, new or unproven medications, and placebo. Investigators should design research to make an accurate diagnosis before definitive treatment or to develop prognostic indicators for selection of optimal treatment of the patient's disease.

Studies of Course and Outcome

A study may include a patient as a subject in research unrelated to the disease or condition being treated if the study is unlikely to interfere with the welfare of the patient or the treatment regimen and the patient otherwise satisfies the prerequisites of a subject.

Studies of Normal Behavior

Research with subjects who are mentally competent, fully informed adults nevertheless imposes ethical responsibilities for the safety, dignity, and rights of these subjects. Such rights include respect for their autonomy and capacity to volunteer.

physical exam-
and assent by
ontrol" sub-
children
sonably
be

'ith in this principle and in other principles
nsideration in *Ethical Principles in the Con-*
's and in *Ethical Principles of Psychologists*,
gical Association.[8,9] Determining whether
study should include review of records
h the treating physician, other staff who
..y members (all with consent of the patient).

..0: *Ethical Responsibility—Physical and Mental Discomfort*

The scientific investigator has the obligation to minimize as much as possible all undue physical and mental discomfort of the subject. When it appears that a research study may have resulted in undesirable consequences for the subject, the investigator shall make every reasonable attempt to detect them and to assure adequate follow up treatment to remove, correct, or relieve those consequences. All clinically significant adverse effects having implications for the research protocol must be promptly reported to the IRB.

Commentary

In scientific investigations of subjects involving physical and/or mental discomfort, the nature of the anticipated physical and/or mental discomfort should be explained to the subject in advance. Furthermore, the investigator should be reasonably certain, on the basis of existing knowledge, that the anticipated physical and/or mental discomfort will not have long-term adverse consequences.

PRINCIPLE 7: *Ethical Considerations in Evaluating Potential Research Study Benefits and Risk; Research Procedures*

1. Scientific gains expected from research studies shall be weighed against the reasonably anticipated risks involved. At the time the research study is undertaken and throughout its performance, there should exist a scientific basis for a reasonable belief that the research study will ultimately produce scientific knowledge which will benefit patients in the future.
2. The scientific investigator shall not use a research procedure if it is likely to cause disabling or lasting harm to subjects, or if the reasonably anticipated benefits to a patient are outweighed by reasonably foreseeable disadvantages.

Subjects of Limited Mental Capacity

1. Children may be subjects in a neuropsychopharmacologic research study if the IRB considers the study to expose the subject to risks that are only minimally

greater than the risks of ordinary life experience, includi
inations and blood tests. Consent of their parent or guardia
the child is necessary. Children may also be included as "normal
jects in comparison studies. In general, research studies of drugs
shall not be undertaken unless similar studies in adults have proved r
safe.

A drug that has been proved to be safe but ineffective in adults ma
evaluated in children if there is a reasonable basis for expecting it to be effect
in children. In some specific disorders that are unique to children, such a
childhood autism, prior demonstration of drug efficacy in adults may be irrel-
evant. Research studies in these uniquely pediatric disorders are not foreclosed
under this principle because of the lack of such a disease process in adults.

2. A research study with children or with adult subjects who are mentally incom-
    petent requires additional considerations because of the limitations of the
    subjects, including their inability to understand fully the procedures and im-
    plications of the research study and to communicate their feelings and responses
    clearly to the investigator.

Pharmacologically Inert Substances

The scientific investigator who proposes to use a placebo as part of the methodological requirement of a study shall justify both the necessity and ethical considerations of the procedure as it relates to the specific illness or particular research
problem. This approach shall be reviewed by the IRB or qualified review body.

Commentary

The report and recommendations by the NCPHSBBR on research involving children
were published in the Federal Register in 1978.[10] In 1983, additional protections for
children involved as subjects in research, including requirements for permission by
parents or guardians, were prescribed in the Federal Register.[11]

The use of a placebo in severely ill patients, such as very disturbed and/or
severely deteriorated chronic schizophrenic patients who present gross thought disorders and hallucinations, should be reviewed by the investigator. The use of a
placebo control group in evaluating treatment in conditions with a tendency toward
spontaneous remission may be appropriate. Thirty to forty percent of patients diagnosed as acute schizophrenics, for example, may show moderate to marked
improvement with placebo. In nonpsychotic conditions, such as anxiety and depression, the "superiority of standard existing drugs over placebo is of sufficiently
modest extent to make the administration of placebo to some patients in a study
justifiable, particularly if there are explicit provisions for removing from the study
patients whose clinical condition worsened".[12]

Subjects in treatment studies should be monitored closely so that fluctuations
in clinical state can be tracked to insure that any clinically significant change is

detected. Determining whether a clinically significant deterioration has occurred often requires repeated observation to ensure that the research subject is not exposed to undue risk. Such patients should be treated as expeditiously as possible.

PRINCIPLE 8: *Informed Consent*

The Requirement of Informed Consent

Research studies with human subjects require their informed consent. If a subject lacks capacity to consent, the scientific investigator shall obtain the consent from a person legally authorized to give consent on behalf of the subject or shall take appropriate legal action.

Informed consent as used in the context of these *Principles* is the agreement obtained from a subject (or from an authorized representative) to participate in a neuropsychopharmacologic research study. The basic elements of informed consent are:

1. An explanation of the procedures to be followed, including an identification of those that are experimental.
2. A description of the reasonably foreseeable attendant discomforts and risks and a statement of the uncertainty of the anticipated risks due to the inherent nature of the research process.
3. A description of the benefits that may be expected.
4. A disclosure of appropriate and available alternate procedures that might be advantageous for the subject.
5. An offer to answer any inquiries concerning the procedures.
6. A statement that information may be withheld from the subject in certain cases when the investigator believes that full disclosure may be detrimental to the subject or fatal to the study design (provided, however, that the IRB has given proper approval to such withholding of information).
7. A disclosure of the probability that the subject may be given a placebo at some time during the course of the research study if placebo is to be utilized in the study.
8. An explanation in lay terms of the probability that the subject may be placed in one or another treatment group if randomization is a part of the study design.
9. An instruction that consent may be withdrawn and participation in the study may be discontinued at any time.
10. An explanation that there is no penalty for not participating in or withdrawing from the study once the project has been initiated.
11. A statement that the investigator will inform the patient of any significant new information arising from the experiment or other ongoing experiments which bear on the patient's choice to remain in the study.

12. A statement that the investigator shall provide a review of the nature and results of the study to those subjects who request such information.

Current FDA regulations for the protection of human subjects require that the subject be informed that the FDA may inspect the records. Thus, the subject should be informed about the extent to which confidentiality of the records identifying subjects will be maintained.[7]

Subjects Who Lack The Capacity to Consent

1. When a patient is mentally incompetent or too young to comprehend, informed consent must be obtained from one who is legally authorized to consent on behalf of the proposed subject. As the study progresses, the investigator also shall keep the person who consents on behalf of the subject informed of any major changes in the research protocol or significant side effects.
2. If a mentally incompetent or incapacitated subject is capable of exercising some judgment concerning the nature of the research study and participation in it, the investigator shall obtain the assent of the subject in addition to the consent of the person legally authorized to consent. Supplemental guidelines for research involving those institutionalized as mentally disabled were published in the Federal Register in 1978.[13]
3. When the subject is a child who has reached the age of some discretion, and the subject is otherwise mentally competent, the scientific investigator shall obtain the subject's assent in addition to the consent of the person legally authorized to consent.[11]

Patients unable to give informed consent pose special problems. The scientific investigator assumes additional ethical responsibilities to the patient-subject who, because of lack of capacity, may not be able to make rational judgments concerning participation or withdrawal from the research study.[14]

Consent of Prison Inmates and Other Especially Vulnerable Groups

1. If potential subjects are involuntarily institutionalized or subject to some legal restraint, investigators should take special precautions to assure the subjects the opportunity to obtain full information about the research study, including the right to refuse to participate or to withdraw from the study at any time without penalty. Guidelines for conditions under which research involving prisoners is permitted were published in the Federal Register in 1978.[15]
2. When an investigator proposes to select as subjects individuals who are involuntarily institutionalized, who are under some legal restraint, or whose personal circumstances are such that their need for volunteer compensation or course accreditation (students) may cloud their caution or judgment, the final approval concerning such a research study shall reside with the appropriate, qualified reviewing body.

Commentary

Informed consent of the research subject is an ethical prerequisite. This *Statement of Principles* establishes the ethical requirements of consent but takes no position on the legal sufficiency of the principles.

The authority of a person to provide informed consent on behalf of one who lacks capacity varies from state to state. Parental consent is usually required when children comprise the subject group in well-designed neuropsychopharmacologic experiments. However, the parent or court appointed proxy has no moral right to give consent for the child to participate in an experiment that has no specific etiologic, diagnostic, or therapeutic goals for the disease presented by the child, except in those cases where there are no reasonably foreseeable risks. With regard to persons who are mentally incompetent, some states may require informed consent from the closest living relative; some states may insist on approval from a court. It is the scientific investigator's responsibility to determine the appropriate person to give consent.

This principle does not contend that persons who may be vulnerable to undue influence must be automatically excluded as potential subjects. Such decisions should be made by an appropriate IRB on a protocol-by-protocol basis.

Documentation that informed consent was obtained is required. The use of forms that incorporate the twelve listed elements that are signed by the investigator and the subject is presently the standard procedure. An alternative procedure involves the utilization of an individual not involved in the research study who is present at the time consent is secured. Such an individual assists the subject by explaining the risks and benefits to the subject and certifies that informed consent has in fact been obtained. Utilization of such an individual may facilitate the explanation of risks and benefits in a manner appropriate for the subject, or for the person giving consent on his or her behalf. This procedure provides subsequent proof of the occurrence of informed consent.

A person who is incarcerated as a result of a criminal conviction should not be disqualified from being a subject in a neuropsychopharmacologic research study merely because he is a prisoner. Furthermore, a prisoner should not be denied the opportunity to participate in a research study evaluating an illness that may have been directly or indirectly associated with the prisoner's incarceration. For example, a prisoner with a history of heroin addiction that resulted in illegal activity and subsequent incarceration should have the opportunity to participate voluntarily in research studies of treatment with narcotic-blocking agents. If such a research endeavor were successful, the prisoner would then have gained a definite benefit from the particular experiment. However, the relative isolation of the prisoner from society and the inherently coercive environment of the prison impose on the scientific investigator the additional obligation to take all practical measures to ascertain that the prisoner understands that he/she is free to refuse to participate and that the prisoner has full information about the study and its possible effects on him or her.

Careful consideration should be given to studies with residents of a poverty area whose need for paid volunteer fees may outweigh their caution or with college students who may participate in a drug research study if it is perceived as a requirement to a course or because of faculty pressure. Every potential subject is responding to some pressures; however, there is a difference between gross external pressures brought about, for example, by prison officials or teachers and internal pressures which are complex and vary among individuals. It may be difficult or impossible for the scientific investigator to be aware of and to evaluate complex internal pressures in a potential subject. The investigator should make special efforts to eliminate or decrease external pressures or reject potential subjects who have been under substantial external pressures.

PRINCIPLE 9: *Subject's Right to Decline or Withdraw*

Right to Decline Participation and Right to Withdraw

The investigator shall respect the freedom of the individual subject, or in the case of those who lack capacity to consent, the person legally authorized to act on the patient's behalf, to decline to participate in a research study or to discontinue participation at any time without penalty.

Reviewing Body

The IRB and the individual investigator are responsible for insuring that the research protocol protects the subject's freedom to participate and withdraw. The IRB shall determine whether or not the research procedures protect the subject from deceit or any type of undue influence.

Commentary

In studies with mentally competent individuals, the subject may withdraw from the research project at any time. However, patient-subjects unable to give informed consent pose particular problems. The scientific investigator assumes additional ethical responsibilities to the subject who, because of lack of capacity, may not be able to make rational judgments concerning withdrawal from the research study. These additional responsibilities require exceptionally careful attention to a patient-subject's rejection of a particular experimental treatment.

Regardless of the research subject's mental competency, the investigator may be uniquely able to anticipate adverse consequences from the continuation of an experiment. Study participation may alter the subject's judgment so that he/she is no longer a good judge of the appropriateness of continuing to participate. It is the investigator's responsibility to withdraw the patient from the study if such a situation appears imminent; this responsibility includes subjects receiving either active drugs or placebo.

PRINCIPLE 10: *Information*

Confidentiality

The scientific investigator is responsible for maintaining the confidentiality of information and for not improperly releasing information pertaining to subjects in the study. This responsibility includes not only information specifically protected by law, which may not apply to all subjects, but also information that affects the privacy and dignity of subjects. When there is a likelihood that others may obtain access to such information derived from the research, the investigator, in obtaining informed consent, shall explain this possibility and the plans for maintaining confidentiality to the subject or, in the case of those lacking mental capacity, to the person who provides consent on behalf of the subject.

Explanation to Subjects

1. Information about foreseeable side effects of pharmacologic agents used in research should be given to the subject and/or the person who consented to the subject's participation.
2. After the data are collected, the investigator should provide a review of the nature and results of the study to those subjects who request such information. When scientific or humane values justify delaying or withholding information, the investigator incurs a special responsibility to take reasonable precautions that this action does not result in damaging consequences for the subject.
3. After termination of studies involving those who lack the capacity to consent, such as mentally incompetent persons and young children, the investigator shall reveal, on request, important and pertinent results to the person who provided consent for the subject.

PRINCIPLE 11: *Ethical Obligations of Investigator for Follow-Up Treatment of the Patient-Subjects*

Responsibility for Follow-Up Treatment for the Patient

The scientific investigator shall take reasonable steps to see that the patient is treated in the most appropriate manner. These steps may include the continuation of a research program if such a procedure is possible. If not, the best alternative should be sought.

REFERENCES

1. Reatig, N. Federal regulations affecting psychopharmacology research in the United States. In Burroughs, G.D. and Werry, J.D. (eds.) *Advances in Human Psychopharmacology*, Vol. 2. Greenwich, CT: JAI Press Inc., 265–314, 1981.

2. Department of Health, Education and Welfare. *The Institutional Guide to DHEW Policy on Protection of Human Subjects.* DHEW Pub. No. 72-102, December 1, 1971.

3. Department of Health, Education and Welfare, Office of the Secretary. Protection of Human Subjects. Amending Subtitle A of Title 45 of the Code of Federal Regulations by adding Part 46. *Federal Register* 39(105):18916, May 30, 1974.

4. Department of Health, Education and Welfare, Office of the Secretary. Protection of Human Subjects: Belmont Report: Ethical Principles and Guidelines for the Protection of Human Subjects of Research: Report of the National Commission for the Protection of Human Subjects of Biomedical and Behavioral Research. *Federal Register* 44(76):23192, April 18, 1979.

5. Department of Health and Human Services, Office of the Secretary. Protection of Human Subjects. Title 45 of the Code of Federal Regulations, Sub-Part 46. *OPRR Reports,* Revised June 18, 1991, Reprinted March 15, 1994.

6. Department of Health and Human Services, Food and Drug Administration. Protection of Human Subjects. Title 21 of the Code of Federal Regulations. *Federal Register* 46(17), January 27, 1981.

7. Department of Health and Human Services, Food and Drug Administration. Protection of Human Subjects. Title 21 of the Code of Federal Regulations, Parts 50 and 56. April 1, 1994 Edition.

8. Ad Hoc Committee on Ethical Standards in Psychological Research. *Ethical Principles in the Conduct of Research with Human Participants.* Washington, DC: American Psychological Association, 1973.

9. American Psychological Association. Ethical principles of psychologists and code of conduct. *American Psychologist* 47(12):1597–1611, 1992.

10. Department of Health, Education and Welfare, Office of the Secretary. Research involving children. Report and recommendations of the National Commission for the Protection of Human Subjects of Biomedical and Behavioral Research. *Federal Register* 43(9):2084, January 13, 1978.

11. Department of Health and Human Services, Office of the Secretary. Additional protections for children involved as subjects in research. *Federal Register* 48(46):9814, March 8, 1983.

12. Bishop, M. P. and Gallant, D. M. Observation of placebo response in chronic schizophrenic patients. Arch. Gen. Psychiatry 14:497–503, 1966.

13. Department of Health, Education and Welfare, Office of the Secretary. Protection of Human Subjects: Proposed regulations involving those institutionalized as mentally disabled. *Federal Register* 43(223):53950, November 17, 1978.

14. Gallant, D. M. Psychopharmacologic research in severely chronic schizophrenic inpatients. *Psychopharmacology Bulletin* 6(4):4–12, 1970.

15. Department of Health, Education and Welfare, Office of the Secretary. Additional protections pertaining to biomedical and behavioral research involving prisoners as subjects. *Federal Register* 43(222):11341, November 16, 1978.

HIV-Related Research

Individuals who are HIV positive and who participate in research efforts may require some special consideration particularly when considering such issues as confidentiality, neuropsychiatric impairment and competence to give consent, consent for long-term storage and possible future use of tissues and samples, and preconsent for autopsy. These issues have been summarized here by Igor Grant, M.D., Professor and Vice Chairman, Department of Psychiatry, University of California, San Diego.

Confidentiality. There are some special issues in regard to guarding confidentiality in research involving seropositive or "at risk" individuals. These are: 1) the potential for *social harm,* if serostatus is inadvertently disclosed. For example, disclosure that a person is seropositive, or, perhaps, even disclosure of the fact that a person has participated in a study on HIV, whether as a control or as a seropositive, might raise risks of noninsurability or even job discrimination; 2) *Legal harm.* Inadvertent disclosure of seropositivity might possibly expose a participant's illegal or socially disapproved activities which are linked to seropositivity, such as an injection drug use and homosexual behavior. In certain settings, e.g., the military, this can lead to adverse occupational consequences.

For these reasons, to protect participants in HIV-related research from possible subpoena of research records, it is recommended that investigators obtain a certificate of confidentiality from the National Institutes of Health. Such a certificate protects investigators from subpoena of documents that may expose participants to social or legal harm.

Neuropsychiatric impairment and competence to give consent. Some persons with HIV dementia or HIV associated psychosis may not be competent to consent to research procedures. At the same time, enrollment in a research protocol, particularly involving experimental treatments, may be beneficial to such a participant. Investigators may wish to seek permission from family members or others authorized to provide consent on behalf of the participant. In such an instance, care must be taken not to disclose serostatus inadvertently.

Consent for long term storage and possible future use of tissues and samples. The long term storage of fluids and tissue samples may be desirable in neurobiologic research on HIV. Investigators need to inform participants if there is an intent for long term storage and for use of such samples in possible future studies beyond those currently planned.

Preconsent for autopsy. For research on etiology and pathogenesis of HIV associated neuropsychiatric disorders, postmortem studies on brain or other tissues may be desirable. In most instances, it is desirable to have a separate preconsent for such an autopsy, which specifies if the brain will be taken. It is desirable that participants in such research inform their next of kin or significant others about the participant's desire to donate postmortem tissue for research.

Index

*Page numbers printed in **boldface** type refer to tables or figures.*